WORKING WOMEN IN RECESSION

WORKING WOMEN IN RECESSION

Employment, Redundancy, and Unemployment

by
RODERICK MARTIN
and
JUDITH WALLACE
Trinity College, Oxford

OXFORD UNIVERSITY PRESS
1984

Oxford University Press, Walton Street Oxford OX2 6DP
London New York Toronto
Delhi Bombay Calcutta Madras Karachi
Kuala Lumpur Singapore Hong Kong Tokyo
Nairobi Dar es Salaam Cape Town
Melbourne Auckland
and associated companies in
Beirut Berlin Ibadan Mexico City Nicosia

Oxford is a trade mark of Oxford University Press

Published in the United States
by Oxford University Press, New York

© Roderick Martin and Judith Wallace 1984

All rights reserved. No part of this publication may be reproduced,
stored in a retrieval system, or transmitted, in any form or by any means,
electronic, mechanical, photocopying, recording, or otherwise, without
the prior permission of Oxford University Press

This book is sold subject to the condition that it shall not, by way
of trade or otherwise, be lent, re-sold, hired out or otherwise circulated
without the publisher's prior consent in any form of binding or cover
other than that in which it is published and without a similar condition
including this condition being imposed on the subsequent purchaser

British Library Cataloguing in Publication Data

Martin, Roderick
 Working women in recession.
 1. Women—Employment—Great Britain
 2. Unemployment—Great Britain
 I. Title   II. Wallace, Judith
 331.4'137941   HD6135

ISBN 0-19-878006-0
ISBN 0-19-878005-2 Pbk

*Typeset at the Alden Press
Printed in Great Britain by
Biddles Ltd, Guildford*

PREFACE

Our first debt is to the women in the five areas who twice gave up their time voluntarily to be interviewed at length during a trying period of their lives: without their active and full participation the study would have been impossible: we hope that our study helps to bring attention to their views. We are also very grateful to the managements of the five companies who co-operated in the project: the project inevitably involved the use of employees' time, without direct benefit to the managements concerned — although we hope that they will regard increased awareness of the effects of the recession on manufacturing industry as beneficial. To preserve confidentiality we can only express our appreciation to them in general terms. Thirdly, we would like to thank the officials of the Manpower Services Commission, especially the Regional Manpower Intelligence Units in the South East, Midlands, and North West, and the managers of the Job Centres in the areas in which the case studies were carried out: they gave valuable help in locating suitable research sites, and in providing important background information on local labour-market conditions.

In addition to the authors a number of other people played a significant role in carrying out the research reported. We are especially grateful to Dr Jennie Dey, who was a Research Officer on the project between September 1980 and July 1981: Dr Dey played a major role in the field-work and the preparation of the second questionnaire. We are also grateful for the work of Mrs Pauline Wilkins, who was a research Officer on the project between February and August 1980. For computing assistance we are grateful to Mr Martin Range, Dr Clive Payne, and Professor Christopher Wallace. The secretarial work has been carried out by Mrs Wendy Eadle, Mrs Stella Wood, and Mrs Pat Rogers: we are very grateful to them for their commitment to carrying the project through. The typescript of the report which formed the basis for the book was prepared on the word-processor by Mrs Stella Wood; we are especially grateful to Mrs Wood for her rapid mastery of word-processing, which greatly eased production of the report and subsequent book, and to Mrs Rogers for completing the revisions speedily.

The Department of Employment, Research Division, Social Science Branch, was responsible for the initial conception and funding of the research project, *Female Unemployment: Redundancy Studies*, which forms the basis for the present volume. Throughout the Department played a valuable and helpful active role. At the Department we are especially grateful to Ms Ceridwen Roberts, the Liason Officer for the project, for her support, encouragement, and constructive criticism, to Mr Francis Butler, and to Mr Peter Brannen, Chief Research Officer, Social Science Branch, for his careful shepherding through of the project.

Finally, the project would have been impossible without the active help of the President and Fellows of Trinity College, Oxford, especially the Estates Bursar, Mr J. F. Wright, and the Domestic Bursar, Dr R. J. L. Popplewell. We are very grateful for the College's willingness to undertake the administration of the initial research contract, and for providing accommodation and other facilities without which carrying through the project would have been immeasurably more difficult.

Although the research reported upon was funded by the Department of Employment the Department bears no responsibility for the views and opinions expressed. Responsibility for any errors of fact or interpretation rests with the authors.

Trinity College, Oxford Roderick Martin
February 1984 Judith Wallace

CONTENTS

Chapter 1 Introduction: Female Employment, Redundancy, and Unemployment   1

1.1 Background Literature 1.1.1 Women and Employment 1.1.2. Women and Redundancy 1.1.3. Women and Unemployment 1.2. Research Strategy and Tactics 1.3. The Women Interviewed 1.3.1. Age and Family Circumstances 1.3.2. Social Background 1.3.3. Length of Working Life 1.3.4. Occupation 1.3.5. Economic Situation 1.4. Conclusion

Chapter 2 Female Employment Experience and Attitudes to Work   52

2.1. Women and Employment 2.2. Job Choice and Occupational Career 2.3. Current Attitudes to Work 2.4. Family Influences Upon Women's Attitudes to Work 2.5. Conclusion

Chapter 3 Women and Redundancy   103

3.1. Reasons for the Redundancies 3.2. Long-Term Labour-Force Changes 3.3. Management Decision-Making on Redundancy 3.4. Management-Union Relations 3.4.1. Industrial Relations before the Redundancy 3.4.2. Management-Union Relations during Redundancy 3.5. Redundancy Agreements 3.6. Women Workers' Responses to Redundancy 3.7. Redundancy Pay 3.8. Conclusion

Chapter 4 Women in the Labour Market   151

4.1. Post-Redundancy Experience in the Labour Market 4.2. Job Search 4.2.1. The Timing of Job Search 4.2.2. Methods Used in Job Search 4.2.3. Female Handicaps 4.3. Post-Redundancy Employment Experience 4.4. Retraining, Homeworking, and Own Business 4.5. Conclusion: Women in the Labour Market

Chapter 5	Women and Unemployment	223

5.1. Length of Time of Unemployment 5.2. The Economic Impact of Redundancy and Unemployment 5.2.1. Women's Post-Redundancy Financial Status 5.2.2. Uses Made of Redundancy Money 5.2.3. Predicted Long-Term Financial Situation 5.2.4. Economies 5.3. Activities 5.4. The Effects of Unemployment on Family Life 5.5. The Effect of Unemployment on Social Life and Social Contact 5.6. The Effects of Unemployment upon Health 5.6.1. The Effect of Unemployment on Physical Health 5.6.2. The Effect of Unemployment on Mental Health 5.7. Women's General Attitudes to Unemployment 5.8. Attitudes Towards Government 5.9. Conclusion

Chapter 6	Conclusion: Working Women in Recession	279
	Appendix	290
	References	291
	Index	294

1

INTRODUCTION: FEMALE EMPLOYMENT, REDUNDANCY, AND UNEMPLOYMENT

As late as 1976 it was still possible to conclude that women were sociologically invisible participants in industrial life, as Richard Brown did in his survey of the treatment of women in industrial sociology.[1] Since the mid 1970s sociological interest in women's employment issues has expanded rapidly.[2] The increase in the number and visibility of women in employment in the 1970s, and the growing influence of the feminist movement, led to widespread political and academic interest in issues involving women and work. The Equal Pay Act (1970), the Sex Discrimination Act (1975), and the establishment of the Equal Opportunities Commission indicated political concern with improving women's position in employment — although there remains widespread controversy over the practical effects of such legislation.[3] The feminist movement has been especially strong in British sociology, the British Sociological Association establishing its own Standing Committee on the Equality of the Sexes. Political and academic interest were combined in the Department of Employment's programme of research on Women and Employment, of which the present book is a product.[4]

Despite the increased research effort being put into research on female employment issues, the amount of published empirical evidence in women in employment is limited.[5] Published evidence on the effects of the present recession on women is almost non-existent. The present study is presented as an exploration in depth of the experience of groups of working women who were declared redundant in 1981–2, based upon extensive interviews. In this introductory chapter we place our study in its intellectual context by indicating some of the issues raised by previous writers, outline the research strategy followed, and discuss the main features of the sample of women interviewed.

1.1 Background literature

Our study is concerned with women's experience and attitudes in three areas —

employment, redundancy, and unemployment. We therefore briefly review major issues raised in relevant previous writing in the three areas in turn.

1.1.1 Women and employment

In the last decade neo-classical models of the labour market have been undermined by empirical research showing the limitations of the 'rational maximizing' assumptions of labour-market behaviour which underlie neo-classical models, and the resilience of institutional rigidities. Neo-classical models have been substantially replaced by alternative theories of segmented labour markets.[6] Alternative explanations for the segmentation process (employer strategy, work-group closure) and for the location of different groups within particular segments have been put forward. Women are generally located within segments where employment is insecure, earnings are low, promotion opportunities few, and collective organization weak. Their access to more valued labour markets is restricted by the strategies of groups already controlling those markets, by their own limited qualifications, training, and experience, and by domestic responsibilities.

The variant of segmented labour-market theory most widely used to explain women's position in the labour market is dual-labour-market theory.[7] This model postulates two separate labour markets — a primary labour market, in which jobs are secure, relatively well rewarded, and tied to promotional or career ladders, and in which labour is highly organized and solidaristic, and a secondary labour market, in which jobs are insecure, poorly paid, and lacking in opportunities for promotion, and where union activity is weak. There are few points of access into the primary labour market, mainly at the beginning of an individual's work career, subsequent access being restricted by employer and trade-union policies based upon both overt and covert methods of social closure. Moreover, women do not share equally in access to the initial points of entry.[8] Women workers are characteristically recruited into the secondary labour market, especially on their re-entry into the labour market following a period of concentration upon child-rearing.

Several general criticisms have been made of dual-labour-market theory, including its difficulty in analysing the role of public-sector employment. Most importantly, the model is very loosely defined, many jobs possessing attributes characteristic of both labour markets, for example employment security, but limited opportunities for promotion. The employment experience of the women we interviewed examplifies the limitations of dual-labour-market theories as explanations for female employment experience. The women were employed in large-scale manufacturing industry and highly unionized, with terms and conditions of employment governed by collective bargaining, and, until the current recession, enjoying employment security. The majority of the women were also low paid and had few opportunities for promotion. However, although dual-labour-market theory has little relevance to the pre-redundancy employment experience of the women interviewed, it is more relevant to the post-redundancy employment experience: the minority of women who obtained jobs following the redundancies found them primarily in the secondary labour market, and re-entry into the primary sector is likely to be difficult, especially for older women.

The Marxist concept of the reserve army of labour has an explicitly political function, linked to the 'marginalization' of the groups constituting the reserve army. The availability of ethnic minorities, immigrants, and women as a potential reserve army of workers whose relative powerlessness or access to alternative sources of income makes them relatively dispensable renders worker control of labour supply impossible, and therefore undermines union bargaining power — especially if accompanied by a de-skilling of the labour process.[9] However, the concept has also been used in a less contentiously Marxist sense, to refer to the restriction of recruitment of women into market employment to periods of economic expansion, or to occupations in which, for whatever reason, less-marginal workers are reluctant to seek employment. Hence the expansion of female employment in the UK in the 1970s was due both to an overall expansion in labour demand and, more particularly, to the expansion of the service sector, where the abilities required were regarded as particularly suited to women and the organization of work made part-time work acceptable and inexpensive to employers. During recession unemployment might be likely to affect women disproportionately because of their concentration in sectors with a high elasticity of demand for labour (and a low level of unionization). In addition, competitive pressures during recession might lead employers to introduce technological change more rapidly.

Empirical evidence for the role of women as a reserve army of labour is limited, and based largely on experience in the two world wars, when women were recruited to perform work previously done by men, only to be expelled from their jobs when the war was over to give place to returned soldiers. Although the government, media, and men encourage women to withdraw from the labour market during recessions, the encouragement has been largely ineffective, apart from the special circumstances of the two world wars. As Milkman has shown, despite media propaganda and direct employer and union action to expel married women from the labour force during the 1930s, the number of women in the labour force in the United States increased slightly between 1930 and 1940.[10] Female employment opportunities were protected by the sex-typing of occupations, clerical jobs and jobs in service industries increasing whilst traditionally male jobs in extractive and manufacturing industries declined. Similarly in Britain in the late 1970s: women's employment share rose between 1977 and 1981, when unemployment increased. In 1977 the female employment share was 38.8 per cent, and unemployment 7.4 per cent, in 1979 39.0 per cent when unemployment was 5.1 per cent, and in 1981 40.1 per cent when unemployment was 9.7 per cent. The decline of manufacturing industry, primarily a male employment sector, between 1979 and 1981 resulted in an increase in the female employment share.[11] Sex-patterned segmentation of jobs thus inhibits male encroachment upon female jobs. The effects of social convention are reinforced by economic considerations: as long as unemployment rises and falls in cycles of reasonably short duration, the inconvenience and expense of training workers who have acquired even minor skills — and associated induction costs — will inhibit any major encroachment by one occupational group upon the territory of another's during recession. A further factor inhibiting encroachment is the tendency of industries to have a geographical pattern, and likewise the problems of geographical mobility for unemployed workers.[12]

Although sex-patterned segmentation of the whole labour force has probably operated to protect, or even to enhance, the female share of employment overall, experience in manufacturing industry has been different. Female workers are segregated vertically, at the lower end of the qualifications and skill hierarchy, and horizontally, in the more labour-intensive sectors.[13] In the labour-intensive sectors the effects of the recession have been exacerbated by technological change and competition from Third World countries, for example in clothing, textiles, and electronic assembly. The sex patterning of jobs in manufacturing industry has therefore operated to the disadvantage of women workers, especially women manual workers, resulting in a more rapid loss of female, compared with male, jobs. Hence in the three OPCS occupational categories covering manufacturing industry (groups xi, xii, xiii) female employment fell by 4 per cent between 1977 and 1979, and a further 14 per cent between 1979 and 1981, compared with figures of 1.4 and 11.5 per cent for men for similar periods.[14] If changes in the number of part-time shifts had been taken into account the decline in female employment would probably have been relatively greater.[15]

Theories based upon labour-market segmentation or the role of women as a reserve army of labour do not, in themselves, explain female employment experience. However, economic changes, especially changes in the structure of employment, sex-role stereotypes, the policies of employers and trade unions, and the attitudes of the women themselves combine to explain women's employment behaviour.

In previous paragraphs we have been concerned with structural explanations for women's place in the labour market. In addition, there has been a limited amount of research on how women evaluate their employment, and some comparison between their evaluations and those of men doing similar types of work. Such research suggests that women place a higher value upon some categories of the experience of employment than men who perform similar work tasks, and less value than men upon others. For example, it has been suggested that women workers in low-status occupations are more likely to mention the rewards of sociability and companionship, and less likely to mention a sense of accomplishment.[16] Blauner argues that women in the textile industry, working in unskilled or semi-skilled jobs, are less dissatisfied than men, because 'work does not have the central importance and meaning in their lives that it does for men, since their most important roles are those of wives and mothers.'[17]

These results do not necessarily show that, given identical work experiences, women would evaluate them differently to men since gender-based segmentation of the work-force means that women's jobs are rarely directly comparable to men's. However, it is impossible to predict women's reactions to job loss simply by adjusting known data for men to allow for the different profiles of men's and women's jobs, since gender and job-status effects on job satisfaction interact. As Crosby showed, gender differences are less in high-status than in low-status categories. It is therefore necessary to assume that reactions to employment and unemployment will differ according to both gender and occupation. The evaluation of both employment and unemployment will depend upon the existence of alternative 'compensatory' categories of experience, which are likely to differ according to gender. It is not necessary to assume, and we are not assuming, that the basic goals or values of men and women differ — nor is it necessary to assume that they are the same.

1.1.2 Women and redundancy

Our project is the first major British research project concerned with redundancy and unemployment amongst women: there is therefore no directly relevant research to provide comparative data. Redundancy studies have traditionally either concentrated exclusively on men or studied people who have turned out to be men. The two significant exceptions are Daniel (1972), and Wood (1982).[18] Daniel's research was based on the more extensive field-work, and led him to conclude that

> women fared better than men following their redundancy. They had experienced less difficulty in finding a satisfactory new job. Their new jobs compared more favourably with the old... where they had changed their type of work this had tended to be from choice and the majority expressed a preference for the new job in comparison to the old... nevertheless while women suffered less than men, in general they still felt they had lost more than they had gained.[19]

However, Daniel's research was carried out in south-east London in 1968–70, where the level of unemployment was 1.5 per cent (0.5 per cent for females) in November 1970; female employment opportunities were expanding with the growth of the service sector, especially in London. Daniel's sanguine conclusions are hardly likely to be valid over a decade later, especially for women outside the London region.

Wood's paper is based upon field-work carried out in 1972–3, involving a smaller number of respondents than Daniel's research did: his conclusions echo those of Daniel — 'despite their attachment to their jobs... they did not appear to value specific employments as particularly important. They had a flexible orientation and confidence that they could always find work which was roughly equivalent to what they were currently doing.'[20] Wood goes on to suggest that women would probably react to redundancy in a relatively accepting way even in the present very different economic conditions.

The relevance of previous studies of women's experiences in and attitudes towards redundancies is therefore limited. The studies were undertaken when unemployment was low, the women interviewed correctly believing that alternative employment opportunities were available. Nevertheless, previous research raised the issue of the existence of gender-specific experiences of, and attitudes towards, redundancy. It has been suggested that women are likely to adopt a more fatalistic attitude towards redundancy than men do, because their attitudes towards employment differ, and their investment in specific jobs is less. However women have been active in opposition to redundancies, as is shown in Judy Wadjman's study.[21] Moreover, women are not unwilling in principle to oppose redundancies, especially when they believe that opposition can be effective. Like those of men, women's attitudes towards redundancies are conditioned by their previous socialization, especially at work, the attitudes and behaviour of the managements involved, and their labour-market position. In general, redundancies exemplify labour weakness, whether male or female, unionized or non-unionized.[22]

1.1.3 Women and unemployment

Research upon unemployment has also traditionally neglected the position of women: women have usually been ignored or treated as the spouses of unemployed men. In their recent survey of the literature on unemployment, Hayes and Nutman (1981) comment:

The place work occupies in the life of women has dramatically changed over the years. These changes are not reflected in the many studies of unemployment reported in this book. In the majority of cases these studies examined only the effects of unemployment of men. Wherever possible we have included studies which have embraced [sic] women, and we believe that the models and explanations that we have developed are equally applicable to both men and women who have experienced unemployment.[23]

The neglect of women in previous research has not been total. The classic Pilgrim Trust study, *Men Without Work*, includes a discussion of female unemployment especially in areas with traditionally high levels of female employment, as in Leicester and Blackburn.[24] Similarly, Daniel (1974) covers women as well as men, although there is little analysis of the specific issues involved in female unemployment, women being only a small minority of the unemployed at the time of his research.[25] However, such exceptions do not undermine the conclusion that research into female unemployment has been seriously neglected: the only major empirical work devoted to female unemployment has been the programme of work recently commissioned by the Department of Employment, of which the present project is a part.

Although there has been little previous research into female unemployment, there is a long tradition of relevant research and comment on male unemployment. Unfortunately — or fortunately — the majority of post-war studies of unemployment were conceived and carried out in a very different economic environment from that of the early 1980s. From the end of the war to the late 1960s, Britain experienced almost full employment — unemployment levels of 2 per cent or below were, for the most part, accounted for by people moving between jobs and a small residue of people who were disabled or unable to adapt to steady employment. Unemployment was essentially a 'welfare' issue and not one of general social concern — the problems of unemployment were the subject of those interested in improvements in manpower planning to minimize frictional unemployment, the proper organization of relief measures to tide people over periods between jobs, and how to motivate the supposedly 'work-shy'. It was not until the 1970s, when cyclical periods of depression began to deepen and lengthen and recoveries failed to provide sufficient jobs to fulfil demand that unemployment came to be viewed as a social and economic problem which was both diffuse and pervasive. Confidence that unemployment would diminish sharply with improved levels of economic activity has been undermined, improvements in output in the early 1980s being achieved through higher productivity, not through increased employment.

Hill's 1973 study of unemployment, begun in 1971 when the unemployment rate was only 2.5 per cent, was originally conceived with the intention of shedding light on the phenomenon of 'long-term unemployment in situations of full employment' by providing a profile of the long-term unemployed in three English towns.[26] In the event, between the conception of the enterprise and the commencement of field-work the rate of unemployment rose to 4.7 per cent — a situation of full employment no longer existed. The section of Hill's study dealing with attitudes to employment and unemployment had originally been designed to provide explanations for a lack of motivation to work; it soon became apparent that it was impossible to disentangle the social and psychological pre-conditions of unemployment from the demoralizing effects of long-term unemployment.

In response to the rising unemployment rate of 1971 and 1972, Daniel undertook a national survey of 1,500 unemployed workers drawn from the Department of Employment's register of the unemployed with the intention of providing general demographic information on an increasing unemployed population — a small section of the survey explored personal feelings about being unemployed.[27] Daniel encountered the opposite problem to Hill's — the unemployment rate dropped from 4.7 to only 2.5 per cent by the time the survey was started in 1973, and his findings, to a far greater extent than those of Hill, refer to people who were either between jobs or belonged to a small residue of chronically unemployed. His findings on the attitudes of the unemployed reflect those of people facing a temporary period of unemployment, or of people whose way of life was not basically work oriented. Their emphasis on the economic aspects of unemployment is hardly surprising in that context.

In the 1960s and early 1970s it was possible to view the unemployed as suffering either from individual disabilities, which made it difficult to hold down employment, or from inefficiencies in the operation of labour-market institutions, resulting in gaps between jobs. Beveridge himself had seen an unemployment level of 3.0 per cent as a working definition of full employment. Since 1975 unemployment has remained above 4 per cent, and since 1980 above 10 per cent. Unemployment has become an expected — even perhaps accepted — feature of economic life. The scale and character of unemployment have therefore changed.[28] The larger number of unemployed are drawn from a wide range of social groups: the unemployed worker is as likely to be a young girl who has just left school as a middle-aged male manual worker, with wife and children to support. Both class and gender influence orientations to employment and unemployment. The growth in the number of workers unemployed, and their social diversity, has led to the need for more extensive, and more sophisticated, research than was carried out in the 1960s and early 1970s. In practice, unemployment research in the 1980s has profited more from the unemployment studies of the 1930s than of the early 1970s.

The sociological studies of unemployment in the 1930s — Jahoda and Lazarsfeld's *Marienthal*, Bakke's *The Unemployed Man*, and the Pilgrim Trust's *Men Without Work* — remain classics.[29] Their relevance has been underlined by Jahoda's recent review, *Employment and Unemployment: A Social-Psychological Analysis*, which consolidated the empirical research of the 1930s into a single theoretical framework.[30] Jahoda isolated five significant aspects of the experience of unemployment involving psychological deprivation: changes in the experience of time, the reduction of social contacts, the lack of participation in collective purposes, the absence of an acceptable status and its consequences for personal identity, and the absence of regular activity (p. 39). She omits the psychological deprivations of poverty, although these were stressed in the Marienthal study and were strongly present in other studies of the 1930s, and remain relevant in the 1980s. In varying degrees the impact of all five dimensions of the experience of unemployment (and the loss of earning status) will vary depending upon the availability of alternative resources, which in turn will depend upon the sex and marital status of the individual. Miles (1983), using Jahoda's five dimensions, showed that the impact of unemployment upon men depended upon their access to compensatory categories of experience.[31] However, Miles was concerned only with men; there was no attempt to draw a comparison between the alternative categories of experience available to men and those available to women. Jahoda herself comments:

Many women know from their own experiences or those of their mothers the depressive effect of being isolated without personal status and social identity, deprived of wider experiences than the highly emotionally charged family relations permit, and outside the communal purpose of the larger society... [nevertheless] unemployment hits [women] less hard than men psychologically speaking because an alternative is available to them in the return to the traditional role of housewife that provides some time structure, some sense of purpose, status and activity even though it offers little scope for wider social experiences.[32]

Jahoda's conclusion neglects the effects the experience of employment has upon the women themselves: for individuals, the clock cannot be turned back, and it is misleading to refer to a 'return' to a previous role. The previous role is unlikely to exist if children have grown up, and expectations and attitudes are likely to differ as a result of the experience of employment. Hence, as German research has shown, long-term unemployed women had 'a less rational or explicit time structure, were more isolated in terms of having fewer friends and acquaintances, were more often resigned, and somewhat less emotionally stable' than women who stayed in work.[33] Moreover, the alternative role of housewife is less attractive to women who have no children at home. As we indicate in Chapter 5, many of the unemployed women we interviewed felt that they had time on their hands and were more isolated than when in employment, although they did not feel that they lacked a role.

Everyone who has become unemployed after having a job will interpret his/her experience of unemployment partly by contrasting it with their pattern of life when employed. Their evaluation of the state of unemployment will take into account the absence from their daily routine of a 'job' – as well as other aspects such as loss of income and additional free time. The impact of job loss will depend to some extent on the value placed upon the job that was lost. We invited the women to place their own evaluation upon their jobs and to contrast their work routine and environment with the routine and environment in which they now spend the eight hours (or less for part-timers) that they would previously have spent at work.

Unemployment affects individual well-being; it also affects family life – the unemployed workers's position in the family and his/her relations with other members of the family. Previous writers have been mainly concerned with three issues in particular: the effect of increased poverty on family life, the effect of increased proximity when the unemployed worker was at home all day, and the effect on self-esteem of role change, which could involve either simply loss of the role of breadwinner or, if the husband became unemployed and the wife still worked, a switch in the gender-based division of family roles, with the husband becoming the housekeeper and the wife becoming the breadwinner.

In the 1930s studies there was, not surprisingly, an emphasis on the tensions that increased poverty caused in family relations. In Marienthal, both men and women had gone out to work, and the closure of the factory meant that both husband and wife ceased working at approximately the same time: problems caused by changing roles within the family, if they arose, were not investigated – it appeared to them that both men and women 'were all in the same predicament together.' The economic effect of the loss of both incomes in households normally reliant on two was extreme. In general, the tensions and unhappiness brought about by the problems involved in trying to exist on limited and dwindling resources caused a deterioration of relations within the family. Incidents which would be relatively minor if the family were comfortably off were sufficient to start quarrels — 'typical complaints were about the children ruining their shoes playing soccer and the like.' 'Generally in happy marriages, minor quarrels appear more frequently than before — in marriages that were already unsettled difficulties have become more acute.'[34] Similarly, there was no mention of increased contact bringing families together in *Men Without Work*. On the contrary: 'the children may get on a man's nerves if he is at home all day.'[35]

In the 1930s studies attention was focused on the effects of loss of male income on male independence, and male injured pride on being unable to maintain a customary pattern of life. In the 1970s there was increasing concern with the shifting 'balance' in family roles, and of the 'feminization' and loss of sexual identity of the male. For example, Marsden (1982) devotes a section to workers as housewives: 'I'm here and the wife's out at work. It's a complete reversal. It's ridiculous.'[36] Sinfield (1981) suggests that, to avoid a change in roles within the family, some women will not go out to work when their husbands are unemployed.[37] The recent emphasis on this aspect of unemployment may be the result of changes in the preoccupations of the unemployed, or of social researchers. Whether widespread or otherwise, it indicates the importance of differences in gender — and possibly of class — in family reactions to unemployment. According to this view, unemployment among married women would restore a balance previously upset. The major effects of unemployment on family life suggested by previous writers — the increased tension caused by the strain of poverty, the harmful effects of over-proximity when additional members of the family are home all day, the unwelcome feelings of dependence caused by having to rely on members of the family for money, and even loss of the status of provider with the family — are all relevant to the female as well as to the male experience of unemployment.

Unemployment could have positive, as well as negative, aspects. Occasionally, especially for families of several children with only one breadwinner, social-security payments are comparable to earnings. In the absence of an economic necessity for employment, redundancy could provide the opportunity for breaking a habit of performing a job that had few, if any, real rewards. 'Frustrated by the lack of meaning in the tasks allotted to him and by the impersonality of his role in the work organization, the alienated worker turns to non-work life for values and identity': unemployment may provide an opportunity to develop this more meaningful non-work activity.[38] Anthony has argued that the nineteenth and twentieth centuries have seen an exaggerated importance attached to work: 'a more realistic view [is] that work has to be done, that its performance often produces rugged and admirable qualities, but that the search for deeper satisfactions must be conducted in other directions.'[39] The possibility that there might be positive aspects of unemployment has been given little attention. The question was hardly considered in the studies of the 1930s, concentrating as they did upon unemployment among the working class.

Although there was a strong tradition of thought that manual work in mass-production industries was dehumanizing, the poverty that accompanied unemployment among low-income earners was even more dehumanizing: it was hardly relevant to view unemployment in the light of a release from hard and unpleasant work, — the alternative, grinding poverty, was even less pleasant. Where redundancy payments are sufficiently large to alleviate the financial impact of unemployment, even among low-paid workers, it is not unreasonable to consider the possibility that unemployment could have positive aspects — especially for manual workers approaching retirement age. For women whose husbands are earning substantial incomes and whose families have grown up, the financial impact of unemployment may not be crucial — redundancy could help them to break a habit and make a choice for the better. Pahl (1982) suggests that for many workers in industry the alternative to full-time employment is not total unemployment, but a more flexible work pattern; the major result of unemployment is the loss of the rigidly structured time pattern associated with low-status work in large organizations.[40] On the basis of research among communities on the southern banks of the Thames Estuary, he suggests that male manual workers are content with seasonal employment that provides a reasonable standard of living, and would prefer not to be tied to a lifetime of regular industrial employment in work which is often boring, dirty, dangerous, and noisy. He argues that a regular, eight-to-four, five-day-a-week work rhythm is unnatural and, in terms of the experience of the past few hundred years, atypical. However, he confesses that his conclusions are based on the experience of workers in a region where seasonal work patterns are more common than in other parts of the country and might not apply to communities in large industrial towns where urban geography and social patterns have evolved around regular, permanent employment. Moreover, the ability to make full use of the time made available by the lack of full-time employment is influenced by access to contacts in the community, which are often facilitated by full-time employment.

On the basis of research into male unemployment it is possible to indicate the possible effects of unemployment upon women: evidence presented in Chapters 5 and 6 below indicates the extent to which expectations were justified. Consideration of differences in male and female unemployment underlines the importance of distinguishing between work as 'employment' and work as 'task'. For men 'work' is held to be almost synonymous with 'employment'. On the other hand, nearly all adult women work at a task, but fewer than 50 per cent are 'employed'. Work, in its broader sense of productive or creative activity, could be described as the prime source of status and function for both men and women (although others have argued that a married woman's status is determined by her husband's work).[41] It is less reasonable to suggest that 'employment' is the prime source of status and function for the majority of women. Employment may be an economic, but it is not yet a moral, imperative for women to the extent that it is for men. In our study being employed means receiving pay for prescribed physical or mental activity, being included in certain categories of relationships (even the self-employed have customers, clients, or colleagues), and possessing occupational status. The last places a man and a single woman in society — a married woman to some extent shares her husband's status.

1.2 Research strategy and tactics

There were two major distinctive features of the research strategy: the carrying out of a set of linked case studies; and the interviewing of the same workers before and after redundancy in each case study. The research design was therefore complex, involving two sets of interviews — and a third postal questionnaire — in each of five research sites. The purpose of this section of the introduction is to outline the overall research strategy and methodology, and some of the practical difficulties encountered in its implementation: more detailed discussion occurs where appropriate in subsequent chapters, and in the Appendix.

The case-study research sites were selected according to a combination of industrial and regional criteria. From previous research it was known that experience of redundancy would differ between industries, as different industries experienced different levels of change in product markets and technologies. Redundancy has been concentrated in manufacturing industry, especially in the engineering sector: it has been less common in the public sector and in service industries. The case studies were therefore drawn from manufacturing industry, one from each of clothing and electronics, and three from the engineering sector. It was also believed that experience of unemployment would be heavily influenced by the level of unemployment in the local labour market. We therefore sought research sites in areas that had different levels of unemployment — high, low, and rapidly changing. Reflecting these requirements research sites in the North West, the South East, and the Midlands were sought. Combining the two sets of criteria, the five case studies were carried out in the following industries and regions: clothing (South East) (case study A), electronics (North West) (case study B), engineering (Midlands) (case study C), engineering–clerical (North West) (case study D), and engineering–clerical (Midlands) (case study E).

In addition to satisfying industrial and regional criteria it was hoped that each case study would involve interviews with approximately 100 women. We were therefore primarily interested in large-scale redundancies. The number of large-scale redundancies involving large numbers of women was relatively small during the period of field-work (1980–1). As a result of wishing to interview a relatively large number of women in each case study we have not carried out research in the sectors employing the largest number of women, because women were primarily employed in small production units in those sectors (outside the public sector). In 1980 the following were the ten largest employers of female labour (with the percentage of women employed in the industry as a percentage of all female employment): professional and scientific services (29.6 per cent); distributive trades (14.6 per cent); miscellaneous services (11.2 per cent); public administration (8.0 per cent); insurance, banking (7.1 per cent); transport and communications (3.5 per cent); food, drink, and tobacco (3.3 per cent); electrical engineering (3.1 per cent); clothing and footwear (2.7 per cent); and textiles (2.1 per cent). We carried out case studies in numbers 8 and 9 (electrical engineering and clothing/footwear). The remaining case studies were carried out in different sectors of the engineering industry. Although the sector was not one of the ten largest employers of women, it did employ substantial numbers of women. Moreover, the three engineering case studies covered manual, clerical, and a small number of professional/administrative employees, making it possible to contrast the experience of different occupations within the same industry (and the same region, since the manual engineering workers and one of the clerical groups worked in the same region). Finally, although the engineering industry was not one of the largest sectors of female employment, it was a major sector experiencing economic contraction in 1981–2: it was therefore more representative of female redundancy and unemployment than it was of female employment. Since the study was concerned with redundancy and unemployment, this was highly desirable.

The variety of redundancy situations we could cover was determined by the actual distribution of large-scale redundancies: we could not investigate what was not happening. Large-scale redundancies were concentrated in manufacturing industries, relatively few occurring in the service sector or in the relevant parts of the public sector. Job loss in services and in the public sector is a gradual, cumulative, and almost invisible process, resulting in lower levels of labour demand and the contraction of employment opportunities. Research into this process requires a longer time scale than was available to the present project, and a different type of research strategy, focusing more upon managerial responses to changing market conditions and less upon the experience of women themselves. Moreover, since the major impact of job loss by attrition is the contraction of employment opportunities and the denial of opportunities to women who might have expected to obtain employment, but did not, it would have been difficult to combine with research into the experience of unemployment on the part of women who had previously been in employment. For these reasons our project is concerned with the manufacturing industries where most of the large-scale redundancies have occurred, and in practice with plant or unit closures.

The industrial distribution of the research sites made it likely that the majority of our respondents would be full-time employees. In 1980 only 21.0 per cent of women employed in the clothing industry worked part time, and 18.4 per cent of female employees in electrical engineering, the proportion in other sectors of engineering being even lower. This contrasted with 45.4 per cent in professional and scientific services (including education) and 41.9 per in the distributive trades. Our expectations were confirmed, the large majority of our respondents being full-time workers, except in the clothing industry case study, where a large minority were part-time workers. This again renders the case study more representative of redundant and unemployed women than of employed women, since full-time women workers were more likely to be declared redundant than part-time workers, partly because reduced labour requirements in industries employing large numbers of part-time staff could be accommodated by a reduction in the hours of work, and partly because some part-time workers were not covered by redundancy legislation.

The second major feature of the research design was the following through of the same group of women from pre-redundancy until as late as practicable following the redundancy. This involved three questionnaires, two administered personally, and a third brief postal questionnaire. The first interview was carried out at the place of work before the redundancy, the second approximately three to six months after leaving the employment where first interviewed. The postal questionnaire was completed between seven and twelve months after redundancy. The first interview was used to obtain a picture of the rewards derived from work before it was distorted by hindsight following redundancy. At the same time it was also possible to discuss the redundancy process itself. The second interview was concerned with women's behaviour in the labour market, and the impact of unemployment upon economic circumstances, health, social relations, and social attitudes, including attitudes to employment. The postal questionnaire was concerned to establish any changes in employment between the second interview and as late as possible in the project's schedule.

In carrying out the strategy we encountered three major practical sources of difficulty: timing, response rate, and access. Timing proved a major practical difficulty, response rate a significant but surmountable one, and access a surprisingly minor one.

By far the major practical difficulties stemmed from the time constraints within which the project operated. Within a two-year project the practical maximum period allowable for field work was a year, an allowance in practice exceeded. Time constraints influenced the range of redundancy situations that could be examined, the time that could be allowed to elapse between redundancy and second interviews and between second interviews and postal questionnaires, as well as the amount of analysis possible of the data gathered. The effect of time limitations on the types of redundancy studied was twofold. First, it was impossible to examine redundancies in which job loss was a gradual process, involving the disappearance of jobs through attrition. (As well as, of course, making it impossible to examine job loss through 'natural wastage' and the non-filling of vacancies.) Secondly, all the large-scale redundancies notified to us at the time we were seeking case-study sites involved product-market changes — there was no case study involving technological change alone. Moreover, all case studies were either total or unit closures: there was no example of the 'thinning out' of a labour force whilst continuing operations. This has limited our ability to discuss the extent to which women are likely to suffer disproportionately from redundancy compared with men (although see our discussion of case study B below, pp. 113—15). These limitations in coverage were due simply to the types of redundancy occurring during the initial stages of our field-work.

Shortage of time also limited the period of time that could be allowed to elapse between first and second interviews. Redundancies are very fluid situations, as indicated in Chapter 3 below: rigid time-tabling is impossible. Women were interviewed a variable length of time before leaving their jobs, depending upon the gap between the announcement of the redundancy and its implementation. In some instances, particularly but not exclusively for the clerical workers in the last two case studies, individual leaving dates were staggered over a period of weeks or even months. However, to minimize the disruption in the plants concerned and to economise on the research staff's travelling time, the initial interviews in each case study were carried out in one period of week(s). We succeeded in our objective of allowing a period of four to six months to elapse between the women leaving the pre-redundancy job and the second interviews in the three earlier case studies, but were unable to do so for some individuals in the two later case studies. The same constraints limited the time between the second interview and the postal questionnaire.

The second major practical difficulty was encountered in ensuring an adequate response rate. It was originally intended to attempt to obtain approximately 400 interviews in stage one in four case-study sites. However, the number of redundancies involving over 100 female employees was very small, and we therefore adjusted our expectations downwards. To increase the number of respondents we undertook a fifth case study (E). The number of women involved in the five redundancies studied totalled 626. But the response rate achieved varied substantially between case studies. Table 1.2.1 indicates the distribution of respondents. The major difficulties were encountered in case studies A and C, for very different reasons.

In all five case studies we had the full co-operation of management and unions. However, in case study A this co-operation was a mixed blessing, since a very substantial number of the women employed felt that they had been let down very badly by both local management and their trade union. The women were unable to oppose the redundancy effectively, or to improve substantially upon the terms of the redundancy agreement. However, they were free to refuse to co-operate with a research project supported by the institutions that had betrayed them. There was therefore a systematic refusal to take part in the project. In the circumstances it is surprising that it proved possible to interview as many women as were interviewed (and that those who were interviewed were willing to express themselves critically, indicating that our respondents were not solely those under management influence). In case study C there were two major problems. In C1, a small feeder plant, many of the women involved were considerably upset by management's handling of the redundancy, especially by management's inability to provide precise leaving dates, and insistence upon

Table 1.2.1
Distribution of respondents

Case study	No. of respondents			No. of women		Respondents as percentage of total work-force[b]
	Full-time[a]	Part-time	Total	Refused interview	Absent at time of interview	
A	28	23	51	44	0	54
B 1	22	5	27	9	3	69
2	26	15	41	11	2	76
C 1	21	0	21	31	0	40
2	45	0	45	5[c]	1	16
D	38	5	43	11	8	69
E	44	7	51	6	7	80

(a) Full-time — 31 hours or more.
(b) Total female work-force at the time of the interviews. The run down leading up to the closure had in each case started before the interviews took place. The distribution of employees between full- and part-time work may also have been distorted as labour was shed.
(c) There were 229 female shop-floor workers: see text.

transferring employees from the feeder plant to the main plant against employees' wishes. (The issue blew up to everyone's surprise the day before the interviews were scheduled to begin.) It is therefore hardly surprising that the women involved were reluctant to co-operate in what was seen as a management-sponsored research project, despite trade-union support. In C2, the major plant, the difficulty derived simply from plant management's inability to release what were seen as key workers from their work, as they wished to avoid disrupting production at all costs: workers directly engaged on the production process could be released only in unusual circumstances. There was little surplus labour to fill in for workers released from the production process, since manning levels had already been very substantially reduced to improve productivity before the redundancy took place.

In view of the problems of wastage usually encountered in panel studies, the number of respondents interviewed in the second stage of the project was satisfactorily high. As Table 1.2.2 shows, the overall number of second interviews achieved was 196.

A small number of respondents refused to be re-interviewed when asked at the first interview. However, the major reason for failing to obtain second interviews were total disinterest in re-employment because of age, impossibility of making contact because of movement away from the area, bereavement, internal transfer within the group without being declared redundant, or leaving work too closely to the time of the second interview. (For further details see below, pp. 155–6.)

The problem of access proved less difficult than anticipated; we were very pleased at the ready co-operation we received from management and unions in very difficult circumstances. As indicated earlier, the major difficulties in

Table 1.2.2
Distribution of respondents: second interviews

Case study	No. of respondents at 2nd interview	Still at work; redeployed	Left district	Permanently retired	Working	Unemployed	Refused (no reason)	2nd interview as percentage of 1st
A	42		3	3	3		12	82
B	41		1	6	3	5	4	60
C	53	8		1	1			80
D	31	2	3		3	3	3	72
E	29	15	2			2		57
Total	196	25	9	10	10	10	19	70

obtaining access arose from the concentration of redundancies involving large numbers of women in a relatively small number of industries. In the areas in which we were primarily interested a number of approaches proved abortive, for very good reasons. The case studies initially projected in the clothing industry were not carried out because one of the plants was taken over by another company in the same group at the last minute, and a second plant was sold as a going concern also at the last minute. An initially encouraging response from a major employer in the communications industry was withdrawn because of serious difficulties in industrial relations. Since our project had little direct benefit either for the management or for the workers concerned in the redundancies studied we were very pleased at the ready access gained.

Although access was granted in principle without major difficulties the handling of relations with plant-level management required considerable tact. Access was, of course, granted in all cases by senior management, who were not involved in day-to-day production management problems. Also, our project appeared more relevant to personnel management than to production management. During plant run-downs day-to-day problems are unusually difficult because of fundamental uncertainties about the future. The extent to which our interviewing disturbed production depended upon the relative tightness of production constraints: the disturbance was greatest where production difficulties were greatest, which varied from case to case. In all cases the initial interview lasted from thirty minutes to an hour, during which time the women were released from their jobs. This was seen as a serious difficulty in one case study (C), and a lesser but still significant difficulty in another (A). Since the union representatives involved saw the project as of potential benefit to their members, relations with unions were less problematic throughout.

1.3 The women interviewed

The impact of redundancy and unemployment is likely to vary with the family circumstances, social background, commitment to employment, and economic situation of the women involved. Such factors will affect both the direct consequences of redundancy, economic and social, and the indirect consequences. For example, redundancy leads to the loss of the social, as well as economic, satisfactions derived from work. The extent to which 'social' satisfactions can be derived from other activities is influenced by the alternative roles available to women, especially within the family. This will be influenced by such factors as age, marital status, age and number of children, and size of household, as well as factors directly linked to market employment.

The basic research strategy for the project was the examination of female redundancy and unemployment through linked case studies, selected to represent a range of industries, occupations, and labour markets: since the criteria used were criteria for the selection of case study-sites, not for the selection of a specific population of respondents, the respondents interviewed do not comprise a sample of a specified total population. For example, we would have included a larger proportion of part-time workers if we had been concerned to sample the female labour force. However, the sites selected resulted in our interviewing women likely to be similar in many demographic characteristics to the majority of redundant women, for example in age. Moreover, the sites selected resulted in our interviewing women for whom the significance of job loss might be thought to be greatest, since their contribution to household income was substantial, and the availability of alternative roles was limited: we were thus concerned with a 'critical' case.

The remainder of this section provides a more detailed outline of our respondents, divided into five sections: age and family circumstances; social background; length of working life; occupation; present financial circumstances. Relevant comparative data is provided where possible.

1.3.1 Age and family circumstances

The majority of women were aged thirty-five or over, as is shown in Table 1.3.1.1.

Table 1.3.1.1
Age of respondents (by company)

Age	Firm					
	A (%)	B (%)	C (%)	D (%)	E (%)	Total (%)
15–24	16	0	8	12	8	8
25–34	10	15	26	19	18	18
35–44	29	41	35	28	27.5	33
45–54	20	37	27	28	31	29
55–59	25.5	7	1.5	14	16	12
Missing			3			1
N	51	68	66	43	51	279

Note: Percentage rounded to nearest whole number throughout.

The age categorization has been adopted to correspond to the different stages in the adult female life-cycle: 15–24 the pre-child-bearing period, 25–34 the period during which women are most likely to be bearing children and bringing them up at home, 35–44 covering the rearing of school-age children, and a remaining period of post-child-rearing. It is significant that our respondents were, on average, older than the total working female population, as Table 1.3.1.2 shows. Hence, only 26 per cent of our respondents were aged under 35, compared with 41 per cent of the total female working population, and 47 per cent of all women aged between 16 and 59. Conversely, it is hardly surprising that 41 per cent of our respondents were aged 45 +, compared with 33 per cent of all working women and 31 per cent of all women aged 16–59.

Table 1.3.1.2
Age of respondents compared with female working population and total female population

	Redundant women (%)	Total female working population (%)	Total female population aged 16–59 (%)
16–24	8	18	24
25–34	18	23	25
35–44	33	26	21
45–54	29	23	20
55–59	12	9	11

Sources: Martin and Roberts, p. 16.
Census 1981: Great Britain: Economic Activity, pp. 16–17.

Mature age, then, was a characteristic of the female work-force in at least four out of the firms studied, with a much higher representation in the older age brackets than is normal for the female work-force as a whole. In all four firms reduced demand and greater competitiveness within the industry had resulted in a need to cut back on employee numbers, which had been done at the expense of younger workers. Recruitment in these firms had almost ceased in the years preceding the redundancy. The total work-force in all firm B's factories had been reduced from over 6000 in 1971 to 1860 in 1981. Firm D's numbers had been reduced from 2000 in 1968–9 to 350 in 1982.

In previous years all four firms had in their heyday recruited and trained a number of school-leavers each year, these programmes had virtually ceased several years before the redundancy. In firm B, where the product had become obsolete and closure anticipated for many years, younger women had accepted redeployment elsewhere in the company. Older women had tended not to take this opportunity, in some cases because increased age and deteriorating eyesight had made them less able to acquire the skill necessary for piece-work assembly on a new product, in other cases because most of the opportunities for redeployment were on alternating shifts, 6.0-a.m. to 2.0-p.m. and 2.0-p.m. to 10.0-p.m., which did not suit married women. In firms D and E a gradually dwindling share of the market had caused these firms to cut back in employee numbers over the years by ceasing to recruit young workers. In firm A there had been very little recruitment for several years. As well as being a characteristic of 'dying' firms, a mature-aged and long-serving work-force, according to firm E's personnel officer, made a factory 'appropriate for redundancy', presumably because the high redundancy payments that long service usually attract would soften the blow of unemployment. This would be especially appropriate in areas of high unemployment (which applied in the case of firm E) where even young workers would have difficulty in securing re-employment.

The age distribution was as expected on the basis of previous research: redundancy is an age-related process for both men and women. Table 1.3.1.3 compares the age distribution of our respondents, who were of course all female, with the age distribution of the 10 per cent sample of notified redundants analysed by Jolly et al. on behalf of the Department of Employment, which included both men and women.[20] For comparison we have included the distributions for the three industries from which our respondents were drawn.

Table 1.3.1.3
Age of respondents compared with age of 10 per cent sample of redundants (1975)

	Redundant women (%)	Clothing and footwear (%)	Electrical engineering (%)	Vehicles (%)	All 10% sample (%)
16–24	8	10	8	5	7.5
25–34	18	17	18	18.5	18
35–44	33	22	21	20	20
45–54	29	30	25	21	25
55–59(64)	12	21	28	35.5	29
N	279	1184	2799	3379	34667

Source: Jolly et al., p. 107.

The figures are not directly comparable, since the DE figures quoted do not include workers under aged 20, who are not eligible for statutory redundancy payments, and our sample had no women aged over 59. The major differences relate to the heavier concentration of our respondents in the 35–54 age range, and the smaller proportion of respondents aged 55 +. This latter result is partly a function of the gender composition of the two groups: since the compulsory retirement age for women is five years earlier than that for men it is inevitable that a group of redundant respondents aged 55 + composed of women would be smaller than a similar group made up of male and female respondents, other things being equal. However, it is also likely that the dates of the two surveys are important: 1975 and 1981–2. In 1975 substantial numbers of redundancies were voluntary redundancies, redundancy compensation being used in practice as a means of easing early retirement:

Redundancy seemed to be acting as a social mechanism to remove voluntarily from the labour force older people nearing retirement after long service by means of comparatively generous compensation. This appears to be a quite satisfactory and unexceptionable way of matching the supply and demand of labour, and it is at one with the current measures to encourage voluntary early retirement where the (particularly financial) conditions are right.[47]

In our study we were concerned with compulsory redundancy, following long periods of attrition and, in case study B, a voluntary redundancy scheme: the relatively benign explanation possible for the age distribution of redundant employees in 1975–6 is not possible in 1981–2.

As would be expected, in view of their mature age, the majority of the women were married: 74 per cent, compared with 73 per cent of all working women and 71 per cent of all women of working age.

Table 1.3.1.4
Comparative marital status

	Redundant women (%)	All working women (%)	All women 16–59 (%)
Married	74	} 65	} 68
Separated	2		
Divorced	6.5	} 8	} 7
Widowed	3		
Single	14	28	24
Total	100		
N	279		

Source: Calculated from *Census 1981: Great Britain: Economic Activity,* Table 4B, pp. 134–5.

The proportion of divorced women amongst the redundant women is higher than amongst working women as a whole, or amongst the total female population in the age group. This would be expected on the basis of the greater age of the redundant women, and possibly also because of the economic pressure on divorced women to be in full-time rather than in part-time employment.

The difference between our respondents, the female employed population, and women as a whole, was even more pronounced with regard to the number of dependent children than with regard to age. 'Dependent' children could be defined either as those needing supervision, or as those who are economically dependent. The mother's role set, and the availability of alternative roles, will be affected where children require adult supervision; the household financial position will be affected where children are economically dependent. The age of 15 was taken as a somewhat arbitrary cut-off point for economic dependence, with 12 representing a legal milestone in the need for supervision and 5 the normal age of school entry. Comparative figures are available only for women with children aged 4 and under and 15 and under. Only 2.5 per cent of our respondents had children aged 4 and under compared with 18 per cent of all women of working age and only 26 per cent of our respondents had a child aged 15 or under, compared with 54 per cent of all women of working age.

Comparison between the number of economically dependent (student and pre-school) children of respondents, of women in employment, and of women of working age shows that the women interviewed had fewer economically dependent children than either women in employment or women in the age group as a whole. The relatively small number of children needing supervision was obviously an important factor in the availability of the women for full-time employment, and helps to explain their relatively sanguine attitudes towards the problems involved in reconciling domestic and work roles. On the other hand, the presence of economically dependent children could be an

Table 1.3.1.5
Comparative numbers of economically dependent children

No. of children	Respondents (%)	Women of working age (16–59) (%)
0	64.5	55
1	23	19
2	10	18
3	1	6
4 +	1	2
Total	100	100

incentive for women to go out to work to augment the family income. The age distribution of respondents' children is therefore clearly important and warrants a more detailed examination.

Table 1.3.1.6 shows the percentage of respondents with children in different age categories, the categories being chosen to represent pre-school (4 or under), the age at which children cannot be left unsupervised (12 and under), required school attendance age (15 and under), and age of pre-adult-hood (17 and under).

Table 1.3.1.6
Age distribution of respondents' children

	Age				
No. of children	⩽ 4 (%)	⩽ 12 (%)	⩽ 15 (%)	⩽ 17 (%)	All ages (%)
0	97.5	85	74	67	34
1	2.5	12.5	18	19	20
2		2.5	7.5	10	26
3		0.4	0.4	3	12
4			0.7	0.4	5
5				0.4	1
6					2
7					0.4

Table 1.3.1.6 succinctly summarizes the age distribution of respondents' children: only 2.5 per cent of respondents had at least one child of pre-school age, 15 per cent had at least one child 12 and under, 26 per cent had at least one child aged 15 and under, and 33 per cent had at least one child aged 17 and under. With ageing families, the household sizes of the respondents tended to be small, 40 per cent living in two-person households. On the other hand, there were very few single-person households.

To summarize, the majority of our respondents were aged over 35, in the second part of an interrupted working life. They were mainly married, but did not have children of pre-school age. The majority had children, and a substantial minority had economically dependent children, although their ages were such as not to require maternal supervision.

1.3.2 Social background

Social attitudes and behaviour are conditioned by the beliefs and expectations acquired over a lifetime, from family of origin, education, work experience, and friends. This applies to attitudes and behaviour in employment, redundancy, and unemployment as well as in other areas of social life. It was obviously impossible to examine the social and cultural background of our respondents in detail. However, social-class background, customarily associated with occupation, is a major influence upon attitudes and behaviour. We have therefore examined the occupations of both fathers and mothers. Moreover, since women are often held to derive their social-class position from their husbands' occupations, we have examined husbands' occupations.[48] Finally, education is important, both in providing formal qualifications and training, and in conditioning attitudes. We therefore present the data on the education of our respondents.

Analysis of the social background of our respondents inevitably involves the classification of occupations, both those of our respondents and those of their parents. There are several well-developed scales for the analysis of male occupations: we have chosen to follow that constructed by Hope and Goldthorpe for the Oxford Social Mobility Study.[49] However, there is no such scale for female occupations: even in Anthony Heath's unusual discussion of female social mobility he does not attempt to develop a scale appropriate for analysing female occupations.[50] As Martin and Roberts emphasize, the customary classifications of social class and socio-economic group are not very satisfactory bases for classifying women's jobs because most of the more common women's jobs fall into a limited number of categories.[51] Despite its limitations, for the analysis of social background we have used the Hope—Goldthorpe scale, as the most convenient method of summarizing our data comparatively: a more specialized categorization is presented below, in a more detailed discussion of the occupations of our own respondents.

As Table 1.3.2.1 shows, there was a general tendency for the occupational status of women to be linked to that of their fathers. Hence 52 per cent of women in occupational status 1 (professional/administrative) and 43 per cent of women in status 2 (supervisors) had fathers in the two higher occupational categories, as compared with only 24 per cent of respondents in status 3 (lower-grade clerical), 17 per cent in status 4 (semi-skilled), and 19 per cent in status 5 (unskilled) with fathers in the two higher occupational categories.

Despite differences in detail, the major conclusion is the similarity in background of our respondents except for those in professional, administrative, and supervisory occupations, who were disproportionately likely to have fathers in similar occupations: clerical and manual female employees were very similar to each other in father's occupation.

Table 1.3.2.1
Respondents' occupational status by fathers' occupational status

Respondents' status	Father's occupational status					
	Professional/ Administrative (%)	Managers/ Supervisors (%)	Clerical and Skilled manual (%)	Semi-skilled manual (%)	Unskilled manual (%)	Row totals
Professional/ Administrative	29 24	23.5 10	18 5	6 1.5	23.5 5	$N = 17$ 100 6
Manager/ Supervisor	29 19	14 5	7 2	14 3	36 6	$N = 14$ 100 5
Clerical/ Skilled	6 19	18 27.5	24 26	23 21.5	29 21	$N = 62$ 100 23
Semi-skilled	6 33	11 32.5	18 37	29 52	35 47	$N = 115$ 100 43
Unskilled	2 5	17 25	28 30	23 21.5	30 21	$N = 60$ 100 22
N Row percentage	21 8	40 15	57 21	65 24	85 32	268 100
Column percentage	100	100	100	100	100	100

($P = 0.009$).
Notes: (a) The occupational scale used is the Hope–Goldthorpe scale.
(b) The upper figure in each pair gives the row percentage; the lower the column percentage.

A similar picture emerges from an examination of the occupational status of daughters by father's occupation: the occupational status of daughters of fathers in status groups 1 and 2 was substantially higher than the status of daughters of fathers in other status groups.

Since we were interested in parental influences upon women's working lives we also asked respondents about their mothers' occupations. A surprisingly small number of women, 48 per cent, reported that their mothers had worked after the birth of the respondent, reflecting the relatively recent growth (at least in the twentieth century) of female participation in market work. As Table 1.3.2.2 shows, mothers of respondents had worked primarily in unskilled or very slightly skilled occupations – 76 per cent.

There is thus evidence of substantial social mobility if the occupations of daughters are compared with the occupations of mothers: 65 per cent of

Table 1.3.2.2
Occupational status of working mothers

Occupational status	Working mothers (%)
1	4.5
2	6
3	9
4	35
5	42
Missing	3
N	133

respondents fell into the low-status categories 4 and 5, compared with 76 per cent of working mothers. The contrast is sharper if attention is focused only on the least skilled group (cleaning): 22 per cent of respondents, but 42 per cent of respondents' mothers, were employed as cleaners.

Women employed in supervisory and managerial occupations were significantly more likely to have husbands in such occupations than any other group. Hence 64 per cent of women in status group 1 and 67 per cent of women in status group 2 had husbands in status groups 1 and 2. However, the comparable figure for clerical workers was only 39 per cent, for skilled and semi-skilled manual workers 25 per cent, and for unskilled manual workers 24 per cent. Moreover, as Table 1.3.2.3 shows, the occupational status of husbands of clerical workers was very similar to the occupational status of husbands of manual workers: hence 36 per cent of clerical workers, 34 per cent of semi-skilled manual workers, and 30 per cent of unskilled manual workers had husbands in status group 3. Interestingly, a majority of men in occupational status group 1 had wives in non-manual occupations (63 per cent), substantially more than any other status group. Comparable figures for other groups were: 2, 35 per cent; 3, 28 per cent; 4, 21.5 per cent; and 5, 23 per cent. There is thus substantial evidence of social homogeneity between wives and their husbands in status group 1, and to a lesser extent 2, and heterogeneity amongst the other groups, including clerical workers.

Comparison between the occupational statuses of our respondents and the occupational statuses of their parents and husbands shows that our respondents had higher statuses than their mothers, but lower statuses than their husbands or fathers. Table 1.3.2.4 summarizes the occupational statuses of all respondents, married respondents, working mothers, fathers, and husbands.

Husbands tended to have higher occupational statuses than fathers, with 63 per cent of husbands in the top three occupational categories compared with 41.5 per cent of fathers. This would be expected on the basis of changes in the overall occupational structure in the period covered by our data.

The majority of the women interviewed had left school at the minimum

Table 1.3.2.3
Occupational status of wives and husbands

	Husband's occupational status					
Respondents' status	Professional/ Administrative (%)	Manager/ Supervisory (%)	Clerical/ Skilled manual (%)	Semi-skilled manual (%)	Unskilled manual (%)	Row totals (%)
Professional/ Administrative	50 23	14 5	7 1.5	7 2	21 9	$N = 14$ 100 7
Manager/ Supervisor	44 13	22 5	11 1	11 2	11 3	$N = 9$ 100 4
Clerical/ Skilled	18 27	20.5 24	36 25	16 17	9 11	$N = 44$ 100 21
Semi-skilled	8 27	17 43	34 51	24 55	17 46	$N = 96$ 100 46
Unskilled	6.5 10	17 22	30 21.5	22 24	24 31	$N = 46$ 100 22
N Row percentage	30 14	37 18	65 31	42 20	35 17	209 100
Column percentage	100	100	100	100	100	100

($P = 0.006$).

Notes: (a) The occupational scale used in the Hope–Goldthorpe scale.
(b) Table refers only to married women with husbands in employment.
(c) The upper figure in each pair gives the row percentage; the lower the column percentage.

Table 1.3.2.4
Comparative occupational status

Category	Hope–Goldthorpe Scale	All respondents (%)	Married respondents (%)	Working mothers (%)	Fathers (%)	Husbands (%)
1	75–61	7	7	4.5	7.5	14
2	58–47	4	4	6	14	18
3	46–38	23	21	9	20	31
4	37–33	46	46	35	23	20
5	31–18	20	22	42	30.5	17
Other				1.5		
Don't know		0	0	1.5	4	
N		279	209	133	279	209

school-leaving age, which for many women had been 14. Only a small number had sat any public examinations or undertaken formal post-school training before entering the work-force. Tables 1.3.2.5–6 show the age at which respondents left school and the public examinations they had passed.

Table 1.3.2.5
Age at which respondents left school

Age	Respondents (%)
14	25
15	52
16	17
17	3
18	3

($N = 279$)

Table 1.3.2.6
Public examinations passed by respondents

Examinations passed	Respondents (%)
None	78
CSE (not Grade 1)	7
CSE Grade 1 or GCE O Level	10
GCE A Level	2
Clerical and commercial	2
Other	1

($N = 279$)

Post-school vocational education mostly took the form of part-time commercial courses (paid for privately) to learn shorthand, typing, and office practice. However, three women had done City and Guilds Catering Courses and five had done City and Guilds Sewing Machinist Courses. One of the more senior clerical workers had completed a Bachelor of Arts degree, and six women had served their time as apprentices, but had subsequently left to raise a family and had not been able to re-enter their trades (hairdressing, printing/bookbinding, and one motor mechanic.) The five industrial nurses had, of course, gained nursing certificates.

Table 1.3.2.7 shows the type of post-school education undertaken.

Altogether eighty-six (31 per cent) women had done some vocational training and a further seventeen, who had done no vocational training, had taken self-improvement courses.

Decisions about leaving school and undertaking further education are likely to be influenced by parents' class and income. There was a correlation between

Table 1.3.2.7
Respondents' further education

Course	Respondents (%)
Vocational	
Commercial (shorthand/typing etc.)	25
Apprenticeships	2
City and Guilds machinist	2
Nursing	1
City and Guilds catering	1
BA (only one completed)	1
Higher-level clerical (Accounting/Institute of Personnel Management/Management	1
Total (percentage)	33
N	93
Self-improvement and Hobby courses (percentage)	8
N	23
None (percentage)	63
N	176
Total N	292*

*Thirteen had taken more than one course.

age of leaving school and father's occupational status ($P > 0.001$) and a slight correlation ($P = 0.101$) between vocational education and father's occupational status, with children of higher-status fathers more likely to stay longer at school and to do some type of further vocational training. Tables 1.3.2.8–9 show the correlation between age of leaving school and father's occupational status and the correlation between father's occupational status and respondents taking one (or more) vocational training courses.

Decisions made about secondary and further education were not always those that the women themselves had wanted. They were asked if there had been any

Table 1.3.2.8
Age at which respondents left school (by father's occupational status)

School-leaving age	Father's occupational status					Missing	Row totals
	1 (%)	2 (%)	3 (%)	4 (%)	5 (%)		
14	5	15	23	21	36		25
15	38	47	54	60	48		52
16	24	27	16	17	13		17
17	9	10	3	1			3
18	24		3		2		3
N	21	40	57	65	85	11	279

($P = 0.001$)

Table 1.3.2.9
Further education (by father's occupational status)

	Father's occupational status				
	1 (%)	2 (%)	3 (%)	4 (%)	5 (%)
Vocational training	48	40	26	29	27
N	21	40	57	65	85

($P = 0.101$)

kind of early training or education they had wanted to do but had been unable to do: 33 per cent answered yes. Table 1.3.2.10 lists the types of vocational training that the women said they would have liked to have done.

Table 1.3.2.10
Vocational training respondents wished to do but could not

Vocational training	N
Nursing	18
Hairdressing	12
Shorthand/typing	9
Teaching	7
Continue with secondary education	6
Nursery nurse	4
Designer	4
Computing	3
Commercial art	3
Secretarial	3
Catering	3
Dressmaking/tailoring	3
Police Force	3
Librarian	2
Motor mechanic	2
Radiographer	1
Vet.	1
Lab. assistant	1
Personnel officer	1
Air-hostess	1
'Other'	4
Total	91

Women saying that they had not wished to undertake vocational training sometimes meant that they had not considered further education or training as a serious possibility at the time. Several commented: 'They didn't have anything like that for girls like us in those days', or, 'You just went straight from school to the factory and didn't think about it, because that's what everyone did.'

Only eleven (12 per cent) of the ninety-one who would have preferred to train said that they had been unable to do so because they had sat and failed qualifying examinations: thirty-three (36 per cent) gave poverty as a reason, and twelve (13 per cent) said that their parents had refused permission.

In conclusion, the majority of women interviewed came from manual-working-class backgrounds, although a small number had fathers in professional, administrative, supervisory, and management positions. Women in professional, administrative, and supervisory jobs were likely to have fathers in occupational status groups 1 or 2, but clerical workers were only slightly more likely than manual workers to do so. In general clerical workers were similar to manual workers in social background, as indicated by their fathers' and husbands' occupations. Only a minority of respondents reported that their mothers had gone out to work after their birth, the large majority having jobs falling in occupational status categories 4 and 5. The majority of respondents had left school at the minimum school-leaving age, without obtaining formal qualifications. A minority had undertaken post-secondary vocational education, by far the most common being commercial subjects: this minority was disproportionately drawn from women with fathers in higher occupational status groups. A large minority of women (33 per cent) said they would have liked to have undertaken vocational training on leaving school but had not been able to do so.

1.3.3 *Length of working life*

Over half our respondents had been in market employment for twenty years or more, as Table 1.3.3.1 shows.

Table 1.3.3.1
Length of working life (by firm)

	A	B	C	D	E	Total cumulative
0–4	100	100	100	100	100	100
5–9	91	100	96	96	96	95
10–14	79	100	85	77	94	89
15–19	69	96	70	72	80	78
20–4	52	74	49	46	64	62
25–9	40	46	29	34	44	43
30–4	26	25	12	27	24	23
35–9	14	9	6	11	18	13
40 +	10	0	1.5	9	12	4

The table indicates a considerably longer period in market employment than working women in general, as would be expected in view of the age distribution of our respondents. Women in case study B, North West electronics, had spent an especially long time in market employment. The table shows the total length of time in market employment, which was not of course continuous; nevertheless, it indicates a considerable commitment to market employment.

The majority of women interviewed had had at least one break in their working life (69 per cent), but relatively few had had more than one break. Table 1.3.3.2 shows the number of breaks in employment by firm.

Table 1.3.3.2
Number of breaks in working life (by firm)

	A (%)	B (%)	C (%)	D (%)	E (%)	Total (%)
None	37	15	41	37	29	31
1	39	47	39	60.5	61	48
2	10	23.5	11	2	8	12
3	8	9	6	0	2	5
4 +	6	6	3	0	0	3
N	51	68	66	43	51	279

($P = 0.002$)

The major finding is that the women in North West engineering (clerical) and Midlands engineering (clerical) had fewer breaks than the manual workers did. This was not because they were younger than the manual workers — there was little difference in age between respondents in case studies D and E and other respondents. Instead, there is a suggestion that clerical workers are more committed than manual workers to jobs which, as we show in Chapter 2 (pp. 90–5) they regard as intrinsically interesting. It may well be more difficult for clerical workers in large-scale organizations to accommodate interruptions to market employment than for manual workers, without losing their occupational status. (And, of course, clerical workers are less likely to be subject to redundancy.) These suggestions are reinforced by an analysis of the number of breaks in working life by occupational status: no woman in a professional or administrative occupation had had more than one break in employment, and only 12 per cent of clerical workers had. Frequent breaks in market employment were concentrated in occupational status group 3 (semi-skilled manual workers), 34 per cent of whom had had two or more breaks.

The length of time spent out of the labour force was short, as Table 1.3.3.3 shows.

Hence 80 per cent of respondents had been out of work for five years or less at their last break, indicating a return to work as soon as children had reached school age, or sooner. We were interested to see if there had been a change in the length of time spent away from work, with a 'speeding up' in the process of returning to work amongst younger age groups. However, since our respondents were heavily concentrated in the age group 35 +, and the amount of time off work was so limited, no significant variation was found. Those respondents who had had more than one break in employment were likely to have had only relatively short breaks: 70 per cent of respondents who reported having had

Table 1.3.3.3
Length of breaks in employment

	Last or only break (%)	Penultimate break (%)
No break	31	80
Under 1 year	18	8
1–2 years	18	6
3–5 years	14	–
6–10 years	11	6
10 +	9	–
N	279	279

two breaks from work had spent two years or less out of work on their penultimate period out of work.

As expected, the major reason for leaving market employment was pregnancy, as Table 1.3.3.4 shows. However, a substantial number had also left market employment for other reasons, including redundancy.

Table 1.3.3.4
Reasons for ceasing market employment

	Last or only break (%)	Second-last break (%)
Pregnancy	50	16
Redundancy	6	–
Moved from district	3	1
Ill health	3	1
Marriage	2	–
Care for sick parent/relative	1	0.4
Did not like job	1	1
Other	2	0.4
No break	31	80
Missing	1	–
N	279	279

Hence 50 per cent of women had left market employment to have a child, 72.5 per cent of all respondents who reported having interrupted their employment career. The other major reason for interrupting employment was redundancy, mentioned by 8.5 per cent of women who had interrupted their working careers.

As would be expected on the basis of their age and length of time in paid employment, the women interviewed had had considerably longer service with their then current employer than working women generally. Table 1.3.3.5 shows length of service by firm.

34 Working Women in Recession

Table 1.3.3.5
Length of service in present job (by firm)

	A	B	C	D	E	Total
0–4	100	100	100	100	100	100
5–9	73	100	72	81	81	82
10–14	61	99	44	51	65.5	65
15–19	38	53	23	37	38	37.5
20–4	32	27	9	18	18	20.5
25–9	24	18	4.5	9	6	12.5
30–4	12	8	0	4	4	6
35–40	6	1.5	1.5	0	0	2
40+	6	0	0	2	0	1

Thus 82 per cent of women had been employed in their present job at least five years, and in the North West electronics firm all respondents had been: 65 per cent had been employed in the same job for ten years or more, and 20 per cent for twenty years or more — 32 per cent of workers in plant A and 27 per cent in plant B. In comparison, only 19 per cent of all working women had been with their current employers for ten years or more, and only 6 per cent for twenty years or more.

In short, if commitment is measured by length of time working, the women interviewed were very highly committed to market employment.

1.3.4 Occupation

In analysing the occupations pursued by our respondents we used two occupational classifications, related to different aspects of jobs. The first was a modification of the Hope—Goldthorpe scale, involving the collapse of the higher categories in the original Hope—Goldthorpe scale, and the elaboration of the lower categories. This scale is referred to subsequently as 'occupational status'. The second was a fuller classification, constructed inductively on the basis of type of occupation, as type of occupation was thought to locate respondents in a particular job market and hence might affect future employment prospects. For example, it was thought that experience of electronic-assembly work would be helpful in finding future employment in the electronics industry, and experience of engineering-assembly work might not, although both occupations fall in the same occupational-status category. The following paragraphs explain the categorizations used, and the location of our respondents in them.

Table 1.3.4.1 outlines the occupational-status classification used, the equivalent Hope-Goldthorpe grading, and for illustration the most common occupations followed by our respondents. The table is not fully satisfactory, since vertical segregation may mean that women placed in the same broad job category as men may not have the same tasks, conditions, or pay: this is especially likely to be so in the group of jobs classified as 'clerical'. However, it is valuable for comparisons among women.

Table 1.3.4.1
Occupational-status gradings

Status	Hope-Goldthorpe grading	Occupation	Respondents (%)	(N)
1 Administrative/ Professional/ Supervisory/	61–47	Administrator, supervisor, nurse, computer programmer	11	31
2 Clerical	46–38	Secretary, typist, clerk telephonist, cashier and wages clerk, data analyst	23	65
3 Manual semi-skilled/service higher grade	37–33	Machinist, assembler, inspector, technical assistant, cook	43	120
4 Manual slightly skilled	28–27	Hand-sewer, underpresser, trimmer, caterer, storeperson	17	47
5 Unskilled	18	Cleaner	6	16
			100	279

In short, 35 per cent of our respondents were non-manual and 66 per cent were manual workers. This classification is the basis for any table referring to occupational status (unless stated otherwise).

The fivefold classification of occupations into status groups derived from the Hope–Goldthorpe scale provided a satisfactory means of differentiating respondents. However, the classification was of only limited value, since 43 per cent of respondents were clustered in the largest category, group 3. Moreover, occupational status, as measured by the Hope-Goldthorpe scale, is based on the general desirability of jobs; it may or may not be relevant to labour-market experience. Accordingly, we constructed inductively a fuller classification, classifying the occupations followed on the basis of type of occupation. Table 1.3.4.2 shows the groups devised, and the distribution of our respondents between the groups.

It is important to stress that the classification of groups is not a vertical scale, but the grouping together of occupations sharing certain characteristics. Subsequent tables referring to 'occupations' refer to this grouping.

The first three case studies were primarily concerned with manual workers, of different types, case studies 4 and 5 primarily with clerical workers, although there were very small numbers of workers from the 'other side' of the manual/non-manual line in each case. Hence there were five non-manual workers interviewed in Company A, three in Company B, and eighteen in Company C; conversely, there were six manual workers (cleaners and caterers) interviewed in Company D, and fourteen in Company E. Table 1.3.4.3 presents the distribution of respondents within each firm by occupational status, and Table 1.3.4.4 within each firm by occupation.

Table 1.3.4.2
Distribution of respondents (by type of occupation)

Occupation	Respondents (N)	(%)
1 Nursing	5	2
2 Catering	13	5
3 Administrative	10	4
4 Clerical	73	26
5 Computing	5	2
6 Machine-sewing	36	13
7 Hand-sewing	24	9
8 Electronic assembly	56	20
9 Engineering assembly	27	10
10 General services (cleaning, stores)	30	11
N	279	102 (rounding)

Table 1.3.4.3
Occupational status (by company)

Occupational status	Company A N (%)	B N (%)	C N (%)	D N (%)	E N (%)	Total N (%)
Professional/ Administrative Supervisory	1 2.0	1 1.5	9 13.6	9 20.9	11 21.6	31 11.1
Clerical	4 7.8	2 2.9	9 13.6	27 62.8	23 45.1	65 23.3
Semi-skilled	23 45.1	56 82.4	37 56.1	1 2.3	3 5.9	120 43.0
Slightly skilled	23 45.1	5 7.4	9 13.6	3 7.0	7 13.7	47 16.8
Unskilled		4 5.9	2 3.0	3 7.0	7 13.7	16 5.7
Total N	51	68	66	43	51	279

Women tend to work in occupations that are segregated, both horizontally and vertically, from those of men. They are clustered in a minority of occupations in which the majority of workers are female, and in those occupations that they share with men they tend to cluster on the lower rungs of the promotional ladder. The 1971 Census showed that, although a quarter of all women were employed in manufacturing industry, half of those were employed in only four industries: food and drink, clothing and footwear, textiles, and electrical engineering. Of those occupations that are represented in our five case studies,

Table 1.3.4.4
Occupation (by company)

Occupation	Company					Totals
	A N (%)	B N (%)	C N (%)	D N (%)	E N (%)	N (%)
Nursing			1 1.5	1 2.3	3 5.9	5 1.8
Catering	2 3.9	1 1.5		3 7.0	7 13.7	13 4.7
Administrative			5 7.6	3 7.0	2 3.9	10 3.6
Clerical	4 7.8	2 2.9	11 16.7	32 74.4	24 47.1	73 26.2
Computing					5 9.8	5 1.8
Machine-sewing	24 47.1	1 1.5	11 16.7			36 12.9
Hand-sewing	21 41.2		3 4.5			24 8.6
Electrical assembly		56 82.4				56 20.1
Engineering assembly			27 40.9			27 9.7
General services		8 11.8	8 12.1	4 9.3	10 19.6	30 10.8
Total N	51	68	66	43	51	279

the 1971 census shows that 96 per cent of all machine- and hand-sewers were women, as were 84 per cent of electrical assemblers, 99 per cent of typists, secretaries, and shorthand writers, 91 per cent of nurses, over 91 per cent of canteen assistants and 76–90 per cent of office cleaners.[52] Although there is a slightly lower degree of horizontal segregation among clerical workers, only 70 per cent of whom were women, a high degree of vertical segregation existed in this occupation, including in the two factories in our study which employed significant numbers of clerical workers.

Legislation on equal opportunities and the social changes that led to it may to a small extent have broken down the horizontal segregation that existed in 1971, although Hakim's research suggests otherwise.[53] In one of the five case studies, Company C, this legislation had opened up to women engineering-assembly jobs previously available only to men, and similarly had encouraged men to apply for machining and trimming jobs which had previously been done by women. Process work had therefore become integrated in this firm, and the average wage for women in this firm was substantially higher than that of female operatives in the two firms in which manual occupations were still segregated. In the clothing factory (Company A) and the valve section of the electronics factory (Company B), sex barriers still divided shop-floor occupations. In Companies D and E women did not work on the shop floor at all, but only as clerks, cleaners, canteen and warehouse assistants. The following paragraphs explain the occupational structure of the five companies in more detail.

In Company A occupations were divided on the basis of gender, with only females engaged in machine and hand-sewing, and only males engaged in cutting and pressing (using heavy steam pressers). One occupation, underpressing, was open to both males and females. Cutting was traditionally the career grade, and the plant General Manager had started his working life as a cutter. There was also vertical segregation; ten of the eleven supervisors were men, and the single female supervisor had been appointed supervisor *qua* training officer only under pressure. The General Manager, Office Manager, two floor managers, and Works Study Officer were also male.

In Company B both men and women were employed as operators: in October 1981 there were 448 full-time male operators, 395 full-time female operators, and 138 part-time female operators. The valve division, the unit being closed, was also integrated, employing a total of 106 women and 62 men. However, there were major gender differences between different sections of the labour force as a whole: although 46.9 per cent of full-time operators were female, only 22.1 per cent of full time weekly staff (technical assistants, skilled craftsmen, clerical workers) were female, and 13 per cent of monthly staff (charge-hands, managers, senior secretaries). Within the valve division there were similar differences, as Table 1.3.4.5 shows.

Table 1.3.4.5
Occupational distribution in Valve Division (Company B)

	Male	Female	Total	Female (%)
Production	51	104	155	67.1
Weekly staff	30	12	42	28.6
Monthly staff	22	2	24	8.3
N	103	118	221	

There was thus a substantial variation in the proportion of women in the different groups, a very substantial majority of production workers being female, but only a small minority of monthly staff. Amongst production workers men were employed in valve engineering, sealing and pumping, grids and frame grids, chemicals and processing, and, to a lesser extent, glass bulbs and bases: women were heavily concentrated in valve assembly.

In Company C there was substantial vertical job segregation, but relatively limited horizontal segregation. Although detailed figures are not available, there were relatively few women employed in managerial, administrative, and supervisory roles. There was a wide dispersal of occupations amongst female production workers. However, because the present distribution of female employees was based upon a traditional division of labour, with relatively little recent recruitment to provide a means for changing the gender distribution, some sections of the labour force remained predominantly female (sewing, some section of trim), and some predominantly male (e.g. early stages of assembly).

In Company D there were no female operatives, all women being employed in clerical or ancillary services (cleaning, catering, nursing, stores). The male operatives were predominantly skilled tradesmen, mainly AUEW members, or held higher qualifications and belonged to TASS. Among the clerical and administrative staff there was a high degree of vertical segregation. At the time of interviewing, thirty-seven men were employed in administrative and clerical duties, and thirty-eight women. Among the men, only six occupied a status below Grade V, and among the women only six occupied a status above that of Grade V. The all-female canteen staff was managed by a man.

In Company E there were very few women operatives, nearly all women being employed in clerical and ancillary services. Again, there was very marked vertical segregation, of the thirty-three men employed in clerical and administrative duties only seven occupied positions below that of Grade III, but among the forty-one women employed in clerical and administrative duties only two occupied positions as high as Grade III and none went above that grade. (In Company D high-numbered grades denoted high status.) Again, the all-female canteen staff were managed by a male manager.

1.3.5 Economic situation

In understanding the impact of redundancy and unemployment it is obviously important to understand the economic circumstances of the women concerned before the redundancy. This section of the introduction presents data on the incomes of respondents before the redundancy, the incomes of their husbands, the uses to which their incomes were put, and the cost of housing, which was seen as a major long-term financial commitment.

There are serious difficulties in obtaining reliable financial information in the absence of access to individual wage and salary statements. The difficulties are especially great when the interest is in net earnings, rather than in gross earnings which would be derivable from standard occupational-earnings data. The initial difficulties relate to the reliability of information, especially information relating to earnings of people other than the respondents themselves. There are additional problems in interpreting figures of net earnings, owing to uncertainties about individual tax positions, and the extent to which individuals differed in the non-tax adjustments made in calculating take-home pay. Finally, there are difficulties in the use of average weekly earnings, or surveys in the most recent pay period, where earnings vary weekly according to either the number of hours worked (the part-time workers in plant A), the number of pieces worked (piece workers in plant B), or the level of production bonus (in plant C). Since we did not have independent access to individual-earnings data we relied upon individual respondents for their own and their spouses' earnings: where we could check responses against known rates-for-the-job, respondents appeared to answer reliably, although our ability to check respondents' statements about spouses' earnings was very limited. We considered relying upon gross rather than upon net earnings, but decided to use net earnings as the most easily remembered figure ('the bottom line') and as the indicator of *disposable* income: respondents were asked to answer in terms of earnings actually received. Finally, the figures relate to the most recent pay period, translated into weekly terms where respondents were paid fortnightly or monthly; the pay periods chosen are therefore not the same weeks for all respondents. With these reservations, Table 1.3.5.1 shows the distribution of net earnings per week.

Table 1.3.5.1
Respondents' net earnings

(£s)	Part-time (%)	Full-time (%)	Total (%)
0–29	4	–	1
30–39	44	1	9
40–49	42	6	13
50–54	4	11	9
55–59	2	12.5	10
60–64	4	29	24
65–69	2	12	10
70–79	–	19	15
80 +	–	7	6
Missing	–	3	2.5
N	55	236	279

The average net wage for all respondents was £59.10. More meaningfully, the average wage for part-time women was £40.40, with a standard deviation of 9, for full-time women £63.90, with a standard deviation of 12. This compared with average gross earnings for part-time women workers in 1981 of £38.20 (£43.10 for non-manual, £33.00 for manual), and for full-time women workers in manufacturing industry of £76.30. Although issues of earnings relativities are not central to the concerns of the research project, the distribution of earnings conforms to the general pattern of lower hourly earnings for part-time than those for full-time employees.[54] In our study an 'industry' and a 'part-time' effect mutually reinforced each other, the majority of part-time workers being employed in the clothing industry.

Apart from a substantial gap of nearly £14 between the average weekly net earnings of respondents in occupational status group 1 and the overall average, there was very little difference between occupational-status groups in earnings. The range was particularly narrow for full-time workers, as Table 1.3.5.2 shows.

Table 1.3.5.2
Average weekly earnings (by occupational status)

Occupational status	Earnings (full-time only) (£s)	Standard deviation	N
1	76.40	17	28
2	61.10	7	59
3	63.90	11	94
4	58.40	11.5	31
5	59.80	10	5
Total	63.90	12	217

The standard deviation was also small for all except occupational status group 1, and was especially small for clerical workers. In other words, the range of earnings appeared to be very narrow. As we show below, this was because specific industry and occupational variations overrode differences associated with differences in occupational status, not because earnings were similar overall.

There were systematic earnings differences linked to occupation, as Table 1.3.5.3 shows.

Table 1.3.5.3
Occupation and earnings

	Average earnings				
	Part-time (£s)	Standard deviation	Full-time (£s)	Standard deviation	N
1 Nursing	–	–	96.00	27	5
2 Catering	43.40	8	60.00	14	13
3 Administrative	–	–	73.40	14	9
4 Clerical	48.00	15	61.60	7	68
5 Computing	–	–	72.60	11	5
6 Machine-sewing	37.20	8	63.30	13	36
7 Hand-sewing	35.70	7	53.20	12	23
8 Electrical assembly	43.80	9	58.80	9	56
9 Engineering assembly	–	–	73.40	9	27
10 General services	40.10	8	63.10	9	30
Total	40.40	9	63.90	12	

Nursing, an organized profession with restricted entry, attracted the highest average wage, with the highest standard deviation (due to a formal promotional ladder with significant gradings), followed by administration, computing, and engineering assembly, all of which attracted similar wages, approximately £20 lower. Catering, clerical, machine-sewing, electronic assembly, and general services are grouped together, with an average wage approximately a further £10 lower, and hand-sewing, for which the demand has practically disappeared, occupied the lowest rung of the ladder.

For comparative purposes, Table 1.3.5.4 shows average gross weekly earnings for full-time women and men in the industries in which the case studies took place:

Table 1.3.5.4
Average earnings of full-time women 18 and over and of full-time men 21 and over

Manual	Women (£s)	Men (£s)
All manufacturing industries	76.3	124.7
Automotive engineering manufacture	90.1	122.6
Clothing	64.1	96.7
Radio and electronic components	78.1	110.7
Non-manual		
All manufacturing industries	87.3	168.6
Automotive engineering manufacture	89.1	161.8
Mechanical engineering	81.6	168.6

Source: New Earnings Survey, April 1981.

Since the dates of the figures differ, and the coverage of the NES figures and our own are not identical, detailed comparison is inappropriate. However, the NES figures indicate that our earnings data are not implausible, and that the relativities are a reflection of those in the industries concerned as a whole.

Average income did not generally vary with breadwinner status. However, although only 10 per cent described themselves as earning 'extras', their earnings were significantly lower than the rest. Table 1.3.5.5 gives a distribution of the average income of respondents by breadwinner status, excluding the seven women who did not give their income.

Table 1.3.5.5
Women's earnings (by breadwinner status)

Breadwinner status	Average (£s)	Respondents (N)	(%)
Earning own keep	59.70	46	17
Sole breadwinner	61.80	43	16
Joint breadwinner	60.20	151	55
Earning extras or own pocket money	47.00	29	11
Main breadwinner	96.00	2	0.7
Missing data		1	0.4
Total		272	100

In addition, five women who defined themselves as 'earning their own keep' and two women who described themselves as 'joint breadwinners' did not give their income.

Wives' earnings were, as expected, lower than husbands, as Table 1.3.5.6 shows: respondents' incomes are shown for comparison.

Table 1.3.5.6
Husbands' and wives' incomes

Income (£s)	Husbands (%)	Wives (%)
0–19*	5	0
20–45	6	20
46–65	6	54
66–85	21	22
86–105	18	3
106–220	9	1
Missing data	35	0
N	207	207

*The 5 per cent in this category had no income.

The data on husbands' incomes are seriously unreliable owing to the very large number of non-responses, due either to ignorance or to unwillingness to reveal. The non-response rate was slightly higher for husbands in a relatively high-status occupation (non-manual and skilled manual), differential non-response thus biasing the mean income downwards.

On the basis of the responses given, working husbands' average contribution to the family income was higher than that of their wives, the average take-home pay of working husbands being £88.50, whilst that of married women was £59.20. (Single respondents were not included in this figure.) Standard deviation for wives' earnings (including both full- and part-time) was 15, compared with 28 for husbands' income. On average, wives with working husbands contributed 40 per cent of the family income; and full-time wives contributed 43 per cent. However, twenty-two husbands were unemployed. The average wage for wives was 66 per cent that of their husbands. However, the average wage for *all full-time* working respondents was 72 per cent of the average wage for husbands.

Table 1.3.5.7 gives a breakdown of the wife's earning as a percentage of the joint earnings of husband and wife, in comparison with figures for all working women. As Table 1.3.5.7 shows, the respondents made a higher proportionate contribution to joint earnings than working women generally, in both part- and full-time categories. Hence, 71 per cent of part-time respondents contributed 30 per cent or more to joint earnings, compared with only 21 per cent of part-time women workers generally (although the number of relevant part-time

Table 1.3.5.7
Wife's earnings as percentage of joint earnings: respondents compared with all working women

Wife's earnings as percentage of joint income	Full-time		Part-time		All	
	Respondents (%)	All working women (%)	Respondents (%)	All working women (%)	Respondents (%)	All working women (%)
1–9	0	0	0	10	0	5
10–19	0	1	5	34	1	19
20–9	1	10	24	35	5	23
30–9	26	34	52	15	31	24
40–9	61	39	19	4	53	20
50+	12	16	0	2	10	9
N	102	757	21	888	123	1645

Note: Unpublished data made available by J. Martin and C. Roberts.

workers amongst our respondents is only small): even making due allowance for the relatively low incomes of respondents' husbands, and the downwardly biased figures for husbands' earnings, the difference is substantial. There was a similar contrast amongst full-time workers: 73 per cent of respondents contributed 40 per cent or more to joint earnings, compared with 55 per cent of full-time women workers generally. As would be expected, since our respondents were primarily manual workers and routine clerical workers, relatively few contributed more than 50 per cent to joint earnings – 12 per cent, compared with 16 per cent in the *Women and Employment* survey, the 12 per cent including working wives of the unemployed and pensioners. In short, the economic contribution of respondents' incomes to joint incomes was substantial. (The words 'joint income' have been used throughout in place of 'household income' because of the unreliability of data on contributions made to household income by people other than respondents and their spouses.)

In changing household financial circumstances it is necessary to examine patterns of expenditure as well as earnings. Patterns of expenditure obviously vary widely, depending upon the values and preferences of the people involved: it is therefore difficult to compare households. However, housing is a necessary item of expenditure. We therefore asked respondents about housing tenure and levels of expenditure on housing.

The majority of respondents lived in privately owned accommodation, as Table 1.3.5.8 shows. The small number of married respondents living in rented accommodation is noteworthy, especially in view of their relatively low occupational status (14 per cent compared with 42 per cent of all households.) This is of course consistent with an economic motivation to work, a primary economic motivation being house purchase.

Table 1.3.5.8
Housing tenure and marital status

	Single/Widowed/Divorced (%)	Married (%)
Rent-free	37	0.5
Renting	22	14
Mortgage	22	63
Owned outright	10	22
Missing	8	0.5
N	73	206

Although a majority of respondents were owner-occupiers, with mortgage payments likely to be higher than rents for rented accommodation, especially publicly rented accommodation, housing expenditure was relatively low, as Table 1.3.5.9 shows:

Table 1.3.5.9
Cost of housing

£s per week	Percentage
0	32
1–9	16
10–14	13
15–19	14
20–9	9
30–49	7
50 +	4
Missing	5

($N = 279$)

The relatively low figure for housing costs reflects the location of the research sites, the age of respondents, and probably relatively modest tastes. Three of the research sites were located in relatively low-cost housing areas. Moreover, since few respondents were in early married life, it is likely that most houses were purchased before the escalation in house prices of the 1970s.

Married women and householders indicated that their earnings went mainly towards meeting basic household needs. Forty-eight per cent said that their earnings were pooled jointly with those of their husbands (or other joint breadwinners), and not used for special items of expenditure. Forty per cent listed the items in the family budget for which their earnings were earmarked, presented in Table 1.3.5.10. The remaining 12 per cent were young single women still living with their parents who did not contribute to family income except through a fixed sum paid for their board and lodging. This amount was generally under £20 a week, leaving £30–40 a week for personal expenditure and savings.

Table 1.3.5.10
Use of women's earnings

	Percentage*
Pooled for joint use	5.5
Household expenditures	
Food	22
Fuel, telephone	8.5
Mortgage, rates	5
Clothes	3
Durables	3
Children's needs	2
'Household things'	2
Petrol	1
Car	0.4
Everything	8
Other	
'Extras'	4
Holidays	3
Savings	2
Pocket money	2
Children's education	0.4

*Percentage is that of women mentioning each item.
Population = 247 (married women and householders).

The table indicates that earnings were earmarked for items of domestic expenditure, of varying degrees of urgency. In general, earnings were not earmarked for savings and special circumstances but regarded as an element in the routine household budget.

To summarize: the average net earnings of part-time employees was £40.40, for full-time employees £63.90: 88.4 per cent of part-time employees earned under £50 a week, 11.5 per cent of full-time employees earned under £50 per week. The small number of women describing themselves as 'earning extras' earned less, on average, than those who described themselves as joint bread-winners – they were also more likely to be part-time workers. Wives with working husbands contributed 40 per cent of the family income, full-time working wives contributed 43 per cent. In general, our respondents made a higher contribution to household income than respondents in the *Women and Employment* survey, among both part-time and full-time workers. Although the majority of respondents were paying off mortgages expenditure on housing was low. Women's earnings were frequently pooled with those of other members of the household, but where they were earmarked for special purposes the purposes were invariably domestic.

1.4 Conclusion

Since the mid 1970s there has been a rapid growth in political and academic interest in issues concerning women and employment. This interest has resulted in a burgeoning growth of publications in women's studies, and increasing awareness of womens' perspectives on social issues. However, the publication of systematic research on issues concerning women and employment has been slower, and on female redundancy and unemployment barely started. The major focus of previous research on women and work has been on the links between domestic and work roles, and on the way in which work roles complement domestic roles. A less prominent theme has been the different experiences of women workers, as workers. Two alternative, but overlapping, models have been put forward to explain women's position in the labour market — dual labour market theory, and the 'reserve army of labour' theory. In themselves, neither model explains the experience of the women we interviewed. Moreover, neither theory is concerned with a major concern of our work, the subjective meaning of work, redundancy, and unemployment for women.

Earlier research on redundancy and unemployment has paid little attention to the particular experiences and attitudes of women, largely because such work began with the assumption that going out to work was less central to women than to men: loss of employment was therefore less important. Hence Wood has argued that women are more likley to adopt a fatalistic attitude to redundancies than men. Similarly, Jahoda argued that women are less likely to suffer psychologically from unemployment than men because employment is not central to their social identity. However, as Jahoda herself demonstrates, many of the practical consequences of unemployment for women are the same as for men — including increasing social isolation and a loss of sense of participation in collective endeavour. The massive growth of female employment since 1960 has increased consciousness amongst women of employment discrimination, and might in itself be expected to lead to a gradual shift in women's conception of their role. Female unemployment in the 1980s might thus have a very different significance from female unemployment in the 1930s or in the early 1970s. Such differences are especially likely for women employed full time, for whom unemployment is likely to lead to the greatest changes in pattern of life. The women declared redundant in the five redundancies examined are thus a 'critical case'.

The research strategy involved five linked case studies of redundancy, one in the clothing industry, one in electronics, and three in engineering. In each case study women were interviewed after the declaration of a redundancy, but before they left employment, and re-interviewed approximately six months after leaving. In addition, a brief postal questionnaire was sent out. The major problems faced in carrying out the research strategy arose from time constraints: time constraints reduced the number and type of redundancy situations which could be examined, and the time that could be allowed to elapse between the redundancies and the second interviews, and between the second interviews and the despatch of the postal questionnaire. The response rates achieved varied between case studies, major difficulties being encountered in two of the case studies — although substantial numbers of women were interviewed in even the least favourable research sites.

The women interviewed were older than the female working population as a whole, although probably not older than the population of redundant female workers. Slightly more were married than in the female working population as a whole (74 per cent compared with 73 per cent). Very few women had children below school age (2.5 per cent), and relatively few children of school age (25 per cent had children aged 15 or under). Although a relatively small number lived in rented accommodation (14 per cent, compared with 43.5 per cent of all households), expenditure on accommodation was modest. In terms of social-class background, professional and administrative workers were primarily drawn from non-manual backgrounds, the majority of the remainder (including clerical workers) from manual backgrounds.

The average net wages of women interviewed was £40.40 for part-time workers, and £63.90 for full-time workers. The highest-paid occupation was nursing (£96.00), the lowest hand-sewing (£52.23) for full-time workers: differences in hours worked render occupational comparisons for part-time workers of limited value, but hand-sewers were also the lowest paid part-time workers. The women made a larger contribution to joint earnings than the women interviewed in the *Women and Employment* survey, 73 per cent of full-time workers contributing 40 per cent or more to joint earnings, compared with 55 per cent of full-time women workers generally.

The women interviewed had worked for longer than the average for working women in general, as would have been expected in view of their age — 83 per cent had worked for ten years or more. The majority had worked either for the whole of their adult lives (31 per cent) or with one break (48 per cent). The women who had interrupted their working lives had normally done so for five years or less at their last break: only 20 per cent had had more than one break. They had had longer service with their employers than working women generally, 20 per cent having been with their current employer for twenty years or more, compared with 6 per cent of all working women. Although the women interviewed had had extensive working careers, relatively few had acquired formal qualifications: 6 per cent had left school above the minimum school-leaving age; only 10 per cent had GCE or CSE Grade 1 equivalents; 33 per cent had some form of vocational post-secondary training, in nearly all cases part-time commercial training. Daughters of higher-status fathers were more likely to stay on at school, or to acquire post-secondary qualifications, than daughters of manual workers. The degree of occupational segregation varied from work-place to work-place, but was substantial in four of the five case studies: only in case study C was substantial horizontal job segregation not present.

In this introduction we have briefly reviewed the literature relevant to the project and outlined the overall research strategy of the project. We have also presented basic demographic, financial, and employment experience data on our respondents. In the following four chapters we discuss in turn women and employment (Chapter 2), women and redundancy (Chapter 3), women in the labour market (Chapter 4), and women and unemployment (Chapter 5).

Notes

1. R. K. Brown, 'Women as Employees: some comments on research in industrial sociology', in (eds.) D. L. Barker and S. Allen, *Dependence and Exploitation in Work and Marriage* (Longman, 1976).
2. See, e.g., the extensive bibliography given by Professor Sheila Allen, *Women in Local Labour Markets*, prepared for the SSRC Workshop on Research Initiatives on Local Labour Markets and the Informal Economy, 1980.
3. M. W. Snell, P. Glucklich, and M. Povall, *Equal Pay and Opportunities: a study of the Equal Pay and Sex Discrimination Acts in 26 organizations* (Department of Employment Research Paper no. 20, 1981).
4. Other work from the same programme includes Cragg, Ross, and Dawson, 'Draft Report: Unemployment among Women' (unpublished report, Department of Employment, 1981); Q. Search, 'Women and Unemployment: A Qualitative Preliminary Research Report (unpublished, Office of Population Censuses and Surveys, 1979).
5. In S. Delamont's survey, *The Sociology of Women*, published in 1980 there is very little empirical evidence on women in employment (George Allen & Unwin, 1980). Since 1980 a number of books and papers have appeared: see J. West (ed.) *Work, Women and the Labour Market*, (Routledge & Kegan Paul, 1982), as well as specific case studies, such as A. Pollert, *Girls, Wives, Factory Lives* (Macmillan, 1981).
6. F. Wilkinson (ed.), *The Dynamics of Labour Market Segmentation* (Academic Press, 1982); R. Loveridge and A. L. Mok, *Theories of Labour Market Segmentation* (University of Aston Management Centre Working Paper, December 1979).
7. R. Barron and G. Norris, 'Sexual Divisions and the Dual Labour Market', in Barker and Allen, op. cit.
8. See, e.g., P. Brayshaw and C. J. Laidlaw, *Women in Engineering* (Engineering Industry Training Board, 1979).
9. T. Baudouin, M. Collin, and D. Guillerm, 'Women and Immigrants: Marginal Workers?', in (eds.) C. Crouch and A. Pizzorno, *The Resurgence of Class Conflict in Western Europe*, Vol. 2, (Macmillan, 1978); I. Breugel, Women as a reserve army of labour: a note on recent British experience' *Feminist Review*, 1979; S. Walby, *Women and Unemployment* (Lancaster Regionalism Group, 1981).
10. R. Milkman, 'Women's Work and the Economic Crisis: some lessons of the Great Depression', *Review of Radical Political Economy*, 1976.
11. Office of Population Censuses and Surveys, *Labour Force Survey, 1981; Labour Force Survey, 1983*.
12. D. Massey and R. Meegan, *The Anatomy of Job Loss* (Methuen, 1982), part 3.
13. C. Hakim, *Occupational Segregation: a comparative study of the degree and pattern of the differentiation between men and women's work in Britain, the United States and other countries* (Department of Employment Research Paper, no. 8, 1979).
14. Office of Population Censuses and Surveys, *Labour Force Surveys 1979* and *1981*.
15. V. Beechey, 'Part-time Work and the Labour Process' (mimeo, University of Warwick, 1981); V. Beechey and T. Perkins, 'Women's Part-time Employment in Coventry' (unpublished conference paper, City University, 1982).
16. H. Beynon and R. M. Blackburn, *Perceptions of Work: Variations within a Factory* (Cambridge University Press, 1972) p. 62; F. J. Crosby, *Relative Deprivation and Working Women* (Oxford University Press, 1982), p. 55.
17. R. Blauner, *Alienation and Freedom* (Chicago University Press, 1964), p. 81.
18. W. W. Daniel, *Whatever Happened to the Workers in Woolwich?: A survey of Redundancy in South East London* (PEP, 1972); S. Wood, 'Redundancy and Female Employment', *Sociological Review*, 1981, pp. 649–83.
19. Daniel, op. cit., pp. 122–3.
20. Wood, op. cit., p. 675. See also S. Wood and I. Dey, *Redundancy: Case Studies in Cooperation and Conflict* (Gower, 1983), p. 33.
21. J. Wadjman, *Women in Control: Dilemmas of a Workers' Co-operative* (Open University Press, 1983).

22. R. Martin, 'Female Redundancy: Some case studies in manufacturing Industry', *Employment Gazette*, forthcoming, 1984.
23. J. Hayes and P. Nutman, *Understanding the Unemployed: the Psychological Effects of Unemployment* (Tavistock, 1981), p. 3. Whether their view that the Hayes and Nutman model applies equally to men and women it is impossible to say: women are not mentioned later than p. 3 in their book.
24. The Pilgrim Trust, *Men Without Work* (Cambridge University Press, 1938), part iv.
25. W. W. Daniel, *A National Survey of the Unemployed* (PEP, 1974).
26. M. J. Hill, R. M. Harrison, A. V. Sargent, and V. Talbot, *Men Out of Work: A Study of Unemployment in Three English Towns* (Cambridge University Press, 1973).
27. Daniel, 1974.
28. A. Sinfield, *What Unemployment Means* (Martin Robertson, 1981).
29. M. Jahoda, P. Lazarsfeld, H. Zeizel, *Mariental: The Sociography of an Unemployed Community* (Tavistock, 1972, first published 1933); E. W. Bakke, *The Unemployed Man* (Nisbet & Co., 1933). The Pilgrim Trust, op. cit.
30. M. Jahoda, *Employment and Unemployment: A Social Psychological Analysis* (Cambridge University Press, 1982).
31. I. Miles, *Adaptation to Unemployment?* (Science Policy Research Unit, University of Sussex, Occasional Paper no. 20, 1983).
32. Jahoda, op. cit., pp. 52–3.
33. Ibid., p. 53.
34. Jahoda *et al.,* op. cit., p. 86.
35. The Pilgrim Trust, op. cit., p. 146.
36. D. Marsden, *Workless* (Croom Helm, 1982), p. 127.
37. Sinfield, op. cit., p. 87.
38. S. R. Parker, R. K. Brown, and J. Child, *The Sociology of Industry* (George Allen & Unwin, 1967), p. 154.
39. P. D. Anthony, *The Ideology of Work* (Tavistock, 1977), p. 312.
40. R. Pahl, 'Family, Community, and Unemployment', *New Society*, 1982, pp. 91–3.
41. J. H. Goldthorpe, 'Women and Class Analysis: In defence of the Conventional View', *Sociology*, 1983, pp. 465–88.
42. For evidence on the distribution of confirmed redundancies see *Employment Gazette*, June 1983, pp. 245–56, 259. In 1981 there were 72.9 confirmed redundancies per 1000 workers in clothing and footwear, 70.9 in electrical engineering, 147.3 in metal manufacture, and 74.1 in mechanical engineering. The numbers of workers involved were 19 789, 48 166, 47 474, and 57 214 respectively. The figures are only an approximate guide to the distribution of redundancies, in particular under-estimating the extent of redundancies in small firms (Table 5, pp. 252–3).
43. We are grateful to Department of Employment Regional Manpower Intelligence Units for information on the distribution of redundancies.
44. Our initial intention was also to carry out research in retail distribution and education. In both industries we approached the unions, and in retail distribution approached the management of an appropriate firm. Discussion with industry representatives indicated that, although both industries were contracting, they were not contracting through large-scale redundancies. In the education sector job losses occurred through the non-replacement of staff, recruitment by internal transfer within the same employing authority, the non-renewal of annual contracts, and reduction in the use of *ad hoc* part-time staff: there were no compulsory redundancies in schools and voluntary redundancy took the form of early retirement schemes. Although other sectors of education experienced redundancies, none involving large numbers of women occurred at the time we were scheduled to carry out field-work. In retail distribution job loss occurred primarily through natural wastage, an effective method in an industry with a high level of labour turnover, and through reductions in the hours of work. At the time of the field-work a major closure involving compulsory redundancy was announced, but although access was initially granted by senior management operating management did not feel that staff would have the time to be interviewed in the short period before the closure was due to take place. Since the period before

closure included Christmas and a grand closing-down sale operating management's attitude was probably realistic!
45. The age distribution was not a product of sampling bias in the factories concerned. In three plants, B, D, and E, the response rates achieved were 72, 69, and 76 per cent respectively; in plants A and C, where the response rates were lower, there was no sampling bias towards older workers: see Tables 3.1.2.1 and 3.1.2.3, pp. 000 and 000.
46. J. Jolly, S. Creigh, and A. Mingay, *Age as a Factor in Employment* (DE Research Paper, 1980).
47. Jolly *et al.*, p. 8.
48. J. H. Goldthorpe, *Social Mobility and Class Structure in Modern Britain* (Clarendon Press, 1980), p. 288.
49. J. H. Goldthorpe and K. Hope, *The Social Grading of Occupations: a new approach and scale* (Clarendon Press, 1974).
50. A Heath, *Social Mobility* (Fontana, 1981), Ch. 4.
51. J. Martin and C. Roberts, *Women and Employment: a Lifetime Perspective* (HMSO, 1984), p. 20.
52. *Census 1971: Great Britain: Economic Activity* (Part iv) (10% sample), Table 35, pp. 252–5.
53. C. Hakim, op. cit.
54. J. Hurstfield, *The Part-time Trap* (Low Pay Unit, 1978).

2

FEMALE EMPLOYMENT EXPERIENCE AND ATTITUDES TO WORK

One interpretation of female employment is to see it as an extension of domestic roles. Women go out to work for a combination of instrumental and social reasons — primarily money and social contact. Primary identification — and source of satisfaction — lies in family life. Research is therefore focused on the effects of domestic roles on womens experience of, and attitudes towards, employment. This perspective is valuable, but far from comprehensive. The rewards derived from going out to work differ for different groups of women — as they do for different groups of men. Women in high-status jobs have different work experiences and different attitudes to work from those of women in low-status jobs, although only limited academic attention has been given to the attitudes of women to specific jobs.[1] In this chapter we examine women's reasons for undertaking market employment, their occupational histories, why they chose some jobs rather than others, and why they liked some jobs more than others: as such our study follows the tradition of British industrial sociology. The experiences and attitudes of the women we interviewed are not, of course, necessarily representative of all women workers; however, they are probably representative of the views of a substantial group of women workers, namely clerical and manual workers employed in large-scale manufacturing industry, especially those working full time.[2]

This chapter is concerned with women's work histories and attitudes before the redundancies, based upon material gathered during the initial interview. It therefore represents the picture before job loss, providing the basis against which to compare experience and attitudes following job loss. The evidence is also important in its own right, providing unusually extensive documentation on women's work experience and attitudes.

The chapter is divided into four sections: (1) employment; (2) job choice and occupational career; (3) attitudes to work; and (4) family influences upon women's attitudes to work. The chapter concludes with a short summary.

2.1 Women and employment

The concepts of 'work' and 'employment' are inherently problematic. Work can refer to any task undertaken as a means to an end, where the activity itself is not the sole good. As such, the definition rests on the actor's intentions, not on the content of the task: swimming may be 'work', as in the work of a life-saver, or non-work, as on holiday. In this chapter we are concerned with women's attitudes to employment, i.e. work undertaken for financial reward, and throughout the term 'employment' is used for what is colloquially referred to as 'having a job'.

Implicit in the discussion on women's motives for undertaking employment is the assumption that women have a choice, implying that employment is less financially necessary for women than for men. This is so for only a proportion of women. Employment is as financially necessary for single, childless women, who do not receive state support unless they are prepared to work and cannot get it, as for men in the same position; 14 per cent of our sample fell into this category. For the rest of our sample employment was not a financial imperative in the same terms. Nevertheless, it was usually undertaken in response to perceived economic needs; by going out to work the women raised the living standard of themselves and their families. We were concerned, however, to place the financial motive in its context, by looking at the other rewards of employment, and comparisons between employment and other activities. Our purpose in studying women's attitudes to employment was primarily to investigate the value that the women attached to their employment status in general as a basis from which to investigate their experience of unemployment; but the empirical data on female attitudes to employment and work is valuable in its own right.

The women interviewed expressed a strong desire for market employment for the economic, social, and psychological rewards it was seen as bringing. The majority of the women interviewed went out to work for economic reasons, only a small minority not including financial reasons among the reasons given for going out to work. However, a majority of women said that they also went out to work for other reasons, primarily interesting activity and company. A substantial minority recognized that combining going out to work with household responsibilities was too tiring, although the large majority of women felt that they had coped successfully with the stresses involved. Although they expressed a strong preference for employment themselves, the women were ambivalent about the effects of going out to work upon their status in the eyes of others; only a minority of the women felt that they earned more respect from their husbands, children, and community by going out to work. Uncertainty about the 'entitlement' of married women to employment during periods of high unemployment was reflected in their views on the relevance of 'queueing' principles for employment during such periods, where the majority felt that married women should give precedence to single men and women and to married men (other things being equal). Despite this uncertainty, a very substantial majority of the women interviewed intended working until retirement age before the announcement of the redundancy.

54 *Working Women in Recession*

The women were asked to give their main reasons for going out to work and were allowed up to three responses, 55 per cent giving more than one main reason, and 15 per cent giving more than two. As expected, most women gave money as one of their main reasons for going to work, although only 31 per cent gave money as their only main reason for going to work, and 13 per cent gave other reasons only. The other reasons mentioned most frequently related to work providing useful and interesting activity and company.

Table 2.1.1
Respondents' main reasons for going to work (up to three reasons allowed)

Reason	Company				Total
	B (%)	C (%)	D (%)	E (%)	(%)
Money	88	89	83	84	87
Interest, to relieve boredom	26.5	18	58	59	38
Company	26.5	23	23	35	27
'Keeps you in touch'	4	3	7	6	5
Independence/autonomy	12	3	12	4	7
'To be of use to society'		6	2		2
Other	1.5	6	2		3.5
N	67	66	43	51	227

Percentage is that of respondents giving each reason.
Number of reasons given = 378.
The question was not asked in Company A.

Women in case studies D and E were more likely than women in the other case studies to say that they went to work for interest as well as money. This is probably because of the relatively large number of professional/administrative women in these case studies, professional/administrative women being the most likely to give interest as one of their main reasons for working; 67 per cent of women in this status gave interest as a reason, compared with only 34 per cent of clerks and 24 per cent of operatives. This is hardly surprising, status 1 occupations being the ones most likely to require initiative and responsibility. In view of the women's later reactions to unemployment, it is interesting that few said they went to work for the sake of the company it provided; when unemployed it was the company that women said they missed most about their job.

Money was important to the women both as a means of raising their own and their family's standard of living, and as the source of a degree of financial independence for themselves. The majority of women agreed with the view that women needed to go to work for financial independence. Women from Company D were significantly less likely to agree that work was necessary for financial independence, although this appeared to be a specifically local point of view.

Table 2.1.2

Respondents' main reasons for going to work (by occupational status; up to three reasons allowed)

Reason	Occupational status					Total
	1 (%)	2 (%)	3 (%)	4 (%)	5 (%)	(%)
Money	73	90	93	74	88	87
Interest	67	34	24	30	37	38
Company	33	27	24	21	6	17.5
N	30	61	96	24	16	227

N = number of reasons given (378).
Percentage is that of respondents giving each reason.

Table 2.1.3

Responses to *A women needs to go to work because having her own money gives her independence*

	Company					Total
	A (%)	B (%)	C (%)	D (%)	E (%)	(%)
Agree	82	85	86	58	74.5	79
Disagree	14	9	9	29	16	14
No opinion	4	6	4.5	14	10	7
N	51	68	66	43	51	279

($p = 0.035$)

There was no significant difference in responses by occupational status ($p = 0.713$), nor by age ($p = 0.684$), nor by marital status ($p = 0.355$).

The women stated a definite preference for going out to work, 87 per cent saying that they were happier doing so than not, 7 per cent that they would be happier not going out to work, and 6 per cent not knowing. In view of the very large majority preferring employment, it is hardly surprising that there were no significant differences between companies, occupations, age groups, or marital statuses. The overall preference for going out to work was confirmed by responses to questions on the relative merits of employment and alternative activities, household and family work, and voluntary work. Reflecting their importance to our respondents, we discuss household work first, before turning briefly to voluntary work.

A majority of women disagreed with the view that household and family work were more enjoyable than going out to work, as Table 2.1.4 shows. (To avoid 'respondent agreement' bias leading to a systematic tendency towards pro-employment responses the question was constructed to require a negative answer for a pro-market employment response.) Awareness of the rewards of household and family work was more likely to be shown by single than by married (or widowed, divorced, and separated) women, although a minority of married women specifically stated that their views had been different when their children had been little. As would be expected, a large proportion of single women had no view on the matter; however, of those who did, a higher proportion than average thought that household and family work would be more enjoyable than going out to work. This agreed with general impressions based on extensive interviewing that the single women among the respondents showed a slightly greater tendency to be supporters of traditional, family roles for women than married women did. Not surprisingly, only a very small minority, 17 per cent, of separated and divorced women considered household and family work more enjoyable.

A very substantial majority of women also agreed that women need market employment to avoid boredom at home — 71 per cent.

Table 2.1.4

Responses to *Household and family work are generally more enjoyable than going out to work*

	Marital status				Total
	Single (%)	Widowed (%)	Separated/Divorced (%)	Married (%)	(%)
Agree	27.5	12.5	17	18	19
Disagree	27.5	87.5	75	69	64
No opinion	45		8	13	16.5
N	40	8	24	207	279

Table 2.1.5

Responses to *Women need work to avoid boredom at home*

	A (%)	B (%)	C (%)	D (%)	E (%)	Total (%)
Agree	76.5	79	70	58	65	71
Disagree	16	19	26	14	23.5	20
No opinion	6	1.5	4.5	26	12	9
Other	2					0.4
Missing				2		0.4
N	51	68	66	43	51	279

($p = 0.003$)

Women in Companies D and E, primarily professional, administrative, supervisory, and clerical and ancillary workers, were less likely than women in Companies A, B, and C to believe that women needed to go out to work to avoid being bored at home. The view that non-manual workers were less likely than manual workers to believe that women needed market employment to avoid domestic boredom was confirmed by analysis of responses by occupational status, as Table 2.1.6 shows. Differences between women in different occupational statuses in the extent of belief in the need to go out to work to avoid boredom at home was partly a result of differences in demographic composition: higher-status occupations contained higher proportions of younger women, and young women (especially young single women) were less likely to see a need for compensations in work. But it also reflected a general stratification: women in high-status jobs had higher salaries themselves, and also husbands with higher incomes. There was thus a greater range of rewards available to them in their non-work lives, as in their work lives (see below, pp. 239, 242).

Table 2.1.6
Responses to *Women need work to avoid boredom at home* (*by occupational status*)

	Occupational status					Total
	Professional/ Administrative (%)	Clerical (%)	Semi-skilled (%)	Slightly skilled (%)	Unskilled (%)	(%)
Agree	58	58.5	75	79	87.5	71
Disagree	23	18.5	23	15	12.5	9
No opinion	19	20	2	6	–	20
Other		1.5				.4
Missing		1.5				.4
N	31	65	120	47	16	279

($p = 0.002$)

A majority of women agreed with the view that women lost self-confidence through staying at home, and that staying at home led women to feel cut off from the world, as Tables 2.1.7–8 show.
The feeling that work was necessary to maintain confidence and avoid social isolation was especially marked amongst widowed, divorced, and separated women. On the other hand, single women were less likely than married women to believe that staying at home led to reduced confidence (51 per cent compared with 65 per cent) or to social isolation (42.5 per cent compared with 61 per cent). There were no statistically significant correlations with company, occupational status, or age of youngest child.

There was an awareness that combining paid employment with looking after a household was demanding. As Table 2.1.9 shows, 43 per cent of women interviewed agreed that it was 'too tiring'. There was less concern about the strain involved in combining household responsibilities and going out to work in the two primarily white-collar case studies, D and E, reflecting differences between women in different occupations. Women in professional adminis-

Table 2.1.7
Responses to *Women lose confidence if they stay at home*

	Married (%)	Single (%)	Widowed (%)	Divorced/Separated (%)	Total (%)
Agree	65	51	75	79	64
Disagree	29.5	38.5	–	21	29
No opinion	5	10	25	–	6
Other	0.5				0.4
N	207	40	8	24	279

($p = 0.129$)

Table 2.1.8
Responses to *Women feel cut off from the world if not working*

	Married (%)	Single (%)	Widowed (%)	Divorced/Separated (%)	Total (%)
Agree	61	42.5	87.5	58	59
Disagree	31	40	–	37.5	32
No opinion	8	17.5	12.5	4	9
N	207	40	8	24	279

($p = 0.085$)

Table 2.1.9
Responses to *Looking after a household and doing paid work as well is too tiring*

	A (%)	B (%)	C (%)	D (%)	E (%)	Total (%)
Agree	41	51.5	51.5	35	27.5	43
Disagree	41	41	36	35	51	41
Yes, when children small		1.5	3			1
No opinion	18	4	9	28	22	15
Missing		1.5		2		1
N	51	68	66	43	51	279

($p = 0.015$)

trative and supervisory jobs were the least likely to agree that combining the two roles was too tiring (19 per cent), compared with as many as 56 per cent of unskilled manual workers – the women most likely to agree. Fifty per cent of married women agreed with the statement, compared with 37 per cent of widowed, separated, and divorced women; 30 per cent of single women had no view, but of those who did a surprisingly high proportion, 72 per cent, agreed that combining the roles was too tiring. Despite the fairly high rate of agreement with the general proposition, very few women, only 11.5 per cent, said that they were experiencing difficulty themselves in combining the two roles, the most commonly cited difficulties being the need to care for elderly relatives and the lack of help from husbands and children. The contrast between the general and the particular was due to the women's current domestic circumstances — only 2.5 per cent of the women had children under school age. Although family loyalties may have helped to produce more sanguine responses than reality justified, it is possible to conclude that, in general, the women were aware of the difficulties involved in attempting to combine going out to work with household responsibilities, but felt that they coped successfully with them.

Although the women felt that they were coping successfully with their dual role at the time of the interview, the majority believed that the difficulties were considerable when children were below school age. Hence a very substantial majority believed that women should ideally stay at home when their children are below school age — 88.5 per cent. A very substantial majority did not agree that women should stay at home when their children had reached secondary school age — 77 per cent. Such responses would be expected on the basis of respondents' practice: a majority had had a break for child-rearing, but very few had had a gap of more than five years on the occasion of their last pregnancy. The majority of respondents did not think that it was harmful for children to be looked after in a creche or by professional child-minders, although a substantial minority (35.5 per cent) thought that children should be brought up only by their parents or other relatives. Indeed, a majority of women, 53 per cent, agreed that children benefited from their mothers' going out to work by becoming more independent, only 26 per cent disagreeing, the remainder having no opinion. Since there were so few children below school age the issue of child-care facilities did not arise.

Since experience of voluntary work was limited a large number of women had no opinion about the relative merits of paid employment and voluntary work. However, only a small minority agreed with the view that voluntary work was more enjoyable than paid work, although there were marked differences between case studies, women in Company A being more likely to view voluntary work favourably. Table 2.1.10 summarizes the evidence.

Table 2.1.10

Responses to *Voluntary work is generally more enjoyable than paid work*

	Company					Total
	A (%)	B (%)	C (%)	D (%)	E (%)	(%)
Agree	35	21	23	14	18	22
Disagree	41	46	44	23	47	41
No opinion	23.5	34	33	63	35	37
N	51	68	66	43	51	279

($p = 0.008$)

The activities involved in going out to work were thus preferred at a general level to the two major alternative activities generally available, household and family work and voluntary work.

The value of going out to work did not lie in its effect on the respect in which they were held by husbands, children, or the wider community. Only a minority of women agreed with the view that 'your husband respects you more if you contribute to the breadwinning' (30 per cent), a further 1.4 per cent saying that he did so only when there were no children at home. Even fewer women agreed with the view that 'children respect their mother more if she has a job outside the home' (20 per cent). Similarly, only 29 per cent of women believed that people in general respect you more if you go out to work. The issue was not, however, a major one, large numbers of women having no opinion. Morever, although few husbands respected their wives more for their financial contribution to the household, very few had ever opposed their wives going out to work — 14 per cent.

Although few women appeared to believe that going out to work enhanced their status, few had ever had their right to work challenged: only 6 per cent or seventeen respondents reported that anyone had ever questioned their right to work in view of the number of married men unemployed. Although this number was small, it was highly concentrated in relatively integrated occupations ($p = 0.001$). Thirteen of the seventeen women whose right to work had been questioned were employed in the small number of fully integrated occupations (eight engineering assembly workers, three storewomen, one administrator, one in computing): of the remaining four, three were in clerical positions which may have overlapped male/female boundaries, and only one was in a completely segregated occupation (a cleaner). No challenges were reported in either the clothing or the electronics industries. This suggests, although the figures involved are very small, that women's right to market employment is more likely to be questioned where women are employed in integrated occupations, rather than where they are segregated into generally recognized 'women's jobs'.

Although very few women reported that they had had their right to work challenged directly, there was considerable ambivalence, especially amongst married women, about their 'entitlement' to work in a period of high unemployment. We asked women whether they felt that married women should give precedence in the queue for jobs to single men and women or to married men with families to support (assuming that the women's husbands were employed and there was therefore at least one household income).[3] We were especially concerned to establish whether married women themselves might feel constrained in their labour-market behaviour by consciousness of a lesser right to work because they were able to share their husbands' wages. (Similar views might also, of course, influence potential employers.) Three related questions were asked: 'If there is a shortage of work married women should stay at home to give job opportunities to single men and women'; 'If there is a shortage of work married women should stay at home to give more job opportunities to married men?'; and 'Ideally, in a perfect world the husband should be the only breadwinner and the wife should not go out to work?' We also tried to distinguish between their views of what should happen now (during a period of high unemployment) and what they thought should happen in an 'ideal world'.

Many women stressed that individual economic circumstances varied so much that it was inappropriate to discuss queueing principles between social groups in general, and that single men and women should not be given priority on general grounds, but that there might be circumstances in which it would be appropriate to do so. Nevertheless, nearly all respondents were prepared to give a definite answer on whether, as a general rule, married women ought to give preference in the job market to single men and women, and to married men: 53 per cent agreed with the view that if there is a shortage of work married women should stay at home to give more job opportunities to single men and women, and 65 per cent to give more job opportunities to married men. Similarly, a majority believed that married women should give precedence to married men in present circumstances. On the other hand, only a minority of women (34 per cent) agreed with the view that, in an ideal world, the husband should be the only breadwinner and the wife should not go out to work. In other words, the majority felt it was necessary to accord priority to married men during a period of job shortage, but that it was by no means desirable.

We had thought that responses on these issues would vary according to people's own experience and position in the labour market. For example, we had thought that younger women might be less likely to accord precedence, reflecting changing social expectations. Similarly, we had thought that higher-status women might be less willing to accord precedence, reflecting a principled commitment to female employment opportunities. However, there were no significant variations in responses by age or by occupational status. There was a slightly significant ($p = 0.083$) variation by marital status: on the question of the allocation of priority to married men, separated and divorced women were less likely to concede priority than single, widowed, or married women. This may have been due to an awareness of the possible risks inherent in depending upon the continued presence of a breadwinning spouse (or simply to lack of special feeling for married men).

There were, however, significant variations in responses to all three questions by company. Tables 2.1.11–13 show the distribution of answers by company. Women in the two Midlands companies were the least likely to recognize the existence of priorities, Company D (North West engineering, clerical workers) and Company A (South East garment workers, many part time) were the most likely. However, on the issue of the desirability of married women sharing the breadwinning there was much less variation, Companies A, B, C, and D clustering very closely together and only Company E being significantly different, with substantially fewer women in favour of the proposition that the breadwinning role should be reserved for married men.

The results are difficult to interpret. The correlation between attitudes

Table 2.1.11
Responses to *If there is a shortage of work married women should stay at home to give more job opportunities to single men and women*

	A (%)	B (%)	C (%)	D (%)	E (%)	Total (%)
Respondent agrees	65	51.5	38	72	47	53
Respondent disagrees	35	48.5	58	28	53	46
No response			4.5			1
N	51	68	66	43	51	279

($p = 0.007$)

Table 2.1.12
Responses to *If there is a shortage of work married women should stay at home to give more job opportunities to married men*

	A (%)	B (%)	C (%)	D (%)	E (%)	Total (%)
Respondent agrees	74.5	69	58	74	51	65
Respondent disagrees	25.5	31	41	19	47	33
No response			1.5	7	2	2
N	51	68	66	43	51	279

($p = 0.022$)

Table 2.1.13
Responses to *Ideally, in a perfect world the husband should be the only breadwinner and the wife should not go out to work*

	A (%)	B (%)	C (%)	D (%)	E (%)	Total (%)
Respondent agrees	45	40	35	35	14	34
Respondent disagrees	55	51.5	62	58	80	61
'Don't know' and no response		9	3	7	6	5
N	51	68	66	43	51	279

($p = 0.018$)

towards employment priorities in present economic circumstances and attitudes towards economic roles in an ideal world was not as high as expected: for example, women in Company C were more likely to agree that the husband should be the breadwinner and that women should not go out to work in an ideal world than would have been expected on the basis of their replies to the questions on priorities in present economic circumstances. However, in general the data suggest that attitudes towards women's employment in general are linked to company or region rather than to occupation or demographic status.

Hence, examining the deviation of individual case-study response distributions from overall average distributions for the three relevant questions, women in case studies C and E were less 'traditional' in their views than women in case studies D and A. The findings are summarized in Table 2.1.14

Table 2.1.14
Distribution of traditional/non-traditional views of female employment: 'tranditionalism score'

D = + 34	North West (clerical)
A = + 29	South East (manual)
B = + 8	North West (manual)
C = − 21	Midlands (manual)
E = − 42	Midlands (clerical)

It is impossible to explain the distribution of responses between case studies in detail with the limited data available. Nevertheless, there are differences between case studies, associated either with companies or with regions. It is impossible to say whether the attitudes are fostered by experience within particular companies, possibly heavily influenced by specific individuals (through recruitment practices or informal leadership) or specific collective experiences, or by experience of living in a particular region: on balance we favour a regional explanation, 'traditional' attitudes holding less sway in the Midlands than in the North West.

Social attitudes are moulded by discussion with others, and by exposure to general cultural norms and values. We were therefore concerned to investigate women's perceptions of the views of others. Instead of asking about their perceptions of cultural norms and values in general, we asked women what they thought were the opinions of most other women and of most other men on the three questions under discussion. On the one hand we thought that women in this instance might show the well-known tendency of people to believe that others share their own opinions, both because this provided reassurance and because people are more likely to associate with those with whom they agree than with those with whom they disagree. On the other hand, attitudes towards women's employment, especially married women's employment, may be so uncertain during a period of recession that the usual self-reinforcing perceptions might not apply.

Assessment of our respondents' perceptions of the attitudes of most women is difficult owing to a very substantial proportion of 'don't knows': 37 per cent of respondents had no idea of the attitudes of most women to giving priority in employment to single people, and 34 per cent had no idea of the attitudes of most women to giving priority to married men. Significantly, a greater proportion of respondents felt that they knew the attitudes of most men to these questions, the non-response rate on the attitudes of most men being only 26 and

21 per cent respectively. On whether husbands should be the only breadwinners in an ideal world women were more confident of the view of other women than previously: the non-response rate on the attitudes of other women and of other men was only 28 and 26 per cent respectively. The large proportion of 'don't knows' is itself of considerable interest, indicating the absence of a generally accepted cultural norm. This might reflect the fact that queueing principles are not a topic of discussion (especially among women), or that individual circumstances vary so much that a general answer would be meaningless.

On issues of priorities, respondents were more likely to be in favour of priorities themselves than they were to think that most women would be in favour of them; on the ideal division of roles respondents appeared to think that their views coincided with those of most women. Of those who gave a response only 36 per cent thought that most women would believe that precedence should be given to single men and women. On the issue of whether married men should be given precedence a bare majority of women who had an opinion, (53 per cent) thought that most women would agree that priority should be given to married men. On the issue of whether, ideally, the husband should be the only breadwinner, 40 per cent of those who responded thought that most women would agree. It is therefore unlikely that, in general, our respondents felt any great social pressure against working from other women in their social environment. On the other hand, our respondents, by a large majority, felt that most men were in favour of all three propositions. Tables 2.1.15–17 summarize the distribution of responses on the three issues, by company. For the sake of clarity the 'don't knows' have been removed and the percentages given are of only those who expressed an opinion.

Table 2.1.15

Attitudes to *If there is a shortage of work married women should stay at home to give more job opportunities to single men and women*

	Company					All	N	
	A (%)	B (%)	C (%)	D (%)	E (%)	(%)		
Respondent agrees	65	51	40	72	47	53	276	$p = 0.007$
'Most women agree'	42	36	21	46	45	36	177	$p = 0.169$
'Most men agree'	83	86	80	93	86	85	207	$p = 0.217$

In view of these findings it is interesting to look at which women thought most women agreed with them and which did not: i.e. to assess whether women who were in favour of married women's rights were more inclined to believe that other women agreed with them than women who thought priority should be given to single men and women or to married men. Those who agreed with priorities were more likely either not to know the views of other women, or to think that the views of other women were contrary to their own. Those who

Table 2.1.16
Attitudes to *If there is a shortage of work married women should stay at home to give more job opportunities to married men*

	Company					All	N	
	A (%)	B (%)	C (%)	D (%)	E (%)	(%)		
Respondent agrees	74	69	58	80	52	66	274	$p = 0.022$
'Most women agree'	64	58	39	77	52	53	185	$p = 0.170$
'Most men agree'	98	96	89	97	92	94	222	$p = 0.243$

Table 2.1.17
Attitudes to *Ideally, in a perfect world the husband should be the only breadwinner and the wife should not go out to work*

	Company					All	N	
	A (%)	B (%)	C (%)	D (%)	E (%)	(%)		
Respondent agrees	45	43	36	37	15	36	265	$p = 0.018$
'Most women agree'	30	56	33	48	35	40	201	$p = 0.055$
'Most men agree'	65	78	76	77	76	74.5	208	$p = 0.734$

disagreed with priorities were more likely to think that they knew the views of other women, and that they were similar to their own. Conversely, those who agreed with priorities were more likely to think that most men shared their views, and those who disagreed that most men did not share their views. On the issue of whether the husband should be the only breadwinner the large majority of both those who agreed and those who disagreed thought that most women shared their views. Those who agreed thought that most men shared their view, those who disagreed did not.

In view of possible misinterpretations of our questions by respondents, and the complexity of the analysis, too much should not be read into our evidence. However, it suggests that women who support traditional roles are likely either not to know what other women think, or to think that other women disagree with them and hold more radical views. At the same time, women who disagreed with according priorities to single people or to married men were more likely to think that they knew the views of other women, and to believe that they were the same as their own. In other words, women holding less traditional views were more confident that they reflected the views of women in general. (Although if our findings on respondents' own views are accurate they do not do so.) Interestingly, the majority of women who believed that the husband should be the only breadwinner in an ideal world, and the majority of women who disagreed with this view, both thought that the majority of women agreed

Table 2.1.18
Perception of others' attitudes to *If there is a shortage of work married women should stay at home to give more job opportunities to single men and women*

Opinions of most women	Respondents' opinions			Total
	Yes (%)	No (%)	Missing	(%)
Yes	31	14		23
No	28	55.5		40.5
Don't know	41	30.5		36
N	148	128	3	279

Opinion of most men	Respondents' opinions*			Total
	Yes (%)	No (%)	Missing	(%)
Yes	65	62.5		63
No	7	16		11
Don't know	28	21		25
N	148	128	3	279

*$p = 0.028$.

Table 2.1.19
Perception of others' attitudes to *If there is a shortage of work married women should stay at home to give more job opportunities to married men*

Opinions of most women	Respondents' opinions			Total	N
	Yes (%)	No (%)	Missing	(%)	
Yes	44	20		35	98
No	21	53		31	87
Don't know	35	27		33	92
N	181	93	5		279

Opinions of most men	Respondents' opinions*			Total	N
	Yes (%)	No (%)	Missing	(%)	
Yes	77	72		75	209
No	4	6.5		5	13
Don't know	19	21.5		20	55
N	181	93	5		279

*$p = 0.516$.

Table 2.1.20
Perception of others' attitudes to *Ideally, in a perfect world the husband should be the only breadwinner and the wife should not go out to work*

Opinions of most women	Respondents' opinions				Total	N
	Yes (%)	No (%)	Don't know (%)	Missing	(%)	
Yes	62	12	15		29	81
No	17	59	23		43	120
Don't know	21	29	61.5		28	77
N	95	170	13	1		279

Opinions of most men	Respondents' opinion				Total	N
	Yes (%)	No (%)	Don't know (%)	Missing	(%)	
Yes	75	46.5	38.5		56	155
No	7	26.5	8		19	53
Don't know	17	26.5	54		25	69
N	95	170	13	2		279

with their viewpoints, in this instance upholding the general presumption that people tend to perceive others as agreeing with them. There was no disagreement between traditionalists and non-traditionalists on men's views: both agreed that most men favoured traditional views, namely that priority should be accorded to single people and to married men, and that the husband should be the only breadwinner in a family in an ideal world.

We have examined women's conceptions of 'queueing' principles at length because of their obvious importance during a period of high unemployment and competition for work: married women who believed that jobs ought to be allocated to single people and married men first might be inhibited from looking for work after being declared redundant. However, the concept of queueing is only relevant where individuals are competing for the same jobs: to the extent that men and women are employed in different jobs, and operate in different labour markets, the concept of priorities between women and men is irrelevant. (For relevant evidence see below, pp. 191–2.) As we have shown, the majority of women were working in women's jobs (above, pp. 37–9), and, where they were working in integrated occupations, many women were in lower-status jobs, with lower pay, than men. It is therefore likely that women working in women's jobs would not see their continued participation in the labour force as putting the jobs of male breadwinners at risk, even where they believed that, in general, male breadwinners should be given priority. It is perhaps significant that women workers who were in fully integrated occupations, such as the engineering assembly workers in Company C, were likely to accept queueing principles, and would therefore perhaps be influenced in their labour-market behaviour by doing so since they were competing directly with men in looking for jobs similar to those they had had in Company C. Finally, although the significance of queueing principles between women and men may be undermined by job segregation the significance of queueing principles between married and single women remains.

As we have shown by a detailed examination of their attitudes, the majority of women interviewed preferred market employment. This is confirmed by evidence on the length of time women had spent in market employment (shown in Chapter 1, Table 1.3.3.1, p. 31) and on their further intentions. A very large majority of women had intended to work until retirement age (70 per cent) before the announcement of redundancy, and a further group intended to work until retirement age with a break for children (7 per cent). Very few respondents (6 per cent) said that they would stop working when the family ceased to need the money, although the major reasons for undertaking market employment initially were financial — perhaps the women were unable to imagine not needing the money. Despite differences in job satisfaction (see below, p. 81), there were no differences between occupations, or between companies, in the proportions intending to work until retirement age. Similarly, the only difference between age groups was in the number of young women who intended to interrupt their employment to have children.

The women were thus committed to market employment for the economic, social, and psychological benefits it was seen as bringing. But how far did the women see themselves as primarily working women, rather than housewives? Was work seen as rewarding, but secondary? After the redundancy the women were asked how they had viewed themselves before the redundancy, whether as working women who happened to be housewives, or housewives who happened to go out to work. The majority of women — 56 per cent — saw themselves as primarily working women, and 11 per cent as working women only. Women in professional, administrative, and supervisory jobs were overwhelmingly likely to emphasize occupational roles (87.5 per cent seeing themselves as primarily or only working women), followed by clerical workers (77 per cent), whilst women in unskilled manual jobs were least likely to (45.5 per cent). The differences between occupational groups was partly a result of differences between full- and part-time workers: 49 per cent of part-time workers thought of themselves as primarily housewives, compared with only 30 per cent of full-time workers, and the highest proportion of part-time workers was found amongst unskilled workers (73 per cent, compared with only 3 per cent of non-manual workers).

2.2 Job choice and occupational career

The women interviewed had been working for many years, preferred work to the alternative roles available to them, and before the redundancy anticipated working until retirement age. By any criterion work was therefore important to them. The women's commitment to market employment might have been expected to lead to an occupational 'career' involving the selection of jobs according to specific criteria and subsequent movement either between employers or between jobs with the same employer — the latter especially likely since our respondents were primarily employed in the primary sector of the labour market. Such a career might involve movement from jobs with low occupational status to jobs with higher status, or simply movement from worse to better jobs at the same status level. Such movement would be especially relevant for the acquisition of skills and experience ('human capital') useful in securing further employment after the redundancy. This section is therefore concerned with the extent to which the women interviewed had followed an occupational 'career'.

Studies of occupational choice have traditionally used two alternative 'ideal-type' models, one in which job choice is a rational decision-making process, based upon the evaluation of alternative employment prospects in the light of individual values, and, at the other extreme, one in which job choice is the result of a process of drift.[4] Choice of first job is especially important, repeated studies having shown a close link (in occupational status and in financial rewards) between first and subsequent jobs. As Propper argued in her study of clerical workers, 'it is generally argued that the first few years of work are the most important: in these early years the subsequent patterns of labour force participation are to a large extent set. The choice of first job or the first few jobs is therefore crucial.'[5] As Table 2.2.1 shows, the most commonly stated reasons for choosing first jobs were 'default' reasons (40 per cent), followed by family and peer-group influence (24 per cent) and intrinsic reasons (23 per cent).

Table 2.2.1
Reasons for choice of first job

	Percentage
Default	40
Family/peer-group influence	24
Intrinsic qualities	23
Directed	6
Good pay	6
Good conditions	3
Social	2
Prior training	2
Convenience (suited family role)	.4

($N = 279$)
Percentage is that of respondents mentioning each reason at least once.

The main responses included in the 'default' category were 'first or only job available with my qualifications', 'offered job by firm', 'everyone was going there', 'nothing else available', 'took the job temporarily and stayed on', 'I didn't know what I wanted', 'called at the firm on spec', and 'job was handy to where I lived.' The classification of responses presented difficulty (especially the difficulty of disentangling reasons related to 'why' respondents chose their first job from reasons relating to 'how' they chose their first job), and the classification followed may result in exaggerating the number of 'default' responses, and underestimating the importance of convenience. However, the limited relevance of a 'rational purposive' model of occupational choice is obvious.

The process of drift found among young women is also found amongst young men at the same occupational level.[6] It is based partly on a realistic assessment of their position in the labour market. However, for women interviewed this was reinforced by the expectation that the experience of market employment would be for only a limited period. As Table 2.2.2 shows, on initial entry into the labour market only a minority of women had expected to stay in market employment until retirement age or until retirement age with a break for children.

Table 2.2.2
Expected duration of market employment

	A (%)	B (%)	C (%)	D (%)	E (%)	Total (%)
Until retirement age	10	9	23	5	16	13
Until retirement age with break for children	14	3	15	9	10	10
Until had children	25.5	32	18	42	27.5	28
Until married	16	25	20	35	18	22
Other	6	1.5	6	–	4	4
Didn't think about it/don't know	29	29.5	18	9	23.5	23
N	51	68	66	43	51	279

Since the women were recalling their expectations of work life several years earlier memories may be inaccurate. However, the overall picture is clear: employment was not expected to last a lifetime, amongst any group of workers: working life was envisaged as lasting until marriage, or until the birth of first child — what was to come later was not of immediate concern. This expectation contrasts sharply with the amount of time the women interviewed had in fact subsequently spent in employment, and their intentions at the time of the redundancy, when 70 per cent said that they intended to work until retirement age or until retirement age with a break for children.

There was little difference in expectations of working life on initial employment between respondents in different occupations, or in different regions. In particular, there was no indication that women in a community with a long tradition of female employment (case study B) were more likely to envisage a lifetime of market employment than women elsewhere — rather the reverse. However, social background did appear to make a difference: daughters of status 1 fathers were more likely to have anticipated working until retirement, or until retirement with a break for children, than daughters of manual fathers, as Table 2.2.3 shows. Although the number of non-manual fathers is small, and the correlation is not a very strong one, the data indicate one aspect of the pervasive influence of social class: daughters of middle-class fathers were more likely to anticipate an extended working life than daughters of working-class fathers.

Although the majority of respondents had given largely 'default' reasons for choosing their first job, the reasons given for choosing their current jobs were substantially different: more 'active' reasons were given for choosing present jobs than for taking their initial jobs, as Table 2.2.4 shows.

Table 2.2.3

Proportions expecting to work until retirement (by father's occupational status)

Expectation of market employment	Father's occupational status					
	1 (%)	2 (%)	3 (%)	4 (%)	5 (%)	Missing
Until retirement age	9.5	17.5	14	9	13	
Until retirement age with break for children	33	10	9	6	7	
Total	42.5	27.5	23	15	20	
N	21	40	59	65	85	11 (Total 279)

$(p = 0.057)$

Table 2.2.4

Comparison between reasons for choice of initial and current job

	First job (%)	Present job (%)
Default	40	31
Family or peer-group influence	24	13
Intrinsic qualities of job	23	34
Directed by school, job centre, etc.	6	2
Good pay	6	24
Good conditions	3	7
Social	2	5
Prior training	2	9
Suite family role	.4	11
Number of responses	294	364
N	279	279

Percentage is that of respondents who mentioned each type of reason at least once.

The larger numbers of reasons given for choosing present job may be the result of respondents' being able to explain a relatively recent decision better than a decision made several years earlier. It is also likely that their more complex circumstances when deciding on their present job would influence the number of responses given. However, it is significant that evidence of decision by default is less, and the influence of family and peer group is less. The enhanced importance of good pay, and of congruence with family roles, may be expected, the increased importance of intrinsic qualities of the job less so. Table 2.2.5 shows the shift more clearly. The reasons for choosing the first and present job have been divided into 'passive' and 'active' reasons; those respondents (forty-nine) who had never changed their job, i.e. those whose first job was their present job, have been eliminated.

Table 2.2.5
Change of distribution of reasons for choosing jobs

Reasons	Percentage of respondents giving each type of answer	
	First job	Present job
(a) Passive reasons		
Default	42	29
Family and peer-group influence	26	12
Directed	6	2
Total	74	43
(b) Active reasons		
Intrinsic rewards	25	31
Good pay	6	27
Suits family role	0	14
Prior training	2	10
Conditions	3	8
Social	3	5
Total	37	95

There was substantial variations by occupation in the frequency with which 'default' reasons were mentioned for taking present jobs: 'general services' had the highest proportion giving default reasons (40 per cent), alongside computing (two out of only five respondents); more significantly, a relatively high proportion of clerical workers gave 'default' reasons, perhaps reflecting a definition of clerical work as the 'only type of work available' for girls with a higher-than-minimum educational level, for whom factory work was not regarded as good enough. Clerical work was not seen as the beginning of a career.

In previous paragraphs we have discussed the process of job choice, showing a growth in women's 'activism' in job choice between initial entry into the labour force and choice of present job: job choice appeared to be a more intentional process in adult life than in adolescence. We now turn to the specific reasons for choosing current jobs. As indicated in Table 2.2.5, the most frequently mentioned reasons related to the interest of the work itself (31 per cent), followed by 'good pay' (27 per cent). Significantly, relatively few women said that they had chosen their present job because it suited their family role and was convenient, either in hours of work or travel arrangements. More detailed analysis shows substantial differences between occupations, summarized in Table 2.2.6.

The numbers involved do not justify exhaustive analysis. However, there are substantial differences in the importance of intrinsic reasons for choosing jobs: high proportions of administrative, computing, nursing, and clerical employees mentioned 'intrinsic' reasons for choosing their present jobs; machine-sewing, and hand-sewing workers were the next most likely to mention intrinsic reasons; and electronic-assembly workers, engineering-assembly workers, general services, and catering workers the least likely. In this respect female employees are very similar to male employees.[7] Similarly, there were major differences in the extent to which good pay was mentioned as a reason for choosing jobs: the occupation with by far the largest proportion mentioning good pay was engineering assembly (48 per cent), followed by nursing (40 per cent, but only two people), electronic assembly (30 per cent), and general services (cleaning and stores) (30 per cent). Very few clerical workers mentioned 'good pay' (12 per cent) and even fewer hand-sewers (8 per cent). Not unreasonably, women in the best-paying jobs were more likely to mention good pay as a reason for choosing those jobs than women in the worst-paying jobs (hand-sewers).

We were also interested in the issue of the relationship between age and reasons for job choices: it might be expected that pay would be especially important during the years of child-rearing, but that its importance would diminish with age. There was some limited confirmation of the importance of good pay during the child-rearing years: 34 per cent of women aged 35–44 mentioned good pay, compared with 18 per cent aged 15–24 (who were a relatively small group) and no women aged 55 +. Similarly, the age category 35–44 contained the lowest proportion of women mentioning intrinsic reasons – 31.5 per cent, the highest proportion being found in the 55 + age group (42 per cent). (Since only 5 per cent of respondents mentioned good company as a reason for taking their present job, nothing can be said about a possible link between sociability and age.) It is significant that few women mentioned friendly colleagues as a reason for choosing their present job: this factor was not important in causing our respondents to undertake market employment, nor in choosing one job rather than another, despite its importance in explaining why they liked a particular job (see below, p. 87). Especially in manual jobs, women are unlikely to know very much about their future work colleagues, except by general reputation, and it is unlikely that anticipations of a friendly work group would be of major importance in choosing a job, although it could become of central importance subsequently and its loss deeply felt.

The reasons most commonly given for choosing current jobs thus related to interest, 'default' and pay. We now examine the extent to which the women interviewed followed an occupational career, leading to jobs with increased interest and rewards. Unfortunately we did not have the resources to investigate female labour mobility fully; however, we obtained data on up to three jobs

74 *Working Women in Recession*

Table 2.2.6
Reasons for choice of present job (by occupation)

	Occupation									
	Nursing (%)	Catering (%)	Administrative (%)	Clerical (%)	Computing (%)	Machine-sewing (%)	Hand-sewing (%)	Electrical assembly (%)	Engineering assembly (%)	General services (%)	Row totals (%)
Intrinsic qualities	60	15	70	51	60	44	37.5	16	15	20	34
Default		31	20	38	40	11	37.5	32	33	44	31.5
Good pay	40	15	10	12		19	8	39	48	30	24
Family/parent influence		31		16		19	8	7	7	20	13
Suits family role	80	31		1	20	3	8	23	4	20	11.5
Prior training		15		15		14	12.5	4			9
Social			10	5		3	12.5	5		3	8
Conditions				5.5		8	12.5	16	4	3	7.5
Directed				4				5			2
N	5	13	10	73	5	36	24	56	27	30	279

Percentage is that of women giving type of reason.

with previous employers: we also obtained data on first jobs. Two conclusions emerged. First, there was no evidence of 'career' development when initial jobs are compared with present jobs. Secondly, the women interviewed had had relatively few jobs in view of their length of time in the labour force, and they had held their present jobs a relatively long period of time. Additionally, there is no evidence of systematic movement between the jobs which intervened between first and present job, although we do not have the evidence to document this conclusively.

Overall comparison between present job and first job shows a slight tendency for present job to be lower in status than first job, admittedly on the rather unsuitable Hope–Goldthorpe scale used for comparative purposes. The data are summarized in Table 2.2.7.

Table 2.2.7
Comparison of first and current occupational statuses

Occupational status	First job (%)	N	Present job (%)	N
1	2	4	6	15
2	4	10	6	13
3	30	69	18	42
4	44	102	49	112
5	16	37	21	48
Missing	3	8	0	0
N		230		230

The figures refer only to women who had more than one job.

Table 2.2.7 shows the distribution of occupations among respondents at the beginning of their work careers, and at the time of the interview. There is a small increase in the number of women with jobs in the numerically small occupational statuses 1 and 2 (fourteen more), but a greater decline in the number of women in occupational-status group 3 (twenty-seven fewer), and an increase in the proportion of women employed in jobs falling in occupational-status groups 4 and 5. The tendency for the occupations to be lower in status is only slight. However, this may underestimate the amount of downward social mobility, since first jobs may be thought to be the lowest-status jobs obtained during the first stage of a work career, assuming some upward mobility after initial entry into employment. There is thus limited confirmation for the general finding that the jobs women take after a break to start a family are of lower status than those they held in the first stage of their working lives.

In view of their long working lives the women interviewed had worked for a relatively small number of employers. As Table 2.2.8 shows, 17 per cent of women had worked for only one employer, and 18 per cent for only two; at the other end of the scale, 14 per cent had worked for six or more employers. There were differences in the number of employers worked for between companies, and between occupational statuses. As Table 2.2.8 shows, women in Company A had worked for fewer employers than women in any other company, 59 per cent having worked for only one or two employers, compared with 34 per cent in Company B, 22 per cent in Company C, 37 per cent in Company D, and 26 per cent in Company E. There were also differences between occupational statuses, as Table 2.2.9 shows.

Table 2.2.8
Number of employers (by company)

	A (%)	B (%)	C (%)	D (%)	E (%)	Total (%)
1	37	7	8	23	16	17
2	22	27	14	14	10	18
3	10	31	20	21	16	20
More than 3	31	35	58	42	59	45
N	51	68	64	43	51	271

Table 2.2.9
Number of employers (by occupational status)

	Occupational status					Total
	Professional/Administrative/ Supervisory (%)	Clerical (%)	Semi- skilled (%)	Slightly skilled (%)	Unskilled (%)	(%)
1	7	35	12.5	15	6	17
2	30	8	22.5	15	6	18
3	20	16	22	15	37.5	20
More than 3	43	41	43	54	50	45
N	30	63	120	46	16	275

($p = 0.003$)

As expected, clerical workers had worked for fewer employers than manual workers had, reflecting the very positive views they had of their jobs (see below, p. 86) and the rewards that could result from loyalty to a specific firm by movement through an informal hierarchy of jobs, even where job titles remained the same. Even when age is controlled for, clerical workers were more likely than others to have had only one employer. Women went straight into clerical work from school and, because of the popularity of clerical jobs, were likely to stay in them. The firms for which the women worked tended to recruit girls straight from school, and to retain their loyalty by movement through a limited hierarchy of jobs, even though the jobs remained within the same broad job (and pay) category. Interestingly, women in occupational status 1, professional/

administrative/supervisory, were likely to have had more than one employer, possibly demonstrating that some mobility is necessary to gain real promotion. Even amongst manual workers the number of employers worked for was relatively small. Such evidence suggests that women in large-scale manufacturing industry (both clerical and manual) are part of a 'primary' labour market, within which they remain once they have secured a foot-hold, and from which movement into higher turnover occupations in the service sector, especially distribution and hotels and catering, has normally been relatively rare: the redundancies were to change this for manual workers as is shown in Chapter 4 below, pp. 203–4.

The women interviewed had also been in their present jobs a relatively long time. As Table 2.2.10 shows, 64 per cent of women had been in their present jobs for five years or more: this contrasts with the 40 per cent of women interviewed in the *Women and Employment* survey who had worked for their current employers for five years or more, many of whom would have had jobs other than their current ones with the same employer.

Table 2.2.10
Length of service in current jobs (by company)

	A (%)	B (%)	C (%)	D (%)	E (%)	Total (%)
≤ 1 year	4	1.5	20	16	16	12.5
2– 4 years	33	3	33	28	23.5	23
5– 9	20	15	26	16	23.5	20
10–14	16	46	6	16	25.5	23
15–19	10	23.5	11	12	8	13
20 +	16	12	4	12	4	8
N	51	68	66	43	51	279

Women in Company B, the electronics case study, had worked on the same jobs for an especially long time, 81.5 per cent for ten years or more. Long service in the same jobs was also a characteristic of the women in Company A, who were primarily sewing-machinists. Women in the engineering industry, whether manual or non-manual workers, had a more varied work experience; 53 per cent of women in Company C, 44 per cent of women in Company D, and 39.5 per cent of women in Company E had been working at their current jobs for under five years.

In view of the evidence of a lack of 'career' progression, it is hardly surprising that a majority of women interviewed (61 per cent) said that, if they could go back to the beginning of their working life again, they would prefer to have done something different. Respondents were asked, 'if you could go back to the beginning of your working life what would you have done instead, or would you have done the same?' Table 2.2.11 shows the distribution of responses by occupational status.

Table 2.2.11
Preferences for alternative work at 16 (by occupational status)

	Occupational status					Total
	Professional/Administrative/ Supervisory (%)	Clerical (%)	Semi-skilled (%)	Slightly skilled (%)	Unskilled (%)	(%)
Yes	58	37	36	36	94	36
No	39	61.5	62	62	94	61
Don't know	3	1.5	4	2		3
Missing data	1	1	2	1		1
N	31	65	120	47	16	279

($p = 0.009$)

Q. *If you could go back to the beginning of your working life . . . would you have done the same?*

Only a minority of women in occupational status group 1 would have preferred to have acted differently at the beginning of their working lives (39 per cent), compared with 62 per cent in statuses 2, 3, and 4, and 94 per cent in occupational status group 5. Amongst the semi-skilled manual workers, the electronic assemblers were the least likely to have wanted to do anything different (54 per cent did so), and the engineering assemblers the most likely (74 per cent).

The most common career preferred was in a female 'caring' profession, as Table 2.2.12 shows.

Table 2.2.12
Preferred career

	Respondents
Female caring profession (nursing, social work, teaching)	29
Any career, better job unspecified	16
Female skilled occupation (hairdressing, catering)	13
Clerical work	11
Unspecified jobs, offering travel, working with people	13
Profession not elsewhere classified	7
Skill n.e.c.	6
Arts, craft, performing arts	4

($N = 170$)

The data do not purport to convey a picture of what respondents would have done had they been able to go back to the age of 15 or 16, since present circumstances clearly differ from past circumstances. However, the commitment to female caring professions is striking, since respondents were free to name any occupation they wished.

The preference of women in clerical and manual jobs for other occupations may not be surprising, since such jobs were likely to offer substantial rewards, both in material and non-material terms, compared with the jobs the women had. However, a substantial minority said that they had previously worked at jobs they preferred to their present jobs. The preference for former jobs was most common amongst unskilled workers, as Table 2.2.13 shows. Among specific occupations, engineering-assembly workers were especially likely to have preferred former jobs, 56 per cent doing so. The major reasons mentioned for preferring previous jobs were intrinsic ones, mentioned by 64 per cent of those who preferred previous jobs, and social ones, mentioned by 30 per cent. No one preferred a previous job because of better money, or because it fitted in with family roles more conveniently.

The women were also asked what type of job they would like to see their daughters in, partly as an indication of their evaluation of their own working lives, and partly to see if women had specific occupational aspirations for their

Table 2.2.13
Responses to *Did you have any previous job that you preferred?*

	Professional/Administrative/Supervisory (%)	Clerical (%)	Semi-skilled (%)	Slightly skilled (%)	Unskilled (%)	Total (%)
No	77	49	52.5	47	37.5	53
Yes	13	21.5	37	38	56	32
No previous job	10	29	11	15	6	15
N	31	65	120	47	16	279

($p = 0.016$)

daughters. Many women did have occupational aspirations for their daughters, and did not especially wish them to follow in their own footsteps, as Table 2.2.14 shows. The table relates only to women who had daughters, or were planning a family. A large minority of women were happy to leave the choice of future occupation to their daughters, without having any specific aspirations; there was a similar distribution of replies for sons. Substantial numbers would have liked to see their daughters in professional and clerical jobs, relatively few in manual trades. Despite the recession, relatively few wanted to see their daughters in 'any job that was secure'.

In this section we have examined women's job choices and occupational careers before the redundancy. We have shown that women's expectations of duration of employment were relatively limited on initial entry into the labour force, especially among women from manual-working-class backgrounds — in contrast to their present expectations. The most commonly mentioned reasons for choosing initial job did not involve rational comparison between the rewards available from different jobs, perhaps reflecting the view that their working

Table 2.2.14
Career aspirations for daughters

Type of career	Percentage
Whatever occupation she chooses	44
Specified profession	19
Unspecified profession	9
Clerical	12
Specified trade	5
Unspecified trade	0.5
Any secure job	2
Married and not working	4
Don't know	4

($N = 190$)

lives would only be relatively short as well as the limited range of openings available. However, women gave more 'active' reasons for choosing their present jobs than for choosing their initial jobs, although there was a slight drop in the occupational status of present jobs when compared with initial jobs. The majority of women would have preferred to do something different from the jobs they had entered at 15 or 16 if they had the opportunity, 18 per cent showing a marked preference for female 'caring' professions; the only status group with a minority taking this view being status group 1. A substantial minority of women had had previous jobs which they preferred to current jobs, especially amongst manual workers: a majority of unskilled workers had preferred previous jobs, as had the majority of engineering assembly workers. Although as many as 44 per cent of women said that they would be happy with whatever occupation their daughters (or their sons) chose, there was a marked preference for professional and clerical occupations for daughters.

In general the history of the women's behaviour in the labour market was of only limited usefulness in explaining their present 'orientation' to work. General social attitudes towards the gender-based division of roles had changed during their lifetime, as had their own expectations. For the women from blue-collar families in particular anticipation of a short period in employment as a prelude to a lifetime as housewives had given way to the reality of an adult life spent largely in the work-force. There was a consciousness that the first steps they had taken were governed by expectations of the future which were not fulfilled — or that they were taken with inadequate knowledge of the alternatives that would eventually be available to them. An obvious explanation for the passivity which marked the entrance of so many of the women into the work-force was that they expected, wrongly, that their working lives should be short, rather than that they were indifferent to the nature of the employment in which they were ultimately to spend a large part of their lives.

Nevertheless, although many of the women felt that, 'knowing what they do now' they would have acted differently on their initial entrance into the work-force, it would be misleading to infer from this that the women interviewed were dissatisfied with the rewards provided by their jobs. A full examination requires consideration of their attitudes towards the rewards derived from work, and their attitudes to specific jobs. This is undertaken in the following section.

2.3 Current attitudes to work

In this section we outline our findings on what women looked for in jobs in general, and then explore the extent to which their objectives were met by their current jobs. The job aspirations and attitudes of administrative and professional, clerical, and three groups of manual workers are compared with each other. In the first part of the section we examine the importance of different job factors in general terms, and in the second the extent to which the women felt that their objectives were met. The four factors most frequently emphasized as being important in jobs were friendly colleagues, autonomy, interest, and a good rate of pay. In general, the women felt that their jobs were at least reasonably satisfactory, although non-manual workers were substantially more satisfied than manual workers.

Attitudes to work are influenced by primary and secondary socialization, past work experience, present needs (psychological, social, and economic) and awareness of the extent to which needs can be realistically satisfied. It is impossible to say that some aspirations are more primary, basic, or fundamental than others. It is also impossible to establish the relative priority of different job attributes in an absolute sense, since the different attributes are incommensurable, and in practice not assessed against each other in general terms: comparisons are made in specific situations and contexts according to the criteria seen as appropriate, notably in choosing jobs, and in evaluating present jobs. We have discussed choice of jobs in the preceding section (2.2): we discuss evaluation of present jobs below (pp. 86–7). The women were asked how important specific attributes were to them in a job, on a five-point scale ranging from essential to not important: respondents were not asked to place the attributes themselves in rank order. We expected few to be regarded as not important, but that there would be important differences between occupations in the importance attached to different attributes. These expectations were confirmed.

Using hypotheses derived from the extensive previous research into attitudes to work amongst men, we asked respondents about the importance of: a good rate of pay; promotion prospects; interesting work; responsibility; autonomy; friendly people to work with; convenient travel arrangements; security; availability of part-time work; ability to work for a variety of employers; and time off during school holidays.[8] Questions thus covered both the intrinsic and extrinsic rewards from work, as well as external factors which might affect women's ability to combine domestic and work roles, and thus to influence attitudes to work (availability of part-time work, ability to take time off for school holidays).

As a convenient method of summarizing the data, Table 2.3.1 presents the proportion of women in each occupational status group regarding a given attribute as essential or very important. The attribute most frequently cited as essential or very important was thus 'friendly people to work with', the second most frequently cited was autonomy, and the third most frequently cited was

Table 2.3.1

Percentage of women regarding job attributes as essential or very important (by occupational status)

	Occupational status					Total
	Professional/ Administrative/ Supervisory (%)	Clerical (%)	Semi-skilled (%)	Slightly skilled (%)	Unskilled (%)	(%)
Friendly people to work with	58	74	74	77	63	72
Autonomy	71	71	62.5	61	75	67
Interest	84	71	53	57	50	61
Good rate of pay	48	51	53	62	75	55
Variety	58	57	32.5	38	44	43
Easy journey to work	23	38.5	47.5	45	56	43
Security	29	37	49	38	50	42
Responsibility	58	45	22	36	25	33
Promotion prospects	29	31	12.5	8.5	25	19

interest. It is important to stress that the three attributes were the most frequently cited, not necessarily the most important in an absolute qualitative sense. Some attributes may be of central importance for some groups, but totally irrelevant for others. Moreover, one women's 'very important' may be equal in intensity of feeling to another woman's 'important'.

As was expected, the gratifications that the women looked for in their work differed according to their occupational status, suggesting that to some extent the women looked for the rewards that they were likely to find. Interesting work and variety were rated more highly by administrative, professional, and clerical workers than they were by the semi-skilled and unskilled manual workers. Responsibility was rated highly only by status 1. Pay was rated most highly by status 5, the only category who rated pay more highly than 'friendly people to work with'. This category included the cleaners, whose work could hardly have provided any intrinsic interest not already available in their own domestic chores, and who also worked in comparative isolation, often at night, four or five cleaners each 'doing' her own section of the building, with the result that even the rewards of sociability were relatively sparse for this group. Pay, therefore, assumed a higher relative importance for this group.

For administrative and professional women the job characteristic most frequently mentioned as essential or very important was 'interest', the second most frequently mentioned was 'autonomy', with 'friendly people to work with' only in third place, mentioned by substantially fewer respondents. Overall, there

Table 2.3.2
Priority of job attributes (by occupational status)

	Percentage giving a high priority
Status 1	
Interesting work	84
Autonomy	74
Friendly people to work with, variety, responsibility	58
A good rate of pay	48
Good prospects for promotion, security	29
An easy journey to work	23
Status 2	
Friendly people to work with, autonomy	74
Interesting work	71
Variety	57
A good rate of pay	51
Responsibility	45
An easy journey to work	38.5
Security	37
Good prospects for promotion	31
Status 3	
Friendly people to work with	74
Autonomy	62.5
A good rate of pay, interesting work	53
Security	49
An easy journey to work	47.5
Variety	32
Responsibility	22
Good prospects for promotion	12.5
Status 4	
Friendly people to work with	77
Autonomy	64
A good rate of pay	62
Interesting work	57
Variety, security	38
Responsibility	36
Promotion	8.5
Status 5	
Pay, autonomy	75
Friendly people to work with	62.5
An easy journey to work	56
Interesting work, security	50
Variety	44
Promotion, responsibility	25

appeared to be four major groupings of job characteristics for this group: first, interest and autonomy; second, variety, responsibility, and friendly colleagues; third, a good rate of pay; fourth, promotion prospects, security, and an easy journey to work were relatively unimportant. Moreover, the dispersal of response was higher for group 1 than for any other occupation group: interest was essential or very important for 84 per cent, an easy journey to work for only 23 per cent.

Amongst clerical workers, the three characteristics most frequently classed as essential or very important were autonomy (74 per cent), friendly colleagues (74 per cent), and interest (71 per cent); the three least frequently mentioned were promotion prospects (31 per cent), security (37 per cent), and an easy journey to work (38.5 per cent). Friendly colleagues and an easy journey to work were more frequently highly regarded by clerical workers than by women in occupational group 1, as one might expect: the work offered less opportunity for individual creativity, the work environment was inherently more gregarious, and the degree of commitment required to overcome inconvenient travel arrangements was likely to be less common. Although convenient access was more important for clerical than for professional/administrative workers, it was still regarded as essential or very important by only a minority.

Among manual workers the pattern of responses was different. The three attributes most frequently mentioned as essential or very important by semi-skilled manual workers were friendly people to work with (74 per cent), autonomy (62.5 per cent) and equal third a good rate of pay and interest (both 53 per cent). The three least frequently mentioned were promotion prospects (12.5 per cent), responsibility (22 per cent), and variety (32.5 per cent). The rankings of responses amongst workers having slight skills were almost identical. The three most popular were friendly colleagues (77 per cent), autonomy (64 per cent), and a good rate of pay (62 per cent) — interest being fourth (57 per cent). Similarly, the three least popular were promotion prospects (8.5 per cent), responsibility (36 per cent), with security and variety being joint third (38 per cent). The third manual group, the more heterogeneous and smaller one of unskilled workers, was slightly different. The three most popular were autonomy (75 per cent), a good rate of pay (75 per cent), and friendly colleagues (63 per cent). The three least popular were responsibility (25 per cent), promotion prospects (25 per cent), and variety (44 per cent). Although it would be dangerous to press the interpretation too far, three items were essential or very important for a majority of our manual respondents — friendly colleagues, a good rate of pay, and autonomy — and three items were regarded as essential or very important by only a minority — promotion prospects, responsibility, and variety. It is especially significant that autonomy was more frequently stressed than variety, showing a preference for being left to get on with the job over having a more varied job which might involve more detailed supervision and which would probably disrupt the friendly work relations to which so much importance was attached.

Comparison of the importance of job factors suggests a significant difference in the meaning of 'interest' for different occupational groups. A majority of respondents in all occupational groups regarded interest as either essential or very important, although the size of the majority was greater in non-manual than in manual groups. There was little difference between manual and non-manual groups in the importance attached to autonomy. However, there were substantial differences in the importance attached to variety and responsibility, the two factors being stressed much more heavily by non-manual than manual workers. In other words, interest is associated with autonomy by manual workers and with autonomy, variety, and responsibility by non-manual workers.

In previous paragraphs we have been discussing women's attitudes to jobs in general: in the remainder of this section we are concerned with their attitudes to their specific jobs at the time of the interview.

As we have suggested earlier, going out to work was, for most of the women, the result of a choice made on the basis of their economic needs and on an assessment of the alternative rewards available to them in their domestic role. Although the majority of women did not feel completely satisfied with their 'career' choice, or that they had had complete control over the factors that led to it, their responses showed a marked satisfaction with their choice of employment status as an alternative to not being employed. Assessing their jobs in the light of the existing alternative opportunities available to them, and faced with the prospect of losing them, the majority of women said that they liked their jobs – 50.5 per cent said that they liked their jobs very much, 26.5 per cent that they liked them, 18 per cent that they found them reasonable, 5 per cent did not like their jobs very much, and only 0.4 per cent, or one respondent, said that she did not like her job at all. Although feelings towards present jobs were generally positive, there were substantial differences between occupational groups as Table 2.3.3 shows.

Table 2.3.3
Job satisfaction (by occupational status)

	Occupational status					Total
	Professional/ Administrative/ Supervisory (%)	Clerical (%)	Semi-skilled (%)	Slightly skilled (%)	Unskilled (%)	(%)
Liked very much	77	69	35	49	44	50.5
Liked it	10	20	32	32	31	26.5
Reasonably	13	9	28	8.5	6	18
Not much		1.5	5	8.5	19	5
Not at all				2		0.4
N	31	65	120	47	16	279

$(p = 0.001)$

86 *Working Women in Recession*

It is likely that the respondents' perception of the difference between liking a job and liking it only reasonably well are variable and slight. However, there is a clear difference, even at the most general level, between non-manual and manual workers at the extremes: hence 77 per cent of professional/administrative workers said that they liked their jobs very much, as did 69 per cent of clerical workers, compared with 35 per cent of semi-skilled, 49 per cent of slightly skilled, and 44 per cent of unskilled. Similarly, only one non-manual worker (a clerical worker) said that she did not much like her job, compared with thirteen manual workers (and the one person who did not like her job at all was a manual worker). The differences between occupations within the non-manual/manual category were relatively slight: 71 per cent of clerical workers liked their jobs very much, compared with 80 per cent of computing and nursing staff; 33 per cent of electronics assembly workers and engineering assembly workers liked their jobs very much, compared with 50 per cent of general services. There were also differences in job satisfaction by age, younger workers being less likely to like their jobs very much and more likely to like their jobs 'not much'. Overall, it is clear that job satisfaction was least among electronics- and engineering-assembly workers, and that among those groups younger workers was less likely to be highly satisfied (in general terms) than older workers.

In addition to asking the women what they looked for in employment we tried to find out what were the main things they liked about the jobs they had. It would have been possible to pose questions requiring a direct comparison between the rewards looked for and those found, but it was felt that to provide two sets of identical, pre-coded questions would have invited too mechanical a response, with insufficient thought. Moreover, we did not wish to prompt evaluation of attributes irrelevent to their current jobs. The women were therefore invited to volunteer their own comments on the satisfactions they obtained from their present jobs. This led to a wide range of responses, resulting in an initial coding involving forty-three different categories. These were subsequently conflated into six categories: (1) intrinsic, referring to the qualities of the job itself; (2) social, to the companionship of work-mates or to 'dealing with people'; (3) convenience of job for fulfilling family responsibilities; (4) good pay; (5) good conditions: easy-going boss, clean conditions, work not too hard, and similar environmental qualities; and (6) fringe benefits, including pensions and job security. There were also two categories for 'nothing special' and 'nothing at all'. Three of the major categories loosely matched the major pre-coded attributes that the women had looked for in their jobs: intrinsic qualities included interest, responsibility, autonomy, and variety; social qualities and pay had also been included in the pre-coded attributes; however, convenience for fulfilling family responsibilities had only been covered in part by easy journey to work and good conditions and benefits had not been included in the pre-coded questions at all. Table 2.3.4 shows the reasons given by the women for liking their present jobs, by occupational status.

Table 2.3.4
Reasons for job satisfaction (by occupational status)

	Occupational status					Total
	Professional/ Administrative/ Supervisory (%)	Clerical (%)	Semi-skilled (%)	Slightly skilled (%)	Unskilled (%)	(%)
Intrinsic qualities	90	74	52.5	55	44	62
Social	61	61.5	42.5	53	44	51
Suits family role	6.5	3	5	17	6	7
Good pay	6.5	6	13	6	6	9
Conditions		12	15	8.5	19	12
Benefits	3	6	6	2		8
Nothing special	3	1.5	2.5	4	6	3
Nothing at all		1.5	6	2	6	4
N	31	65	120	47	16	279

Percentage is that of respondents mentioning given attribute.

There was a considerable difference between occupational statuses, both in the number of attributes mentioned and the type. Professional and administrative workers were likely to mention a wider range of qualities they liked about their job, and were much more likely to mention intrinsic qualities than lower status workers. Clerical workers had similarly positive feelings about their jobs, but were less likely to mention intrinsic qualities. The semi-skilled, slightly skilled, and unskilled manual workers mentioned fewer qualities, and were much less likely to mention intrinsic qualities. More detailed analysis, by occupation, showed that the engineering assembly workers were especially unlikely to refer to intrinsic qualities (only 44 per cent) and catering (46 per cent) and electronic workers (48 per cent) only slightly more so. However, a majority of hand-sewing and machine-sewing workers mentioned intrinsic qualities as reasons for liking their work — 58 and 67 per cent respectively. The difference between their responses and those of the other 'semi-skilled' workers reflected the nature of their work — the garment makers of Company A were involved in making a wide variety of high-quality garments using batch production methods, and many of the machinists in particular were highly skilled.

When the age distribution of the reasons given for liking jobs is examined, the most interesting finding to emerge is the variation in the importance of 'social' factors (Table 2.3.5). Social reasons for liking their jobs were most likely to be mentioned by the youngest age group (18–24)(68 per cent) and by the oldest age group (55–9)(73 per cent). This may have been partly a positive factor — friendly colleagues and 'a good atmosphere' may have meant more both to young women and to older women, both groups likely to have fewer external domestic commitments than middle-aged women. It may also have been partly a negative factor, in that the other rewards from work were less important.

Table 2.3.5
Reasons for liking current job (by age)

	≤ 24 (%)	25–34 (%)	35–44 (%)	45–54 (%)	55 + (%)	Total (%)
Intrinsic	68	57	55	65	73	62
Social	68	37	46	51	73	50.5
Convenience for family role	4.5	4	8	9	6	7
Good pay	14	8	11	10	3	9
Conditions	4.5	12	9	18.5	9	12
Benefits		6	3	6	6	8
Nothing special	4.5		3	5		3
Nothing at all		10	5			4
N	22	49	92	81	33	277

The majority of women (57 per cent) said that there was nothing about their jobs that they did not like – and only five women had more than one complaint. However, there were very marked differences in the number and type of complaints made by women in different occupations, as is shown in Table 2.3.6. Hence the majority of engineering- and electronics-assembly workers said that there were things about their job which they disliked, the complaints relating primarily to the work itself – that it was boring, monotonous, fiddly, tiring, or dirty. There were, however, fewer complaints from other semi- and slightly skilled manual workers, since their work involved more variety and was carried out under less pressure, especially in Company A. It is perhaps surprising that few women in general services, primarily cleaners, complained about their work, perhaps indicating the importance the women attached to their being able to work without pressure or without close supervision. The largest number of complaints overall concerned the work itself, the second, much smaller, number was over management attitudes and efficiency. Although the figures are too small to be reliable, the complaints about management attitudes and efficiency came mostly from administrative and professional women, who had more contact with senior management, and from groups who worked under relatively close supervision, the hand-sewers in Company A, and canteen workers. The next-largest category of complaints related to other conditions of work and included having to get up early, insufficient tea breaks, and poor environmental conditions. Only two women complained of poor pay.

In addition to asking respondents about what they liked and disliked about their jobs we asked them to rate their jobs in terms of interest, use of abilities, and variety. As Table 2.3.7 shows, the majority of women (84 per cent) found their jobs at the least 'reasonably interesting'. Very few women gave negative responses on any of the three components. Jobs were rated most highly on interest, 56 per cent giving their job a 'good' or 'very good' rating, less highly on use of abilities (46 per cent), and least highly on variety (44.5 per cent). Responses fell most frequently into the 'good' or 'reasonable' category.

Table 2.3.6
Complaints about job (by occupation)

	Nursing (%)	Administrative (%)	Computing (%)	Clerical (%)	Machine-sewing (%)	Hand-sewing (%)	Electrical assembly (%)	Engineering assembly (%)	Catering (%)	General services (%)	Total (%)
Nature of work	20	–	20	10	30	22	57	62	23	17	29
Management's attitude	40	25	20	4	3	18	2	4	15	14	6
Other conditions	–	–	–	11	3	9	2	11	8		7
Insufficient or poor relations with colleagues	–	–	–	1	3	–	–	–	–	3	1
None	40	75	60	74	64	50	39	30	62	65	57
N	5	8	5	69	36	22	56	27	13	29	279

Table 2.3.7
Rating of work

	Very good (%)	Good (%)	Reasonable (%)	Poor (%)	Very poor (%)
Interest	21	35	28	11	5
Use of abilities	15	31	34	15	5
Variety	14	30.5	29	19	8
Average percentage	16	32	30	15	6

($N = 279$)

The results are hardly surprising, as it is normal for people to rate their jobs in fairly positive terms. Of more interest is the wide variation in ratings between occupational statuses, and between occupations. On all three components non-manual workers rated their jobs more highly than manual workers did. Among manual workers the slightly skilled, mostly catering staff and store women, rated their jobs more highly than the semi-skilled and unskilled (cleaners). In the semi-skilled category itself, by far the largest status category, there were differences between the garment workers on the one hand and the valve assemblers and engineering workers on the other, the garment workers rating their jobs more highly on all three components than the assemblers and line workers. The following paragraphs detail the ratings given by each occupational status for each of the separate components: interest, use of abilities, and variety.

Both groups of non-manual workers gave very similar ratings for their jobs in terms of interest, over a third of the women in each category regarding their jobs as 'very interesting', and over 40 per cent rating them as 'interesting'. The majority of women in each of the three manual occupational status groups rated their jobs as either 'interesting' or 'reasonably interesting', although a substantial proportion of unskilled workers (cleaners) rated their jobs as 'uninteresting' or 'very uninteresting'. Table 2.3.8 summarizes the data.

There were substantial differences between occupational statuses in the ranking of jobs in terms of 'use of abilities', including differences between different non-manual occupational status groups. Hence almost half of the women in group 1 (48 per cent) believed that their jobs made 'very good' use of their abilities, but only 14 per cent of women in group 2 (clerical workers). The majority of semi-skilled and slightly skilled workers believed that their jobs made 'good' or 'reasonable' use of their abilities, but 50 per cent of unskilled workers believed that their jobs made poor or very poor use of their abilities, as is shown in Table 2.3.9.

There were also major differences between occupational status groups in the rating of jobs in terms of 'variety'. Hence 35.5 per cent of women in group 1 related their jobs as 'very varied', compared with only 21.5 per cent of women in group 2. Among the manual workers the highest negative rating was amongst the semi-skilled women, 45.5 per cent of whom rated their jobs as 'monotonous'

Table 2.3.8
Rating of interest of job (by occupational status)

	Occupational status					Total
	Professional/ Administrative/ Supervisory (%)	Clerical (%)	Semi-skilled (%)	Slightly skilled (%)	Unskilled (%)	(%)
Very interesting	39	37	10	19	6	21
Interesting	45	41.5	30	32	31	35
Reasonable	13	19	34	36	25	28
Uninteresting	3	3	16	11	25	11
Very uninteresting			10	2	12.5	5
N	31	65	120	47	16	279

Table 2.3.9
Rating of use of abilities in women's jobs

	Occupational status					Total
	Professional/ Administrative/ Supervisory (%)	Clerical (%)	Semi-skilled (%)	Slightly skilled (%)	Unskilled (%)	(%)
Very good use	48	14	10	13		15
Good use	19	48	22.5	38	31	31
Reasonable use	29	28	41	34	19	34
Poor use	3	9	20	13	31	15
Very poor use		1.5	7	2	19	5
N	31	65	120	47	16	279

or 'very monotonous', a much higher proportion than the slightly skilled (19 per cent), and a higher proportion than the unskilled (37.5 per cent). The data are summarized in Table 2.3.10.

Although the majority of women rate their work as good or reasonably good on all three attributes, there are substantial differences between occupational statuses in the proportions rating their work very positively or negatively. Substantial proportions of non-manual workers in occupational groups 1 and 2 rated their work as very interesting, 39 and 37 per cent respectively, and only 3 per cent in each gave their work a negative rating. At the other extreme, 37.5 per cent of cleaners rated their work as uninteresting or very uninteresting. Forty-eight per cent of professional and administrative workers rated their work as making very good use of their abilities, and only 30 per cent as making poor use. On the other hand, 50 per cent of cleaners rated their work as making poor or very poor use of their abilities. Thirty-five per cent of professional and administrative workers rated their work as very varied, the lowest rating on

Table 2.3.10
Rating of monotony at work (by occupational status)

	Occupational status					Total
	Professional/ Administrative/ Supervisory (%)	Clerical (%)	Semi- skilled (%)	Slightly skilled (%)	Unskilled (%)	(%)
Very varied	35.5	21.5	7.5	8.5		14
Varied	32	37	20	49	25	30.5
Reasonably varied	26	37	27	23	37.5	29
Monotonous	3	3	32.5	15	25	19
Very monotonous	3	1.5	13	4	12.5	8

variety being by the semi-skilled operatives, 45.5 per cent of whom rated their work as monotonous or very monotonous.

Overall, work was rated higher the higher the occupational status, with the marked exception of occupational group 4, the slightly skilled workers, who were more satisfied on all dimensions than status group 3. Status groups were of course based on occupational prestige rankings, not upon job attributes. The women in status group 3 had jobs which required both on-the-job training and learned skill, and their hourly and weekly average rates of pay were considerably higher than those of the women in group 4: hence the relatively high ranking of status 3. However, the women employed in the status 4 jobs, catering assistant and storewoman, were allowed considerably more variety in tasks and freedom of movement than the operatives, particularly the valve assemblers and engineering assembly workers, who remained at their bench or on the line and performed the same task repetitively and under the pressure of piece work timing or production bonuses. As Table 2.3.11 shows, the disparity between statuses 3 and 4 is particularly great on ratings of variety, only 27.5 per cent of the status 3 operatives rating their jobs as varied or very varied, compared with 57.5 per cent of women in status 4. The disparity between the statuses 3 and 4 in rating their job on use of abilities (a positive rating by status 3 of only 32.5 per cent compared to 51 per cent for status 4) is more puzzling, but possibly reflects both the higher expectations of the operatives nurtured by their higher pay, and their frustration at the very restricted use made of their acquired skills.

Table 2.3.11 summarizes the relative ratings given to their jobs by the five different occupational statuses. The figures given are the percentages of women in each status giving their jobs positive ratings, i.e. good or very good.

To explore the significant finer variations between occupational statuses in their assessment of jobs we constructed a scale with a numerical value attached to each degree of satisfaction. An arbitrary value of 1 was given to 'reasonable', 2 to 'good', 3 to 'very good', −1 to 'poor', and −2 to 'very poor', the highest possible score being 300.

Table 2.3.11
Proportions of women giving their work a positive rating (by occupational status)

	Occupational status					Total
	Professional/ Administrative/ Supervisory (%)	Clerical (%)	Semi-skilled (%)	Slightly skilled (%)	Unskilled (%)	(%)
Interest	84	78.5	40	51	37	56
Use of abilities	67	62	32.5	51	31	46
Variety	67.5	58.5	27.5	57.5	25	44.5
Average	73	66	33	53	31	49
N	31	65	120	47	16	279

Table 2.3.12
Ratings of jobs on a scale of −200–300 (by occupational status)

	Occupational status					Total
	Professional/ Administrative/ Supervisory (%)	Clerical (%)	Semi-skilled (%)	Slightly skilled (%)	Unskilled (%)	(%)
Interest	217	210	88	142	67	182
Use of ability	208	154	82	132	12	116
Variety	187.5	169.5	31	123.5	37	97
Average	204	178	67	132	39	132

We have discussed differences in relative work satisfaction between occupational statuses. Each status category covered a range of jobs, especially status 1, which covered all administrative and professional occupations as well as supervisors of manual workers, and status 3, which covered the four different manufacturing operations of valve assembly, engineering assembly, hand- and machine-sewing. The numbers of women in specific occupations comprising status 1 are too small to show statistically significant variations in job satisfaction; however, the numbers in status 3 were large enough to show statistically significant and interesting variations in job satisfaction between the electronic and engineering assembly workers on the one hand, and the machine- and hand-sewers on the other. The latter showed a markedly higher level of job satisfaction on all three components of interest, variety, and use of abilities (Tables 2.3.13–14). This difference is not surprising. All of the hand-sewers and most of the machine-sewers were garment workers from Company A and, although most were on piece work, relatively slow time rates were set to ensure high-quality work, freedom of movement was possible since work was done in batch mode, and frequent style and garment changes ensured variety. The pressure of piece-work times, restriction of movement, and monotony of repetitive tasks, were

Table 2.3.13
Proportions of women giving their work a positive rating (by occupation)

	Occupation									Total
	Non-manual				Manual					
	Nursing (%)	Administrative (%)	Computing (%)	Clerical (%)	Machine sewing (%)	Hand-sewing (%)	Electrical assembly (%)	Engineering assembly (%)	Catering (%)	General services (%)	(%)
Interest	60	70	80	82	47	50	34	40	61	47	56
Use of abilities	80	60	80	62	54	46	23	33	54	47	46
Variety	40	70	60	63	25	54	27	26	61.5	43	44.5
Average	60	67	73	69	42	50	33	33	59	45	49
N	5	10	5	73	36	24	56	27	13	30	279

Table 2.3.14
Rating of jobs on a scale of −200–300 (by occupation)

	Occupation									Total
	Non-manual				Manual					
	Nursing	Administrative	Computing	Clerical	Machine sewing	Hand-sewing	Electrical assembly	Engineering assembly	Catering	General services	
Interest	200	190	220	213	126	142	66	69	193	94	182
Use of abilities	200	180	200	161	137	119	42	35	167	73	116
Variety	143	168	200	148	80	104	13	−4	168	83	97
Average	181	179	207	174	114	122	40	33	176	83	131

thus considerably less for the garment workers than for the other manufacturing operatives, so that a higher degree of satisfaction with their work was to be expected.

In short, non-manual respondents rated their occupations very favourably in terms of use made of abilities, variety, and general interest. This conclusion is scarcely surprising for the relatively high status and highly paid occupations of nursing, administration, and computing. However, the very positive reactions of clerical workers was more surprising, possibly indicating that clerical workers compared their jobs favourably with the alternative female jobs which they might realistically have obtained, in view of their generally low levels of formal qualifications. Amongst manual workers, a clear majority found their jobs at least reasonably interesting, although a smaller number regarded them as making good use of their abilities, and a substantially smaller number regarded them as varied. There were important differences between different groups of manual workers, assembly workers in electronics and in engineering being less positive about their jobs than sewers (whether machine or hand), or than catering and stores assistants. The particular discontents of assembly workers were linked to the feeling of pressure generated both by the production system and by the piece-work system and, especially in the electronics industry, the lack of variety. Conversely, both stores and catering (classified as slightly skilled) were relatively varied, free from pressure, and provided ample opportunity for sociability.

In previous paragraphs we have been concerned with the attitude of women towards their work as work. But the attribute the women most frequently mentioned as being essential or very important to their jobs in general was 'friendly colleagues to work with'. As Tables 2.3.15–16 show, the majority of women described the general atmosphere in their work group as good or very good in normal times (84 per cent), and a majority also described the general atmosphere of their factory in the same terms (75 per cent). In general, the women thus regarded both their work groups and their factories as satisfactory, in normal circumstances. However, there was a feeling in Company C that the atmosphere in the factory at large, although not in specific work groups, had deteriorated with a tightening up of supervision in the period preceding the

Table 2.3.15
Perceptions of work-group atmosphere (by company)

	A (%)	B (%)	C (%)	D (%)	E (%)	Total (%)
Very good	35	42	47	61	49	46
Good	39	49	33	31	33	38
Reasonable	23.5	9	17	5	16	14
Poor	2			2	2	1
Very poor			3			0.7
N	51	67	66	42	51	277

($p = 0.090$)

Table 2.3.16
Perceptions of factory atmosphere (by company)

	A (%)	B (%)	C (%)	D (%)	E (%)	Total (%)
Very good	20	34	21	37	41	30
Good	38	54	41	42	45	45
Reasonable	34	4	27	19	12	19
Poor	6		6		2	3
Very poor			1			
Don't know	2	7	3	2		3
N	50	68	66	43	51	278

($p = 0.003$)

redundancy. Moreover, the redundancy itself inevitably led to increased tension in the factories concerned, with an inevitable deterioration in the general atmosphere, especially in Company A.

In short, the three job attributes most frequently mentioned by the women interviewed as being essential or very important to a job were friendly people to work with, autonomy, and interest. As we have seen, the majority of women (84 per cent) regarded the atmosphere in their work group as good, and many informally commented on their friendships with their work-mates: 20 per cent said that most of their friends came from work, and many more said that they had permanent friends at work. A substantial majority of women also regarded autonomy as either essential or very important. As we had not expected this emphasis initially we did not specifically ask women to rate their jobs in terms of the amount of autonomy they were permitted. Finally, most women (61 per cent) regarded interesting work as either essential or very important, and most rated their jobs as at least reasonably interesting. In general the women interviewed believed that their jobs rated at least 'reasonably' on the characteristics which they regarded as essential or very important.

2.4 Family influences upon women's attitudes to work

Non-manual workers were more positive about their jobs than manual workers, especially assembly workers (both electronic and engineering) and cleaners. However, if taken in isolation and without further examination, this emphasis on the occupational determinants of job satisfaction could be misleading: the apparent occupational influences might be the result of differences in the marital status, breadwinner status, family life-cycle, or age of women in different occupations. It might be expected that women with alternative roles available to them might be more demanding of their jobs, married women therefore being less satisfied than single women, and married women who had children least satisfied. If women's desires for activity, involvement, and social interaction are met outside the work-place those attributes of work become less important, and the negative attributes, lack of freedom, monotony, and physical exhaustion more salient. Women who have young children would be most likely to find their needs fulfilled in domestic life and additional work outside the home physically exhausting: it is this group of women that would therefore be the least satisfied with their jobs. Alternatively, since there were only small numbers of women who had young children in our sample, and the majority of women had a break from market employment whilst their children were under school age, it may be that only those women who particularly valued work would be in employment: they would therefore be expected to be highly satisfied. Moreover, women who went out to work to earn 'extras', or whose financial contribution to household income was not indispensable, might be expected to find work more satisfying, their job choices being less constrained by financial circumstances. Finally, research into job attitudes among male workers has shown that job satisfaction increases with age, as workers become reconciled to the often limited rewards work provides for semi- and unskilled workers. Other things being equal, a similar tendency might be expected amongst female semi- and unskilled workers. We therefore examined the relation between marital status, breadwinner status, family life-cycle, and age and job satisfaction. This was possible to only a limited extent because of the restricted overall size of our sample, its demographic homogeneity, and the interrelation between age and other factors, including marital status, breadwinner status, family life-cycle position, and occupation: the inter-correlation between variables is therefore considerable. An index of job satisfaction, derived from four questions discussed individually earlier, was constructed: whether the women interviewed liked their jobs overall, found them interesting, made good use of their abilities, and were varied. Satisfaction scores from 4 to 20 were then computed, the most satisfied scoring lowest. The respondents were then divided into two groups, the satisfied and the rest, the dividing line being a score of 8, representing an average of positive responses to each question. The proportion of respondents with given characteristics falling in the satisfied category was then computed.

There were only slight differences in the probabilities of being satisfied according to marital status, breadwinner status, and family life-cycle position, as Table 2.4.1 shows, and none of the variations was statistically significant. Divorced or widowed women were slightly more likely to be satisfied with their jobs than either married or single women, the latter being the least likely to be satisfied. There were also differences according to breadwinner status, women earning extras being less likely to be satisfied with their jobs than any other group. Finally, women who had children under 16 were less likely to be satisfied with their jobs than either women who had no children or those women whose children were aged 16 or more.

In short, the difference made to the level of job satisfaction by the three 'family'-related factors is small. Such differences as exist are dwarfed by the effects of age and, even more substantially, of occupation. Table 2.4.2 shows the distribution of job satisfaction by age.

Table 2.4.1
Job satisfaction and domestic situation

	Satisfied (%)	N
Marital status		
Married	44	207
Divorced/Widowed	47	32
Single	40	40
Breadwinner status		
Major breadwinner	100	2
Sole breadwinner	44	43
Earning own keep	43	51
Joint breadwinner	44	153
Earning extras	38	29
Family life-cycle		
Children ≤ 15	37	73
Children 16 +	48	110
No children	44	96
Total	44	

Table 2.4.2
Job satisfaction (by age)

Age	Satisfied (%)	N
≤ 24	54.5	22
25–34	35	49
35–44	37	92
45–54	51	81
55 +	51.5	33
Total	44	277

Hence the most satisfied group were the under 25s, followed by the over 55s, and then the group 45–54. This might be expected, on the basis of research into job satisfaction amongst men. Moreover, women aged 25–44 were likely to have the most pressing domestic commitments, and the most easily available alternative roles.

The age differences were much less pronounced than the occupational status differences. As Table 2.4.3 shows, there were major and statistically significant differences in job satisfaction between occupational status groups. Hence a very sharp contrast is drawn between non-manual and manual workers, as would have been expected on the basis of previous discussion. Most notable is the very marked contrast between the high levels of job satisfaction amongst clerical workers and the low level amongst semi-skilled operatives. Equally, there is a marked difference between semi-skilled and unskilled workers, and the slightly skilled.

Table 2.4.3
Job satisfaction (by occupational status)

	Satisfied (%)	N
Prof./Admin./Supervisory	71	31
Clerical	66	65
Semi-skilled	27.5	120
Slightly skilled	40	47
Unskilled	31	16
Total	44	279

The differences in job satisfaction between women were thus primarily related to occupational status, not to domestic circumstances. This may reflect the occupational heterogeneity and the relative demographic homogeneity of our respondents: the range of occupations covered was wide, but the distribution of family circumstances limited. Moreover, there may be a closer link between job satisfaction and domestic circumstances amongst part-time women workers than amongst full-time women workers — although there was no support for this in our research.

2.5 Conclusion

This section has presented the evidence on attachment to the labour market and attitudes to work before job loss, to present the 'before' picture. The evidence is particularly valuable in that we have been able to present the 'before' picture independently of hindsight, especially necessary when hindsight is likely to be heavily influenced by experience of a major event like redundancy. Since the field-work was carried out after the announcement of redundancy, although before its implementation, the views revealed may not be wholly characteristic of women workers in 'normal' circumstances. However, there is no reason to believe that the announcement of redundancy in itself would lead in the very short run to major changes in attitudes towards market employment and work, although subsequent experience of redundancy and unemployment may well do so. In short, we believe that the data accurately reflect the attitudes to market employment and to the specific jobs of our sample, comprising mainly full-time workers in clerical and routine manual occupations in large-scale manufacturing industry.

The large majority of the women showed a strong commitment to market employment if judged by the length of their working career: the average length of time spent in the work-force was twenty-two years. Almost a third of the women interviewed had had no break in their working lives and 80 per cent of those who had broken their working career had done so only once, the majority taking a break for five years or less. Most of the women (70 per cent) had intended to work until retirement age (a further 7 per cent until retirement age with a break for children) if there had been no redundancy.

Most of the women had a strong economic motive for working. Although the figures on total household income are not reliable in detail, the financial contribution made by the women to their household's income was substantial, as might be expected since the sample was drawn primarily from full-time workers with husbands in modestly paid routine non-manual and manual occupations. Eighty-seven per cent of the women said that one of their main reasons for going to work was financial. In addition, 69 per cent gave further reasons for working, the most common being for interest (38 per cent) and for company (27 per cent). On the whole, the women felt that they were happier working than they would be staying at home full time, 86 per cent saying that overall they were happier going out to work than not doing so.

A preference for being in employment rather than being out of employment does not necessarily mean a preference for the routine and the tasks involved in paid employment over the routine and tasks of domestic life; the routine and the tasks involved in going out to work might not be missed. However, the majority of women agreed that women need work to avoid boredom at home, and disagreed with the view that household and family work were more enjoyable than going out to work — although a number of women felt that combining the two roles was tiring. A majority felt that not going out to work would lead to a loss of confidence, and a small majority to a feeling of being cut off from the rest of the world. On the other hand, the women did not feel that being unemployed would lower their status in the eyes of their family or the wider community. On the contrary, the majority felt that they did not have a strong entitlement to work during the periods of high unemployment, and that married women should give priority to single people and to married men where there was competition for jobs.

Although the women interviewed had spent a large proportion of their adult lives in the work-force, there was little evidence of career planning or career development as conventionally understood. Except for the nurses, and some of the clerical workers and sewing-machinists, jobs were not chosen on the basis of natural inclination or prior training, but because they were available and convenient. The most common reasons given for taking their first jobs were 'default' reasons. Moreover, few women had entered their working lives expecting to work until retirement — some had not thought about it and half had thought that their involvement in market employment would be over when they married and had children. The reasons given for taking present jobs were more positive, but there was no evidence of career progression, present jobs tending if anything to be lower in status than first jobs. However, having obtained their jobs the women were sufficiently satisfied with them to stay in them considerably longer than average for people generally, although this was of course partly a consequence of their relatively mature age. Sixty-five per cent of the women had been with the same firm for ten years or more. The women expressed a general satisfaction with their jobs, 50.5 per cent saying that they liked their jobs very much and a further 26.5 per cent that they liked them. Jobs were liked mainly because of the work itself or various aspects of it, and for the company they provided. Nevertheless, many women retained an awareness that their jobs had been obtained through default, and a majority said that, on looking back, they would have preferred a different working career, usually in a recognized profession or trade.

Job satisfaction is impossible to measure in absolute terms because people are only able to judge their jobs from within the limits of their own experience. The women could assess the jobs they had in the light of previous jobs, if they had had them. Since most of the women had spent a period of their adult lives as full-time housewives they were also able to compare the routine and environment of their present jobs with the routine and environment of full-time domestic roles. They could not, however, meaningfully compare their jobs with jobs they had not had. That the women measured the importance of various job attributes in the light of their own experience is suggested by the different emphasis given by women from different occupations to the importance of various aspects of their jobs. Thus women in non-manual occupations tended to rate interest, responsibility, and variety as more important in a job than women in manual occupations did, whereas the importance attached to autonomy (being left alone to get on with the job) and to friendly co-workers, attributes not intrinsic to the work itself, but to the social environment within which work in all occupations was carried out, were less closely linked to occupation.

Although the women evaluated their jobs as satisfactory by context-related criteria, there was less general satisfaction indicated when the women were asked to rate their own jobs by external criteria, chosen by the research team. Women in different occupations expressed different degrees of satisfaction with the interest, use of abilities, and variety involved in their jobs. Women from non-manual occupations rated their jobs higher on all three attributes, whilst women from status 1 rated their jobs higher on use of abilities and variety than women from status 2. Amongst manual workers, cleaners, and women doing highly repetitive piece work gave their jobs the lowest rating, catering assistants, storewomen, and garment workers rating their work more highly on all three attributes.

With the redundancy the women interviewed were to experience a major drop in income, the extent of financial distress resulting depending upon other household financial resources. They were also to lose whatever financial independence market employment had provided. Moreover, as we have shown in this section, they were to lose a valued activity which they had anticipated continuing. Although the reasons for working were mainly financial, there were other substantial rewards. As other writers have stressed, these include social contacts, whose importance was shown in the stress placed upon friendly colleagues as an essential or very important factor in jobs. But work was also valued in itself, as a source of meaningful activity. The extent to which these rewards were simply foregone, or replaced by other rewards, during unemployment is shown in Chapter 5.

Notes

1. See, e.g., the comments of R. L. Feldberg and E. N. Glen, 'Male and Female: Job Versus Gender Models' in the Sociology of Work', in (eds.) R. Kahn-Hut, A. K. Daniels, and R. Colvard, *Women and Work: Problems and Perspectives* (OUP, 1982), p. 76.
2. Since all the studies were carried out in England, and there are important relevant differences between England and other countries in the UK, for example in the proportion of married women working, we do not claim that our conclusions are valid for Welsh, Scots, or Irish women.
3. The issue is of course directly relevant to the position of women in employment. But, at a more general level, it involves the issue of whether priorities of need ought to be taken into account in allocating jobs, in periods of job shortage, rather than relying solely on skill and other criteria of suitability.
4. For a review see (ed.) W. M. Williams, *Occupational Choice* (George Allen & Unwin, 1974).
5. C. Propper, 'An Empirical Enquiry into the Nature of Clerical Work for Young Women' (M.Phil. thesis, University of Oxford, 1981), p. ii.
6. For recent relevant research see K. Roberts *et al.*, 'Unregistered Youth Unemployment and Out-reach Careers Work' (unpublished report, Department of Employment, 1981).
7. For a dated, but classic, review see F. Herzberg *et al.*, *The Motivation to Work* (John Wiley, 1959).
8. For a convenient comparison see H. Beynon and R. M. Blackburn, *Perceptions of Work: Variations within a Factory* (Cambridge University Press, 1972).

3

WOMEN AND REDUNDANCY

For women, as for men, redundancies involve major upheavals in their working lives. In this chapter we examine the process of redundancy in detail, and women's reactions. All five redundancies were caused by declining product demand, although the reasons for the decline and its steepness differed. In two cases redundancy occurred at the end of a prolonged period of labour retrenchment, which is examined in section 3.2. In sections 3.3–4 we examine the redundancy process in detail, concentrating upon management decision-making (3.3) and management–union relations (3.4). The redundancy agreements and their implications for women are outlined in section 3.5. Women's reactions to redundancy, and their evaluations of management and union handling of the process, are discussed in section 3.6; there is no evidence of feminine fatalism. Redundancy payments are discussed in section 3.7. The chapter concludes with a brief summary.

3.1 Reasons for the redundancies

All five case-study redundancies were due to declining product demand, and varying degrees of consequential company reorganization; there were no cases of technological change unaccompanied by product-market changes. However, the three industries, clothing, electronics, and engineering, in which the case studies were carried out experienced different economic fortunes in the 1970s, the companies concerned were in different financial situations, and the specific reasons for the redundancies differed: in this section we outline briefly the reasons for the redundancies. The data are incomplete, in part intentionally so to maintain the anonymity of the companies concerned.

The UK clothing industry, including the outerwear sector to which plant A belonged, experienced a long-term decline in the 1960s and 1970s: exports rose slowly, and imports expanded rapidly. Although exports of mens and boys tailored outerwear rose from £8.7 m. in 1968 to £18.2 m. in 1973, imports rose from £13.9 m. to £63.5 m. over the same period.[1] The trend continued throughout the 1970s: taking 1975 as 100, production of tailored outerwear was 107.2 in 1973 and 76.4 in 1980.[2] Even before the current recession the industry faced a sluggish world demand, whose impact upon the UK industry was exacerbated by four further factors: a trend in fashion away from formal outer-garments towards more casual wear, slower population growth in the UK, declining real incomes leading to a preference for low-cost Third World imports, and the growth of bilateral sector trade agreements restricting access to specific export markets (e.g. the USA).

Company A was engaged in the production and distribution of high-quality garments, distributing its products through its own retail outlets and through other retailers. The company had a substantial export market, representing 65 per cent of group turnover in 1980–1, with particular emphasis on exports to Europe and Japan: in North America and Australia local manufacture was replacing direct exports from the UK, because of customs changes and currency fluctuations. At the beginning of 1981 the company comprised six manufacturing units, as well as wholesaling and distribution networks. The six manufacturing units were located in the South East and the East Midlands, three manufacturing ladies wear, one men's wear, and two both ladies and men's wear. Four of the plants, including the case-study plant A, had belonged to a different company before being taken over by the present owners in the 1970s. The case-study plant A was the plant specializing in the manufacture of men's outerwear.

Owing to its emphasis upon quality and the relative lack of price sensitivity in its sector of the market, Company A survived the long-term decline of the clothing industry noticeably well, as indicated by its expansion through takeover and its continuing flourishing export trade. However, the company faced increasing difficulties in the late 1970s, as the growth in sales revenues failed to keep pace with inflation. The situation deteriorated especially sharply in 1980–1. By 1981 the comapny was able to increase its turnover only at the cost of substantially reduced profit margins: under current cost accounting conventions the company operated at a loss in 1981.

Against this background it is hardly surprising that the company could only maintain its dividend payments by substantially reducing the value of stocks and work in progress. This was especially necessary because of high interest rates. Traditionally, garments were worked for stock in factory A during the slack period in the winter. However, in 1980 production for stock was diverted from plant A to the company's headquarters plant; in 1981 this process was taken a stage further, and plant A closed. Owing to the nature of the production process, the relatively simple technology used, and the small size of the machinery employed (essentially sewing machines), consolidation at the headquarters plant in 1981 was relatively easy to achieve. The building that housed factory A was to be sold.

There were thus powerful financial pressures upon company A in 1980–1, and good reasons for relieving the pressures by reducing the labour force at plant A: since labour costs were so substantial a proportion of total costs, redundancy was the obvious means of reducing costs. Moreover, plant A had the disadvantage of being located over two hours by road away from the headquarters plant and, as a modern building near the centre of a large town, it had attractive resale potential. It was therefore a likely target for closure and sale. This was pre-figured in 1980, when the plant continued operations only with financial assistance under the Temporary Short Time Working Scheme. In 1981 the financial pressures were greater, the headquarters plant had acquired experience in producing the garments usually made at plant A, and plant A's entitlement to financial assistance under the TSTW scheme had been used up. For these reasons the forthcoming closure of plant A was announced in May 1981.

The electronics components industry of which plant B was a part produced goods worth more than £1400 m. in 1980, and employed over 100 000 workers. Output and market size grew by between 10 and 15 per cent p.a. in the late 1970s; approximately 50 per cent of output was exported. The industry is heavily dependent on international trends: both the technology and the markets are international, substantially dominated by the US and Japan. In the late 1970s the UK industry succeeded in maintaining its world-market share, having 6.9 per cent in 1979 compared with 6.8 per cent in 1970. However, the rate of productivity increase exceeded the growth of output, resulting in an overall decline in employment. Hence total employment in the industry fell from 127 000 in December 1979 to 107 300 in March 1981, a decline caused, according to the NEDC Electronics Components Sector Working Party, 'by a combination of increasing capital investment; a shift within the total output to more capital intensive products, and an increasing number of "managed productivity" improvements'.[3]

Company B is the wholly owned subsidiary of a major electronics multinational, based in the Netherlands, engaged in manufacturing electronics components. At the time of the redundancy the company had six major manufacturing sites in the UK. One of four electronics subsidiaries, Company B's capital assets represented approximately a quarter of the multinational's capital assets in the UK. The company's North West electronics plant specialized in the manufacture of valves, video discs, passive electronic components, assemblies for television, domestic appliances, and automobiles, and fine wire, glass, and metal components for transistors. The redundancy involved the closure of the manufacturing unit producing valves.

The subsidiary's financial statement is incorporated in that of its multinational owner. Like other European electronics groups, the company experienced increasingly difficult market conditions in the late 1970s, reflected in declining profits. In 1980 the company achieved a significant sales increase, but a lower trading profit than the previous year; after tax profits were 1.5 per cent of sales in 1980, compared with 1.8 per cent the previous year. Market growth did not keep pace with increasing productivity in the industry, resulting in increased competition, pressure on selling prices, and reduced profits. In the chairman's words,

> This trend is most evident in the field of consumer electronics. In Western Europe especially, where cost levels are high and rising fast, and where moreover Japanese imports continue to increase, this leads to shrinking profit margins, growing losses due to unused capacity and thus to pressure on profitability. In order in this situation to continue operating competitively in the world market and at the same time be able to restore the profitability of certain activities, it is necessary particularly in Western Europe to adjust the industrial structure of our enterprise. Surplus capacity must be trimmed and production plants concentrated in large-scale units...

Trends in consumer electronics had an immediate and direct impact on the electronics components industry.

In brief, 'as a consequence of the structural process of rising labour productivity and of diminished market growth, the number of jobs in our organisation will be reduced in 1981.' The 1980 employment level was already 39 000, or 9.47 per cent lower than it had been in 1974: 373 000 compared with 412 000.

The plants in which jobs were to be lost were determined by the multinational's global strategy. In the 1960s the multinational had encouraged diversification of local manufacturing, in response to local-product markets, manufacturing capability, and labour supply. However, the multinational changed to a policy of greater specialization in the 1970s, with consolidation into more specialized production units: production was seen in international rather than national terms. The multinational's global financial position and production strategy had a direct impact upon plant B. Plant B had expanded as the multinational's major European producer of a component which was superseded in the 1970s; the employment generated by the replacement product was lower. The direct cause of the redundancy at plant B was the almost total collapse of the world demand for electronic valves, requiring the closure of the valve-production units. Plant B had been originally established in 1939 to help meet military requirements for receiving valves. It rapidly expanded during the radio and television boom of the 1950s and 1960s: production rose from 12 million valves in 1947 to a peak of 60 million valves in 1959, to fall steadily to under 3 million in 1981. The development of integrated circuits, and transistorized radio and television sets, completely undermined the demand for valves, only a residual demand by the armed services (and hi-fi buffs) remaining. The expansion and contraction of demand was reflected in trends in employment, and in the development, and closure, of feeder factories. Total employment at the main North West site rose from 2600 in 1946 to over 6000 for most of 1956–71, over half of whom were involved in valve production, over 1000 were employed in six small feeder factories. At the time of the redundancy covered by this study the total labour force employed on the main site had fallen to under 2000, and only one feeder factory remained (see below, pp. 112–14).

The multinational's shift in policy to compete effectively at a time of general recession and the structural changes in the electronics industry outlined above had three consequences for employment at the North West electronics factory in the 1970s. First, the valve programme was closed down as it was financially unprofitable for the company to compete with cheaper, Yugoslav valves. Second, although transistors had been produced in the early 1970s to absorb some of the employees who would otherwise have been made redundant by the contraction of the valve programme, the transistor department was transferred to a south-coast plant as part of the policy of product specialization. Third, the multinational introduced a new video disc to North West electronics in 1980–1 to create jobs for employees affected by the closure of the valve programme. However, the production processes were more fully automated than in the manufacture of valves. Thus, although there are no detailed figures on the transfer of employees from valve to video-disc production, the sixty or so shift workers engaged in the video-disc programme represented only a relatively small proportion of the original labour force employed in valves. In short, in company B the redundancy was primarily due to technological obsolescence, and the impossibility of absorbing all the surplus labour in the production of new products due to increased productivity. The need for restructuring was reinforced by global and national financial pressures on the multinational.

Production in the sector of the engineering industry in which Company C operated reached its peak in 1972: between 1972 and 1979 British production dropped by almost a half. The drop was caused partly by declining exports, which peaked in 1970, and even more by increasing imports. By 1979 over half the domestic product market was held by imported products. Company C's experience mirrored that of the whole industry, the 1970s being a period of declining output, employment, and substantial financial losses. In the late 1970s a new management team was introduced, with specific instructions to 'turn the company round' and to increase productivity to international levels. Even in an expanding market such an achievement would have involved job losses; in a contracting market the job losses were inevitably substantial.

Company C was a major producer of engineering goods covering a wide range of products. The company experienced considerable financial difficulties in the 1970s, requiring substantial government financial assistance. The specific plant at which the redundancy occurred was opened in the mid 1970s, to produce a specialized, quality product, using the latest technology. However, despite considerable critical acclaim, the product never achieved the sales targets anticipated, partly because its launch coincided with the beginnings of a decline in the demand for such quality products, especially ones using relatively large amounts of energy resources. The company's overall financial difficulties made it inevitable that major savings in costs would be necessary; the specific difficulties of plant C's product made it likely that savings would be found at plant C. In the event plant C's product was transferred to another plant owned by Company C, and plant C moth-balled. It was hoped either that another company in the same group would use the plant for a similar product, or that an alternative buyer (probably foreign) would be found. Arrangements were made for the transfer of some of the capital equipment to the new site, and an attempt was made to find alternative employment within the group for some of the redundant employees.

The fourth company, North West engineering (Company D), was engaged in the manufacture of specialized vehicles, used primarily in agriculture, construction, and distribution. The industry experienced considerable difficulties in the 1970s, owing to a contracting UK market, especially in construction, and increasing competition abroad, where the US had always been strong and Japan was a growing competitive presence. Since the firm's products represented a major item of capital expenditure for purchasers, and their life could be extended if required, the product market was always sensitive to financial pressures on potential purchasers. Contracting markets, and slow product renewal, led to substantial losses in the 1970s, and to appeals for government financial help. In place of direct financial help the government sponsored the takeover of the company by a subsidiary of a major national vehicle manufacturer, operating in the same market. With deepening recession rationalization was inevitable following the merger, and in September 1981 the company announced the forthcoming closure of North West engineering:

During the last twelve months the Company had made substantial progress, market share is up, productivity and financial performance has improved, however despite this [the Company] is still a long way from being profitable. This is largely due to the recession in British industry in general, which has led to [our] market falling by 44% over the last two years, and the fact that [the Company] still has excess capacity. For the past year the company has been operating two assembly facilities, when one would have been adequate to cope with the volumes of business available, and those now anticipated in the future. It is the overhead costs associated with these two facilities which is largely responsible for the continuing losses, management has carried out an urgent review of its assembly facilities, their associated resources and support activities. This review shows that the Company's financial position in respect of cash flow and profitability can best be improved by the closure of [North West engineering] and the centralization of all functions at [a Midlands town].

The closure was to be effective in March 1982. The rationalization did not save the company. Early in 1982 the whole subsidiary was disposed of by the vehicle manufacturer as part of a policy of divestment of ancillary activities. The purchaser was the major UK producer of a very similar, rival vehicle to that produced by Company D. The company had remained in major financial difficulties whilst a subsidiary of the motor-vehicle manufacturer, reputedly making a loss of over £13 m. in 1980. It was therefore surprising that a purchaser could be found. However, the objective of the purchaser appeared to be to strengthen an already powerful position in the UK market, to realize property assets, to capitalize upon losses, and to phase out production at a competing firm.

The fifth plant, E, was engaged in the same sector of the engineering industry as plant C, although in the manufacture of components rather than end products. Like Company C, Company E experienced major financial difficulties in the 1970s, and was involved in major company reorganization. However, there was substantial under-utilization of capacity, and in 1981 it was announced that the plant would be closed as a means of reducing the level of fixed costs borne by the company. Production was transferred to the remaining major plants within the group.

The five case-study plants were all attempting to reduce costs to meet major declines in product markets, although the rate of decline, and the availability of financial resources to ameliorate its impact, differed. In four case studies the 1970s had shown a long-term decline in product markets, partly due to import penetration (clothing, engineering). The impact of the long-term decline was reinforced by the increased pressure of competition experienced during the recession, and in the engineering case studies by long-term financial weakness. The same four companies were attempting to reduce overheads by reorganization, and the transfer of capital equipment. In the fifth case study the unit closure was caused by market collapse due to technological obsolescence and the inability to absorb the labour released in the manufacture of new products. All five companies were making major efforts to increase productivity by reducing labour costs and, in four cases, by substantial capital investment programmes in other sectors of the company or plant.

It is perhaps worth stressing that the redundancies were not necessarily concentrated in the least-efficient plants in the companies concerned. In Company B the collapse of the market for valves made the closure of the valve-production unit inevitable, without any suggestion that it had been inefficient. In the remaining four cases the units closed were not regarded as notably inefficient, although the favourable evaluations of the employees involved in the specific plants may be partially discounted. The clothing plant was reputed to be more efficient in producing garments than the headquarters plant, as suggested by the plant being asked to produce the preliminary samples for products due to be produced at the headquarters plant. Similarly, plant C was regarded as more efficient than the plant to which its production was to be transferred, a view confirmed by the very high level of production bonuses achieved at plant C. In Company D the case for closure rested on excess capacity in the industry and the advantages of centralization at the headquarters site, not on relative inefficiency. In Company E management praised the good record achieved by plant E.

3.2 Long-term labour-force changes

Although redundancies are specific events, the final redundancy is often the culmination of an extended period of decline. Compulsory redundancy may be the last stage in a process of declining employment requirements, pre-figured generally by declining product markets or more specifically by limited recruitment or, on a short-term basis, government financial assistance under Temporary Employment schemes. This section contains evidence on changes in the labour force in the case-study plants before the announcement of the redundancies which occasioned our study. The evidence is important in itself, indicating the consequences for a company of successive measures designed to reduce employment levels without compulsory redundancy, and because it helps to explain some of the characteristics of the redundant population relevant for subsequent experience in the labour market, most importantly age. Moreover, we were concerned to assess whether the overall trends affected men and women in the same way. Did long-run decline lead to a lower or higher level of female employment in the company? Such evidence would be directly relevant to understanding the treatment of women in redundancy. Unfortunately, the quality and amount of data available for the case-study plants differs very substantially. The most substantial data available are derived from case study B, where the company used relatively sophisticated manpower-planning techniques, and where financial and product-market constraints were less constricting than in the other four case-study plants. Although differences in the evidence available makes systematic comparison impossible, the following section discusses changes in the labour forces before the formal announcement of the redundancy.

The women we interviewed were older than the female labour force employed in the industries from which the case studies were drawn. Although the age distribution of our sample was not a precise reflection of the age distribution of the total female labour force in the plants studied in the cases where we know the age distribution of the whole labour force, the total labour force was also older than the industry distribution. Table 3.2.1 shows (i) the age distribution of our sample; (ii) the age distribution of the total female work-force; and (iii) the age distribution of the female labour force in the industry for case study A.

Table 3.2.1
Comparative age distribution (Company A)

Age	Sample (%)	Plant (%)	Industry* (%)
15–24	16	13	27
25–34	10	14	17
35–44	29	26	19
45–54	20	27	22
55–59	25.5	20	7
60 +	–	–	8

*Source: EEC Labour Force Survey 1975.

Hence 45.5 of our respondents, and 47 per cent of the workers in factory A were 45 or older, but only 37 per cent of female workers in the industry were. There was a similar bias towards older employees in case-study plant B, as Table 3.2.2 shows.

Table 3.2.2
Comparative age distribution (Company B)

Age	Sample (%)	Industry* (%)
15–24	0	20.5
25–34	15	18
35–44	41	23
45–54	37	26
55–9	7	7
60 +	–	5

*Source: EEC Labour Force Survey 1975.

Whereas 44 per cent of our respondents in factory B were aged 45 or older, only 38 per cent of female employees in the industry were 45 or older. There was a similar bias towards older workers in case study C, as Table 3.2.3 shows.

Table 3.2.3
Comparative age distribution (Company C)

Age	Sample (%)	Plant (%)	Industry* (%)
15–24	8	1	19
25–34	27	14	17
35–44	36	49	24
45–54	28	30	27
55–9	1.5	6	8
60 +	–	–	4

*Source: EEC Labour Force Survey 1975.

Although the age distribution of workers in plant C was biased towards older workers, the difference from the general age distribution was not as pronounced for 45 + as in plants A and B – 36 per cent at plant C, compared with 39 per cent for the industry overall. However, there was a very substantial concentration in the age group 35–44, and a very substantial underrepresentation of the 15- 34 age group. There was a similar bias towards older workers in case studies D and E, as Table 1.3.1.1 (p. 19) shows: since the interviews were conducted almost exclusively with clerical workers, and involved nearly the total relevant population, tables similar to 3.1.2.1–3 have not been constructed. (Industry-specific data on the age distribution of female clerical employees are not easily available, making adequate comparison impossible.)

The ageing labour force in the case-study plants was not accidental. All five plants had been reducing their labour forces though natural wastage and restrictions on recruitment for several years. For example, in plant A there had been very little recruitment for several years, and a training scheme for school leavers had been suspended. Similarly, the three engineering companies (C, D, and E) had all ceased to recruit substantially before the redundancies, although precise quantitative data are not available. Plant C had been reduced from a peak of 5000 to approximately 1500 over a five-year period, plant D from 800 in 1977 to 350 in 1982, and plant E from 2831 to 1219 between July 1980 and April 1982. But the process of long-term run-down was most clearly visible in plant B.

The size of the labour force in plant B (including the feeder factories) fluctuated sharply over the post-war period, in response to changing product markets. In 1979 the level of employment was almost the same as it had been in 1945 — 2693 compared with 2652. However, the labour force had exceeded 6000 in ten years (1956, 1959–62, 1964–5, 1970–1). In the 1970s, the trend was downwards, as Table 3.2.4 shows.

Table 3.2.4
Total labour force trends (Company B 1970–1979)

	Total	Percentage of change
1970	6236	
1971	6041	− 3
1972	4347	− 28
1973	4223	− 3
1974	4392	+ 4
1975	4204	− 4
1976	3238	− 23
1977	2618	− 19
1978	2751	+ 5
1979	2693	− 2

Source: Company records.

Hence in 1979 the labour force was only 43 per cent of what it had been in 1970. In previous decades fluctuations in labour demand had been met by natural wastage and varying recruitment, a viable policy when the overall trend was not consistently downwards, and labour turnover was high. However, in the 1970s the policy became increasingly difficult to operate, with a substantial decline in labour demand accompanied by reduced turnover.

The reduction in labour turnover is shown starkly in a detailed analysis of trends over the period 1979–81. Table 3.2.5 shows the number of leavers through natural wastage and redundancy, as well as the numbers of employees engaged at the main site in 1979–81. In the two-and-a-half-year period there was a 26-per-cent reduction in male and female employees. The number of new employees engaged (which included a small proportion of transfers or pro-

Table 3.2.5

Leavers at Company B main site, as percentage of male and female labour force, 1979–1981

Period	Male leavers as percentage of all male employees			Female leavers as percentage of all female employees		
	Natural* wastage (%)	Redundant (%)	Total (%)	Natural* wastage (%)	Redundant (%)	Total (%)
11 Mar.–9 June 1979	3	0.3	3	4	0.5	4
10 June–8 Sept. 1979	3.5	0.4	4	2	1	3.5
9 Sept.–8 Dec. 1979	2	1	4	3	1	4
9 Dec.–15 Mar. 1980	2	2	4	2	1	3
16 Mar.–14 June 1980	2	2	4	2	2	4
15 June–13 Sept. 1980	2	3	4	3	3	6
14 Sept.–13 Dec. 1980	1	3	4	1.5	1	3
14 Dec.–14 Mar. 1981	1	4	5	2	4.5	7
15 Mar.–13 June 1981	1	5	5	1	3.5	4.5
13 June–12 Sept. 1981	2	7	7	1	4	5
Averages	2	2	4	2	2	4

*This includes leavers through death, retirement, dismissals, and own accord.
Source: Company records.

motions within the company) tended to fall inversely with an increase in the number of leavers, reflecting the company's policy of redeploying personnel where possible. As would be expected in a deteriorating economic situation, the number of men and women leaving through natural wastage declined sharply, whilst the number of enforced redundancies rose.

The result of the long-term decline and reduced natural wastage was an ageing labour force. Unfortunately the company data available on the age structure were not divided by sex, and the ageing process is disguised by expanding recruitment in particular sectors (notably scientists and technologists). However, Table 3.2.6 shows the age distribution of the whole labour force in 1976 and 1979. The contrast between 1976 and 1979 is less striking than expected because the firm's policy on voluntary redundancy was directed towards retaining younger workers, both because of their better eyesight, required for increasingly fine work, and because of their greater flexibility. Moreover, younger women were more willing to work shifts, partly because of greater financial need, than older workers. Accordingly, the firm transferred younger workers out of declining sectors where possible, leaving older workers in the declining sector. Hence the labour force was ageing overall, but the ageing process was concentrated in declining sectors (notably in the valve unit).

The changes in the size of the labour force in company B affected the gender composition directly: the proportion of women employed was substantially lower in 1979 than it had been a decade earlier. Moreover, the level of female

Table 3.2.6
Age distribution of total labour force (Company B)

Age category	Total 1976 (%)	1979 (%)
15–20	5.35	5.38
21–25	10.50	8.71
26–30	11.50	9.46
31–35	13.20	13.01
36–40	11.80	11.97
41–45	12.05	12.68
46–50	10.90	10.43
51–55	14.24	13.56
56–60	7.92	11.33
61–65	2.54	3.37
N	2902	2674

Source: Company records.

employment had fluctuated more sharply than the level of male employment during the decade. Table 3.2.7 shows the number of female employees, and the percentage change from the previous year, compared with that of male employees.

Table 3.2.7
Female employment changes 1970–1979 (Company B)

	Female employees	Percentage of change on previous year	Male percentage change on previous year	Total number of employees
1970	3476			6236
1971	3307	− 5	− 1	6041
1972	2142	− 29	− 19	4347
1973	2107	− 1.5	− 4	4223
1974	2190	+ 4	+ 4	4392
1975	2044	− 5	− 2	4204
1976	1412	− 31	− 15	3238
1977	944	− 33	− 8	2618
1978	1111	+ 18	− 2	2751
1979	1070	− 4	− 1	2693

Hence in 1979 the labour force was only 43 per cent of what it had been in 1970, the bulk of the job losses being amongst the female labour force: women were reduced to 30 per cent of their 1970 strength. Similarly, the year-on-year fluctuations in employment levels for women were greater than for men in seven out of the nine years (and one of the remaining two years, 1974, was a year in which the increase in employment for women was less than the increase for men).

The reduction in the female labour force was associated with an increase in the average age of female as well as male employees. Although company data are not available on the age and gender composition of specific occupations, the majority of female employees were employed as operators (EITB category 7) and the large majority of operators were female. Table 3.2.8 shows the age distribution of operators in 1976 and 1979.

Table 3.2.8
Age distribution of operators (Company B)

	1976 (%)	1979 (%)
15–20	4.04	4.95
21–5	12.24	9.69
26–30	13.23	12.03
31–5	13.66	14.98
36–40	13.66	13.06
45–5	12.42	13.33
46–50	9.00	8.79
51–5	11.74	10.72
56–60	6.96	8.87
61–5	3.04	3.64

The proportion of operators aged 30 or under declined from 29.51 per cent in 1976 to 26.67 in 1979, the proportion aged over 50 increasing from 21.74 per cent to 23.23 per cent over the same period. The changes in the proportions are not large, for the reasons stated above, and the age structure of operators changed less than the age structure of the labour force as a whole. Nevertheless, it is clear that the average age of the operators as a whole was increasing as a result of the decline in company B's employment level.

All five case-study companies were experiencing a long-term decline in their requirements for labour, although the timing, rates, and specific courses of the decline differed. The impact of this decline on female employment in the companies examined differed in predictable ways, depending upon the occupations considered. Where female workers were engaged directly upon production tasks they were disproportionately likely to suffer job losses (compared with men); where they were engaged in service roles they were less likely to experience job losses than men. The immediacy of the impact of product-market decline upon employment levels is obviously influenced by the technology of the production process, but in all three case studies involving manual employees the production process was not such as to require a high minimum-staff level to ensure continuing production: in other words, jobs could be lost as output declined. In the clothing case study the number of part-time employees, and their hours of work, could be varied according to product-market changes; seasonal variations had been customary before the economic difficulties of the late 1970s. In the electronics industry, as shown above, employment levels had varied sharply in response to variations in the demand for valves. In the engineering case study declining demand and rising productivity had reduced the level of both male and female employment without discrimination. In the two case studies involving clerical workers there is some evidence to suggest that job losses are likely to be slower to occur amongst women than amongst men, the difference being due to their role in the division of labour, not to their gender. As Table 3.2.9 shows, in case study E the decline in female employment was proportionately greater only amongst the very small group of direct manual employees: amongst manual indirects and, more significantly for the present argument, amongst staff the decline was proportionately greater among men than amongst women.

Table 3.2.9
Comparison of male and female employment levels (Company E 1980–1982)

	Employee strength (1 July 1980)		Employee strength (23 Apr. 1982)		Percentage decline	
	M	F	M	F	M	F
Staff	368	97	170	63	54	20
Manual indirect	873	58	354	27	59	53
Manual direct	1244	9	565	0	55	100

In short, the effect of long-term decline upon female employment opportunities is obviously dependent upon the location of women in the division of labour. This is especially so because of the high level of job segregation between male and female employees. In the case-study plants the balance between male and female employees is known to have changed in two cases: in case study B the proportion of women employed dropped, and in case study E the proportion of women employed increased, although the time periods covered are not identical. In both cases the changes are easily explicable in terms of the companies' operating requirements, independent of gender. The extent to which the experiences of employees in Companies B and E are typical of female employees generally will of course depend upon the occupational distribution of female employees, and the economic fortunes of the firms in which they are employed.

All five case-study companies were engaged in a long-term process of reducing their labour force. This process had passed through three stages (although not all companies had had voluntary redundancy schemes): natural wastage, restrictions on recruitment, and the filling of vacancies by transfer where possible; voluntary redundancy; and compulsory redundancy. The inevitable result of the way in which the first two stages are normally carried out is that the labour force at the time compulsory redundancies are likely to occur is likely to be a mature one, as in all five case studies. Since re-employment difficulties are likely to be greater for older workers, the result is to exacerbate employment difficulties for groups who are, for other reasons, likely to face greatest difficulty. This is as true for women as it is for men.

3.3 Management decision-making on redundancy

Strategic decisions about redundancy were taken at company or group level in all five case studies: the role of plant-level management was relatively limited. The major strategic decisions concerned which production units to close, where to transfer production and equipment, and, in Company B, which new products to introduce onto the main site. In four of the five cases decisions on the redundancy agreement were also taken at company or group level, the individual plants applying a standard agreement; only in Company A were changes made to the redundancy agreement as a result of negotiations concerning the specific plant. This centralization had important implications for industrial relations, as discussed below (p. 126). In this respect the case-study companies are similar to other companies with whom we discussed redundancies in the course of the project, and to British companies more generally. This centralization is hardly surprising. Ultimate financial responsibility is located at company or group level; managements are concerned to avoid leap-frogging claims; and plant-level management are as likely as plant-level workers to wish to maintain production at their own plants. Moreover, in the case-study companies production could be transferred between sites because of over-capacity in substitutable production facilities.

In the garment case study the decision to close factory A was taken at company level, plant-level management not being involved. The redundancy policy was also determined at company level, although the policy was modified in the course of plant-level negotiations, carried out mainly by the company personnel officer based at headquarters — there was no permanent plant-level representative of the central personnel department. In normal circumstances the links between plant A and other plants in the company were minimal — liaison was maintained by a weekly visit from the headquarters-based Assistant Production Director. Plant A management had traditionally followed a loose, paternalistic policy, involving a generally 'personal' approach to labour management: this involved, for example, a notable flexibility over hours, the fifty-one women interviewed working seventeen different work weeks, designed to accommodate varying family responsibilities. This indulgency pattern, based upon long tradition, was possible in a small firm, concentrating on quality goods, in a medium-sized market town, and desirable as a means of retaining the loyalty of a pool of experienced sewing-machinists.

In the electronics case study local manpower requirements were determined ultimately by the multinational's international strategy. As stated above, the electronics multinational concentrated production of specific components in a small number of production units, whose location was decided on grounds of international competitiveness. Hence the decision to concentrate the production of transistors, which was initially carried out in North West electronics and other sites, in a single UK production unit elsewhere. Such decisions were made at multinational headquarters. The trade unions involved at North West electronics sent a delegation to multinational headquarters, urging an increase in the rate of transfer of new products to North West electronics, to replace the diminishing valve programme. However, the delegation was unsuccessful, in that the new products located at North West electronics could not absorb all the labour released by the run-down of the valve programme. Given the international strategy, there was little influence plant-level trade unions could bring to bear.

In the three remaining cases decisions on product strategy ultimately determined manpower requirements. Such decisions were made at group level in Companies C and E, and at company level in Company D. All three redundancies were governed by the same 'model' agreement, although by the time of its closure plant D had ceased to be a part of the group. The precise manpower levels required could be determined only on the basis of an assessment of future product market demand. In order to minimize the costs of a very extensive redundancy programme the group negotiated a standard agreement, to operate at all companies: no deviation from the agreement was permitted. The group agreement was negotiated by central industrial-relations officials with national officials. Once the 'model' agreement had been accepted at one plant it was difficult for its terms to be changed on subsequent occasions. The terms of the agreement were accepted at one of the company's plants in 1979: the redundancies at Companies C, D, and E were the later stages of a process which had begun over a year earlier, the terms of which were already set.

3.4 Management—union relations

3.4.1 Industrial relations before the redundancy

All five case-study plants were heavily unionized, and almost all respondents were union members. As Table 3.4.1.1 shows, the level of union membership was high, even in the clothing factory and even amongst clerical workers. The major reasons for non-membership were: no appropriate union (2), management position (2), secretary to management (2), temporary employment (1), and in one case, in plant B, disapproval of trade unions. Since all plants were covered by closed-shop agreements, there is no reason to suppose that our respondents were different from female workers in the factories as a whole. The unions involved were the Tailors and Garment Workers Union, the General and Municipal Workers Union, and Transport and General Workers Union, Association of Scientific, Technical, and Managerial Staffs, Association of Professional and Executive Staff, and the Amalgamated Union of Engineering Workers.

Table 3.4.1.1
Union membership (by plant)

	A (%)	B (%)	C (%)	D (%)	E (%)	Total (%)
Ordinary member	92	91	91	81	96	91
Steward/Committee member	8	4	8	7	4	6
Senior steward			1.5			0.4
Non-member		3	1.5	12		2.5
N	51	68	66	43	51	279

The extent to which almost 100-per-cent membership was associated with active trade unionism in the five plants varied. The most elaborately developed system of plant-level trade unionism was in plant C, reflecting the size of the plant and the traditions of the industry in which it operated. At the peak of plant C's operations there had been approximately 100 stewards for 5000 employees; at the time of the redundancy approximately forty stewards for 1500 workers. The T&GWU had previously had a Works Committee of six, but at the time of the redundancy this had been reduced to four (of whom only three were on the main site), employed more or less full time on union business. It was alleged that the union had effectively controlled operations at the height of the plant's operations, but had ceased to do so before the redundancy. Despite nearly 100-per-cent membership there was little plant-level activity amongst ordinary members at plants A and B, and the role of the stewards was relatively limited. But the reasons for the inactivity differed. As indicated earlier, in plant A management had traditionally followed a paternalistic policy, and, although there had been one dispute, there was little tradition of union militancy: management policy and employees' expectations seemed complementary. At plant B there was an elaborate structure of joint consultation within the company, at company, divisional, and plant level, which operated effectively. For collective bargaining purposes industrial-relations issues were handled at company level; following G&MWU tradition the role of plant level officers in negotiations was limited, although important in implementation.

The degree of involvement in plant-level activity reported by our respondents reflected the overall level of activity in the plants: where there were meetings to attend the women interviewed attended them, as Table 3.4.1.2 shows. The data give only an approximate guide to involvement, since the answers are not wholly mutually exclusive: in plant B the number classified as never attending meetings had no meetings to attend; and in plant A some of the 'regular attenders' were recalling regular, but infrequent, meetings held in the past. In plant A there were very few meetings, and the occasional meeting called was largely restricted to office holders or was not generally publicized, in plant B only a minority of work groups held meetings. In plants C, D, and E (the engineering plants) meetings were called and substantially attended. In this

Table 3.4.1.2
Attendance at plant-level meetings

	Company					
	A (%)	B (%)	C (%)	D (%)	E (%)	Total (%)
Regularly	18	15	68	86	76.5	50
Occasionally	4	18	21	5	8	12
Never		32	11		14	13
No meetings to attend	78	34				2
Not a union member		1.5		9		2
N	51	68	66	43	51	

respect there is no reason to believe that our respondents were different from other workers in the plants concerned, male or female.

The women interviewed took very little part in union activity outside the plant, only eight respondents attending branch meetings regularly (primarily stewards).

Table 3.4.1.3
Attendance at union meetings outside plant

	A (%)	B (%)	C (%)	D (%)	E (%)	Total (%)
Regularly	2	3	1.5	7	2	3
Frequently			1.5			0.4
Occasionally	4	10	6	7	8	7
Never	12	71	91	77	90	69
Dont know of any meetings	82	15				19
Not a union member		1.5		9		2
N	51	68	66	43	51	279

The infrequent attendance at branch meetings is hardly surprising, since branch-meeting attendance, especially in the unions to which the respondents belonged, is generally low. We asked respondents whether branch meetings were held at times and places convenient for respondents: 19 per cent stated that branch meetings were held at inconvenient times and places, the highest proportion in any plant being 30 per cent in plant D, North West engineering. The reason for non-attendance was lack of interest, rather than specific difficulties caused by the inconvenient times and locations of meetings.

Although the women interviewed show the same pattern of plant-level involvement and branch apathy as would have been expected of men in a similar situation, there was some evidence that they believed that unions did not look after the interests of women as effectively as they looked after the interests of men, as Table 3.4.1.4 shows.

Table 3.4.1.4
Responses to *In general, do you think the union has been as effective for women as for men?*

	A (%)	B (%)	C (%)	D (%)	E (%)	Total (%)
Yes	63	51.5	74	56	51	59.5
No	35	31	17	30	39	30
Don't know	2	15	9	5	9	9
Not TU		3		9		2
N	51	68	66	43	51	279

($P = 0.046$)

The greatest degree of satisfaction was thus found in company C, where the union involved was the T&GWU. This is not surprising, partly because of the public commitment of plant-level union leadership to sexual equality, and partly because the high level of job integration between male and female employees made any alternative policy difficult to adopt, and impossible to justify. Women were a minority in an effectively integrated plant. Perhaps surprisingly there was more discontent in the plants where women were a higher proportion of the relevant bargaining unit, in plants A and E, i.e. amongst garment workers and female clerical workers. In both plants the explanation probably lies in the direct experience of work and the redundancy.

Table 3.4.1.5 indicates the reasons given for believing that unions were not as effective for women as for men. Although the numbers are small, and therefore the percentage figures should be treated with caution, the reasons given are of interest. The most frequently mentioned reason was simply that male trade-union leaders were not interested in female workers. In company A this view was strongly influenced by the women's experience over the negotiation of the redundancy agreement, in which national union officials took no part and the regional organizer was felt to have been inadequate. This was reinforced by the view that men would have been more willing to resist the redundancy, and in doing so made the union more effective. In plant E there was a similar view that the union had not succeeded in its attempts to improve upon the standard group redundancy terms, and that higher union officials had not provided any help. But workers in plant E were also more likely to give more generally 'feminist' reasons for their views, notably that men received preferential treatment because they were regarded as the main breadwinners, and that women were discriminated against at work: 21.5 per cent of all respondents at plant E providing such explanations. This may be due to the fact that the group included a number of relatively career-oriented women, in secretarial roles where their duties merged into those of administrative and managerial staff, without receiving appropriate recognition in the grading scheme.

Table 3.4.1.5
Reasons for unions being less effective for women than for men

	A (%)	B (%)	C (%)	D (%)	E (%)	Total (%)
Women second-class citizens	4	9	1.5			3
Women discriminated against at work	6	6	3	5	14	6.5
Women discriminated against on redundancy	2	3		12		3
Men more ready to fight	8	3	3			3
Male TU leaders not interested in women workers	16	7	6	7	18	10
'Why aren't you doing old man's cooking?'			1.5			0.4
Men preferential treatment – main breadwinners					8	1
Women less interest in TUs		1.5	1.5			1
Other		1.5	1.5	5		1
No less effective	65	69	82	72	61	70
N	51	68	66	43	51	279

($P = 0.001$)

There is little evidence available on women's perceptions of management–union relations. We were interested in the extent to which women workers had 'co-operative' or 'antagonistic' views of management–union relations. However, we did not feel that the metaphorical questions standard in 'image of the firm' questionnaires would be helpful – and not merely because football-team analogies are peculiarly inappropriate for female respondents. (An alternative 'family' metaphor might have been possible, but carried too many evocative emotional overtones.) Instead, we simply asked 'What do you think should be the unions' relationship with management?' A majority gave broadly 'co-operative' answers, although a minority stressed that unions should put workers' interests first, as Table 3.4.1.6 shows.

The issue raised is unfamiliar, both in generality and in asking about what union–management relations *ought* to be. It is also impossible to know without further investigation how far responses are based on a general ideology of appropriate worker–management relations, and how far on beliefs about the appropriate relations derived from immediate work experience – difficulties customarily encountered in research in this area. Finally, the classifications used in the table represent a very crude simplification of a wide range of responses. Nevertheless it is noteworthy that a substantial number of respondents felt that relations between unions and management ought to be close. However, it is also noteworthy that a very substantial minority of workers in two plants stressed the need for unions to maintain their commitment to the priority of workers' interests. These two plants were those in which there was least satisfaction with the efforts made by union representatives in attempting to prevent

Table 3.4.1.6
Responses to *What do you think should be unions' relations with management?*

	A (%)	B (%)	C (%)	D (%)	E (%)	All (%)
Good terms, friendly	22	19	15		18	15
Close/work in together	18	21	9	40	18	20
Closer than they are	4	1	17	19	8	9
Keep on right side of management to protect workers' interests	4	1	1.5	2	–	2
Open, free discussion, negotiation, each side should try to see each other's point of view everything above board	5	18	24	5	16	15
Union should not be too strong, management should be in charge	0	3	0	5	2	2
Unions should put workers first, not trust management, be aware of conflict of interest not too close to management, not be too ready to agree to management	35	13	6	19	30	19
Don't know/Not interested	10	21	17	0	9	12
No response/Not codable	0	3	8	11	–	4
Other			3			1
N	51	68	66	43	51	279

the redundancies, in one of which there was criticism that union representatives had been too willing to accept management views (plant A). Conceptions of the appropriate character of management–union relations were thus linked to views of the handling of the redundancy process, although it is impossible to indicate the direction of any causal link, if any such causal link exists: the most plausible hypothesis is that general conceptions at the time we were interviewing were influenced by the handling of the redundancy process, rather than the reverse.

None of the five plants had extensive histories of industrial conflict. There had been only one very brief dispute in plant A during its history, in 1977 over a claim for comparability with another plant. The dispute arose over the failure of cutters and pressers to receive a 2-per-cent increase granted elsewhere in the group. The cutters and pressers were out for three days, and won their claim. Cutters and pressers were male: the women machinists did not support the strike initially, but came out after one of the strikers on the picket line had been injured. Although the dispute disturbed the traditional pattern of paternalism at the plant it did not lead to a rise in conflict; according to the stewards, relations with management were good, both on a personal and on a bargaining basis. There was a similar lack of conflict in Company B. The unit due to be closed had never been involved in a dispute, nor had the plant as a whole (except for national disputes involving particular groups in the plants). Industrial relations had been more conflictual in plants C, D, and E, although none of the factories was regarded as especially militant. In plant C the convenor had been subject to disciplinary action for activities outside the plant, but there was no tradition of unofficial disputes, perhaps partly because of the innovative technology and relatively high earnings of the plant: when management became assertive about its prerogatives and earnings dropped, action was inhibited by the firm's obviously difficult product-market situation and by rising unemployment in the area. In plant D the staff unions had only been involved in industrial action once, over a comparability claim with staff at the Midlands plant to which North West engineering became linked in 1977; North West engineering won its parity claim, but did not receive support either from the Midlands staff unions, or from the North West manual unions. Plant E also had a record of good industrial relations, there being no plant-level conflict involving staff-level trade unions.

Only one of the five plants had had experience of compulsory redundancy before the case-study redundancies. However, as shown above, all five plants had been reducing their labour forces for several years, especially Company B. The major means of reducing the size of the labour force in plant A was natural wastage and restricted recruitment. Two companies (C and E) had had voluntary-redundancy schemes, which had not resulted in industrial conflict. The third company, D, had had previous compulsory redundancies, on one occasion the company being taken to an Industrial Tribunal on grounds of sexual discrimination.

3.4.2 Management–union relations during redundancy

Redundancies are situations in which the conflict of interest between employer and employee is acute, especially where the employee concerned is likely to have difficulty in finding alternative employment. This conflict of interest arises both over the principle of job loss, and over the terms of compensation for job loss. It can be mitigated by generous financial compensation or assistance in finding alternative employment, or ignored as unimportant where production units are ceasing operations totally and worker co-operation is irrelevant. For the unions involved there is the initial difficulty of deciding upon the attitude to the principle of job loss and, once a decision has been made, persuading the membership involved to accept it; there is an obvious possible tension between the interests of the union at large, which may involve co-operating with management over specific redundancies as a means of maintaining the overall viability of the firms, and the interests of the workers directly involved, whose interest in the long-term viability of the firm is limited if their jobs are to disappear anyway.

In Company A negotiations over the redundancy were carried out between the group personnel manager and the plant manager and the regional officer of the union and the two (male) stewards: no national-level union official was involved. For the union side, the negotiations were handled primarily by the regional union organizer, the stewards played relatively marginal roles.

The union organizer, the convenor and the superintendents shop steward initially discussed the terms of a redundancy agreement with management, unsurprisingly turning down management's first offer, which was the statutory redundancy payment with no *ex gratia* severance pay at all. An amended package was negotiated, and put to the shop committee by the three workers' representatives. The union organizer and the two stewards met the shop committee, which included two further shop stewards and six other members, three times. The proposed agreement was accepted at the third meeting which finished at 4.30 p.m. on Friday. The agreement was put to a shop floor meeting, but since most of the women were part time, they had gone home: only eight of the fifty-three women interviewed stated that they had attended a meeting, nearly all of the remainder not being aware that a meeting had taken place.

In Company B the redundancy policy was decided at group level, following negotiations between group industrial-relations officers and national union officials. Implementation was left to plant-level industrial-relations staff, within parameters set by group policy. Since the closure was a unit closure, with considerable effort made to find alternative work for those who wanted it, there was little conflict over the implementation of group policy, and data on the process of negotiations at group level were not available to the researchers. However, there is little evidence that the negotiation process substantially changed management policy: the firm was concerned to maintain an image of responsible employer, the electronics industry was financially secure enough to carry the costs of a relatively generous settlement, and the company wished to maintain good relations with its employees elsewhere in the group.

There was a substantial attempt in Company C to organize a campaign to reverse the closure decision. Extensive protest marches were organized, attended by nearly all the workers due to be declared redundant, and meetings were held with representatives of local government and MPs. Alternative uses for the site were explored, including preliminary discussion of the possibility of sale or lease of the site to foreign companies, including Japanese. However, resistance collapsed with a shopfloor vote to accept the company's closure terms. The reasons for the shop floor's acceptance of the closure terms are the subject of controversy. One factor was the extensive feeling that national-level union officials had failed to support the plant convenor, and regional officials, not bothering even to attend plant-level meetings. Secondly, workers were afraid of losing the substantial *ex gratia* and closure payments which the company had made conditional upon an orderly run-down. Such payments were especially significant since they represented a very substantial proportion of the redundancy pay to be received: since the plant was relatively new, few workers had acquired long service with the company. Pessimism about the outcome of any attempt at resistance was increased by the absence of effective opposition to redundancies elsewhere in the group, the serious contraction in the company's product market, and the reputation of top management for inflexible intransigence.

The remaining two companies were part of the same major industrial group as Company C, although their operations were not connected, and they were located in different regions. The agreement covering all three redundancies was the same. By the time of the case-study redundancies the company's policy towards the handling of redundancies was set, and pressure from plant-level unions for variations in the terms in Companies D and E was half-hearted and unsuccessful. In plants D and E factory-level meetings were held, attended by substantial majorities of our respondents: 86 per cent in plant D and 67 per cent in plant E. However, there was no further industrial action, and the standard group terms were accepted.

In the five plants the impact of collective action on the terms of the redundancy agreements was limited. All five cases indicate the difficulties faced by even well-organized factory-level unionism in reacting effectively to redundancies, as both management and unions recognized. Trade unions had little influence in even the best-organized plant (plant C): the role of stewards was reduced to asking management (often unsuccessfully) to deal considerately with hardship cases during the run-down, and to trying to ensure that individual workers did not do anything which would endanger their rights to the *ex gratia* closure payments. Part of this union weakness resulted from the general difficulties facing trade unions during recession. But there were four additional and more specific reasons for the difficulties.

The first source of difficulty was the level at which management decided redundancy policy. The late 1970s witnessed a major expansion in multi-plant company-level bargaining.[4] Redundancies and plant closures are examples *par excellence* of decisions made at company level: industry-level negotiations are obviously irrelevant (except in special circumstances) and plant-level management are normally as likely as plant-level trade unions to wish to keep their plants open. This is shown in the Department of Employment Survey of Workplace Bargaining: in the DE Workplace Industrial Relations Survey 42 per cent of managers of manual workers, and 50 per cent of managers of non-manual workers, reported that negotiations on redundancy took place outside the plant, a further 8 per cent of manual-worker managers and 10 per cent of non-manual-worker managers stating that there were no negotiations at all over redundancy. (This places redundancy after holidays, length of working week, and pensions, but before everything else in terms of the reported extent of extra-plant negotiations on specific issues).[5] The major negotiations on redundancy did not take place at plant level in any of our five cases: all were negotiated at company or at group level. The limited ability of unions to use traditional collective-bargaining pressures at the company level has been commented on previously; events in all five companies confirm this weakness.[6]

The second factor reducing the effectiveness of trade unions in redundancies is the unpredictability of events at plant level: both the unpredictability of the redundancy in the first place, and the timetable of developments. In three of the five cases the timetable for closures was seriously awry: in Company C, for example, during the period from October until May neither plant management nor workers could provide a realistic date for closure, nor for the date at which individuals would leave (although the uncertainty was less personally troublesome for plant management since it was possible for them to leave at a mutually convenient time without loss of redundancy pay, unlike manual workers). Amongst the five case studies, only the electronics company provided a formal warning from management before the formal public announcement, although in two others rumours were circulating amongst significant numbers of workers. The most noticeable aspect of the closure situations was the lateness of the notice received, and the evident surprise it created: 69 per cent of the garment workers, 84 per cent of the North West clerical and ancillary workers in engineering, and 48.5 per cent of Midlands engineering workers first heard of the impending redundancy at the formal announcement. In the fifth case study, of clerical and ancillary workers in the Midlands engineering company, 43 per cent first heard of the impending redundancy in the Saturday evening paper.

Thirdly, management tactics made a substantial contribution to defusing opposition. In the clothing factory the intentional invisibility of the major decision-makers made it difficult for opposition to focus without the support of local management. In the electronics plant the long period of warning, the obvious concern with redeployment, and the operation of the redeployment system itself (reinforced by the obvious technological obsolescence of the product) made collective action neither likely nor sensible. In the remaining three firms, where collective opposition was most likely, management constructed the closure package to maximize the *ex gratia* element, and to reduce the amount paid on the basis of age or length of service. By making the *ex gratia* payments dependent upon an overall orderly run-down management effectively mobilized work-group pressure to conform. In the most highly organized plant an extended reduction in the size of the labour force had already thinned out the stewards' organization. Both formal and informal work-group pressure thus helped to curb potential opposition.

Finally, there is the issue of inter-union co-operation. There was only limited co-operation between the different unions involved in the closures, especially across the manual—non-manual line. For example, in Company C, where there was an attempt to organize opposition, a number of respondents complained that the staff union had failed to support the more militant shop-floor workers. In the North West engineering firm the opposite was the case: all the unions had drawn up and presented to management an alternative plan to closure, but the white-collar-union representatives complained that the shop-floor unions did not give them sufficient support in pressing industrial action to support the plan.

3.5 Redundancy agreements

There were three redundancy agreements covering the five case-study plants.

In addition to the statutory payments, redundancy employees in Company A received enhancement for each year of service on the following scale:

0–4 years with no redundancy pay		1 week
0–4 years with redundancy pay		2 weeks
5–9 years		3 weeks
10–14 years		4 weeks
15–19 years		5 weeks
20–24 years	Plus 1 day per year	6 weeks
25–29 years	Plus 1 day per year	7 weeks
30–34 years	Plus 1 day per year	8 weeks
35–39 years	Plus 1 day per year	9 weeks
40–44 years	Plus 1 day per year	10 weeks

The enhancement amounted to just under one week's pay for every three years of service, with a very small addition for workers with twenty years' or more service. The company agreed to look sympathetically on the request of any employee for voluntary redundancy without sacrificing their statutory redundancy payment, but was not willing to pay any enhancement to voluntary leavers.

The redundancy agreements at the remaining plants were more complex. In plant B the redundancy agreement covered both voluntary and compulsory redundancy. Within limits set by production and commercial requirements, the following principles were normally followed in the selection for redundancy:

Volunteers will be considered but acceptance of their applications will not be automatic. Volunteers should first be invited from holders of jobs affected, but this may be extended to other employees where re-deployment, combined with reductions in total number required, can achieve the business objective.

If there is a surplus of volunteers, the selection should first take account of the Company's business needs; secondly the mutual advantage of selecting employees with documented absence problems (and the like): and, in the last resort, to the employee advantage of selecting long-service employees (first in, first out).

If there are insufficient volunteers and the redundancies are to be compulsory, selection should be based on the business' needs; consistent with this, personal considerations, e.g. absenteeism/sickness records and disciplinary records should be taken into account and, again in the last resort, short-service employees should be selected (last in, first out).

The size of the redundancy payment was based on a combination of age, length of service, and current weekly pay, according to a complex scale. Normal pay included shift premiums, unlike the agreement at Company C. The firm was sympathetic in practice to employees wishing to leave before their redundancy notices expired, but employees leaving voluntarily before their notice lost the firm's severance pay. The basic redundancy terms were standard for all UK subsidiaries of the multinational, and were set out in their booklet on Conditions of Employment circulated to employees in the group. The company's scheme enlarged on the statutory minimum redundancy payments for which the company could claim a state rebate. The main additions were:

i) Employees aged between 16—20 are eligible for severance pay, even if they have not completed a full year of service, whereas under the state scheme the youngest age at which an employee qualifies for a redundancy payment is 20 years, providing he or she has also completed 2 years' service after the age of 18.

ii) While the statutory provisions only start on completion of 2 years' service, the company gives 2 weeks' pay to employees aged 16—40 if they have less than one year's service and 3 weeks' pay for 1 completed year's service. The entitlement for employees aged 41 and above is 3 and 5 weeks' pay respectively.

iii) Employees receive additional graded payments for each year's service above the statutory limit of 20 years.

iv) Employees who are between 55—60 years of age receive an additional weeks' severance pay for each year of service over 31 years of service up to and including 40 years' service, providing they were at least 51 years old on 1 August 1975 and had at that time completed 15 years' service with the company.

v) Under the company's agreeement, half years are used for calculating the number of weeks' severance pay where the scale changes by two or more weeks per age or years of service category.

vi) Employees working less than 16 hours a weeks are also entitled to redundancy payments while they would be disqualified, with certain exceptions, under the state scheme.

The redundancy agreement in the three remaining cases was essentially the same. Since the closures were total, there was no provision for voluntary redundancy, although attempts were made to arrange internal transfers at Company C (especially from the feeder plant) and Company E. Redundancy payments were made up of statutory compensation, plus three types of *ex gratia* payment: for hourly paid, weekly/fortnightly staff, and junior supervision, one week's pay per year of service (not linked to age), with slightly more generous provisions for more senior monthly paid staff; plus payment in lieu of contractual notice; plus twelve weeks' payment on special closure terms, subject to successful completion of an orderly run-down. Plant closures qualified for special financial compensation provided there was full co-operation from all employees to achieve an orderly run-down. It was essential for there to be co-operation with the plans from all bargaining units in order for employees to qualify for plant-closure terms. The company's requirements in respect of co-operation depended upon the task. However, the following were examples of the degree of co-operation essential to the achievement of an orderly run-down and for employees to qualify for plant-closure payments:

Transfer of stock, plant, equipment, records, etc. as required.

Termination of employment in accordance with the closure plan.

Selection to be based on operational needs.

Co-operation on production working arrangements, including the planning and co-ordination of an orderly closure to ensure that the site was left in a secure state.

Acceptance of suitable alternative work as defined.

Full mobility within and between grade categories in accordance with the current operating agreements.

Co-operation with contractors during the run-down period where required to obviate the need for temporary recruitment, e.g. cleaning, maintenance, etc.

Acceptance of retraining on transfers and involvement in any training programmes.

Acceptance of work reallocation to take account of wastage — subject to normal consultation.

No industrial action or disruption.

Acceptance of unavoidable overtime.

The three redundancy agreements were devised to meet different circumstances: the first to minimize the costs of securing an orderly closure, in a highly competitive industry with tight financial constraints; the second to maintain a reputation for good employer practice, and to continue good relations with an existing labour force, in a relatively prosperous multinational; the third to sustain production with a substantially disaffected labour force in a very competitive situation. It is thus difficult to compare them, either with each other, or with other redundancy agreements. However, the principles governing the level of compensation were notably more generous in plant B than in the other four plants. This corresponds with the common-sense assumptions that extra statutory payments are most likely where the company is most able to afford them.[7] The extra-statutory payments made by Company B were in line with those reported as being most common.[8] Finally, it is noteworthy that all five case-study companies did make extra-statutory payments, although only about a third of private-sector firms are reported as doing so. In this context company A was more generous to its employees than it may appear — or than its employees thought.

The redundancy agreements did not, of course make any reference to women: nor is there any evidence that specific efforts were made to accommodate any special difficulties women might experience in redundancy. However, since the occupational experience of women is different from that of men in ways relevant to redundancy the effect of the agreements on women is likely to be different from the effect on men. Two issues are of special importance: the treatment of length of service, and the treatment of part-time work. None of the agreements provided for interrupted service, except for the period of pregnancy leave provided for under the 1978 Employment Protection (Consolidation) Act. Accordingly, length of service provided for did not equal the amount of total service with the company for 23 per cent of employees: this was particularly significant in Companies A and B, both of whom followed a specific policy of encouraging former employees to return after child-bearing, preferring experienced and known employees. Secondly, the agreements treated part-time work differently. Since nearly all female employees at company A were part-time workers, part-time workers were not distinguished from full-time workers. However, Company B and Company C differed in their treatment of part-time workers. Company B's company scheme specifically provided for part-time employees, whilst Company C's agreement followed the 1978 Act in excluding employees contracted to work fewer than sixteen hours per week (except for workers with five or more years' service and contracted to do eight or more hours' work, who were to receive their statutory compensation). Part-time employees working fewer than sixteen hours a week were excluded from redundancy comepnsation (although the effect in plants C, D, and E was limited in practice because there was relatively little part-time work).

3.6 Women workers' responses to redundancy

Responses to redundancy will obviously be conditioned by attitudes towards employment and work, discussed in the second chapter. However, they will also be conditioned by the specific circumstances of the redundancy, and its handling by both management and unions. This section is concerned with the relatively specific and directly linked responses to the redundancy. After examining commitment to the firm we discuss in turn explanations for redundancy, evaluations of management and union handling of the process, and the degree of 'activism' shown in responding.

Before the announcement of the redundancy very few of the women had applied for jobs with other firms, only 13 per cent. The women interviewed had relatively long service with the case-study firms, as was shown in Chapter 1. In all five plants this was more than passive resignation, based on the lack of available alternatives: all five companies were regarded as 'good firms to work for', although changes in working practices were undermining the enthusiasm of employees in Company C. The most notable illustration was in Company A, where employees echoed management's emphasis on the importance of loyalty to the firm, both in belief and action: it is therefore not surprising that employees in Company A were especially distressed by the redundancy, and especially distressed by management's handling of it. Since management had attempted to foster a personal, involved style it was difficult for employees to adjust to their obvious dispensability. Similar disappointed expectations, in a weaker form, were shown in the other case study plants.

There was little evidence of fatalism, feminine or otherwise, in the women's views on the inevitability of redundancy: the majority of women believed that the redundancies could have been avoided. Such views naturally varied from plant to plant, as Table 3.6.1 shows. In all plants except plant B the majority of women believed that the redundancies could have been avoided, the view being most widespread in Company C (where active opposition to the redundancy was greatest). Only in Company B did a majority believe that the redundancies could not have been avoided, the majority accurately perceiving that

Table 3.6.1
Responses to *Do you think the redundancies at X could have been avoided?*

	A (%)	B (%)	C (%)	D (%)	E (%)	Total (%)
Yes	53	28	82	56	55	54.5
No	23.5	53	9	17	22	26
Don't know	22	19	9	26	23.5	19
Missing	1					0.4
N	51	68	66	43	51	279

redundancies were inevitable with the collapse of the valve market. Alternative strategies were believed to be available in the remaining four companies.

The explanations given for the redundancies were varied, but fell into two major groupings: the overall performance of the economy, and management inefficiency.

Table 3.6.2
Respondents' perceptions of reasons for the redundancy

	A (%)	B (%)	C (%)	D (%)	E (%)	Total (%)
Recession/lack of demand	33	21	24	56	14	28
Product obsolete		72		2		18
Bad management	10	3	62	37	41	30.5
Union's/worker's fault	4	7	6	9	6	6.5
Government policy	23.5		4.5	5	6	7
Technological change/rationalization	16	4	21	19	39	19
Overseas competition/loss of markets	8	9	1.5	19	6	8
Other			3		2	1
N	51	68	66	43	51	279

Percentage is that of respondents mentioning category of reasons: up to three choices permitted per respondent.

The women were not asked to rank the explanations in terms of their perceptions of the order of importance, since the question would have been impossible to answer intelligently, and many of the reasons were interrelated: overseas competition, rationalization, bad management, government policy, and declining demand. However, it is clear (and unsurprising) that women in the garment industry emphasized market changes and government policy, in the electronics industry product obsolescence, and in the engineering industry recession, bad management, and rationalization. In Company C management themselves would not be surprised to learn that over half of their workers blamed bad management for redundancy at the plant.

The suggestions made for avoiding redundancies were too varied to compress into meaningful categories, and differed between plants. In Company A suggestions were concerned primarily with diversifying products, and retaining the plant in operation rather than centralizing on the headquarters plant, because of the reputation for quality of plant A. It was suggested that plant A could survive the 1981 down-turn as it had survived previous ones, by the adjustment of schedules, production for stock, and securing government financial assistance. In Company B suggestions included continuing production of valves, since there was still at least a residual market for them, and introducing new products more quickly. As would be expected from the explanations given for the redundancy, workers in Company C concentrated upon the need to improve managerial efficiency as a means of avoiding redundancy. Improving managerial efficiency and introducing new products were the most frequently mentioned way in which redundancies could have been avoided. In plant D it was generally recognized that there was over-capacity in the industry, and that either the Midlands or the North West plant would have had to close. However, it was thought that the Midlands plant should have been disposed of, since it was less attractive than the North West plant. It was also thought that closure might have been avoided if the firm had been less 'top heavy', and had introduced new products earlier. At Company E there was similar criticism of 'top heaviness' and managerial inefficiency — 'it's too top heavy, too many people bleeding the company dry.' In explaining how the redundancies could have been avoided no respondent mentioned work sharing: the major emphases were upon the need for new products, improved managerial performance, and, especially in Company A, temporary measures to cope with normal fluctuations in demand.

We also asked the women whom they held responsible for their redundancies. As might have been expected, the women pointed to government and management, at various levels, as being to blame for the redundancies. However, some women commented that a number of factors were acting in combination: much of the responsibility for redundancies lay in the way in which the system operated, and the allocation of blame was inappropriate. There was no tendency to single out the government, management, or workers alone, as being responsible for redundancies. In short, respondents recognized that there were several reasons for redundancies, some of which were subject to human control, but that no one could be 'blamed' for them.

The amount of warning about the possibility of redundancy differed in the five plants. However, only in Company B did a number of workers claim to have expected the redundancy. Table 3.6.3 shows how the workers first heard of the redundancies. In view of the long-term run-down of the valve division in Company B it is hardly surprising that over 70 per cent in Company B either expected redundancy, or heard about it through rumour. Moreover, management called a meeting before the formal announcement specifically to warn of the impending redundancy. In plants C and E the group's plans for the restructuring of the group were well known, although their precise implications for specific plants were not: it was therefore likely that rumours would be in extensive circu-

Table 3.6.3
Respondents first hearing of redundancy

	A (%)	B (%)	C (%)	D (%)	E (%)	Total (%)
Rumour	20	31	38		43	28
Informally from staff	4		3	9	4	4
Informally from steward		3	1.5			0.1
Formal warning from management		25	9	5		9
Formal announcement	69		48.5	84	6	38
From co-workers after redundancy	8			2	2	2
Expected it		41				10
Newspaper					43	8
Radio					2	0.4
N	51	68	66	43	51	

lation about the possibility of redundancy. However, it is noteworthy that 48.5 per cent in plant C claimed to have first heard of the redundancy at the formal announcement, and 43 per cent in plant E to have first read of it in the newspaper (following an inspired leak in the Saturday evening paper). Although plant D's future was known to be uncertain, a large majority first heard of the redundancy at the formal announcement. In plant A there were only vague, unbelieved, rumours circulating before the formal announcement. The opportunities for 'anticipatory socialization' — or looking for work before large numbers of co-workers were doing so — were thus limited.

Workers at Company A were the most shocked by the redundancy, having expected short-time working, but not closure. 'It was a shock but even now it doesn't seem really true. It seems like a dream. I had expected short-time working.' 'Very upset. No other way to explain it. It suddenly comes out of the blue. In tears, couldn't sit and talk about it. Very shocked.' Similar sentiments were expressed by the majority of respondents, the most concerned being heads of single-parent families or wives with unemployed husbands. In view of the limited value of variants upon 'shock/horror/disgust/indifference', quantitative analysis in inappropriate. Workers in Companies C, D, and E expressed similar feelings about being thought on the scrap-heap after conscientious work.

Sick, absolutely disgusted. I've always been a conscientious worker and I've really enjoyed working here. It helps to keep you happy, young and forget your daily worries. (Company C)

Very disappointed and disheartened. Had hoped it would stop short of closure — we hoped for a successful takeover. Upset. I'd been here since leaving school and hoped I'd had a job for life. (Company D)

Terribly upset, dreadful, I'm not one for changing jobs, I like this job and hoped I'd be here till I retired, would have stayed at the last place if they hadn't closed it down. I pray it will still never happen. (Company E)

On the other hand, some workers, especially at Company D, commented that they felt better than they would have done if they had been individually picked for redundancy:

Very sad. I've enjoyed working here. We have a nice office, nice people. We get on well together. There's been redundancies over the last three years. When the first one came people [were] very very bitter. They felt they had been 'picked on' — it's a different situation now. We're all going together.

Others had mixed feelings:

A bit of a mixture. Relieved, my family were grown up — couldn't have coped it they were small. Annoyed won't get another job easily and wasted, feeling that I've paid into a pension fund that I won't get benefit out of because of inflation. Looking forward to it now for the rest, but I'd have never have left if the firm hadn't forced me out. You get to the stage of life where you accept what you've got and plod on. I think it's a way of forcing women out of work after this equal rights thing — its worked. (Company C)

More positively (and uniquely):

I really felt as if I needed a break and as if they'd done it for me. I feel as if I'm going to do all the things you wanted to do and haven't been able to do before. Visiting friends. I'm going to learn to drive. But I'll still miss my friends at work — but I can always phone them up. I'm one of a big family. I shall go and visit them. (Company A)

At the electronics plant, Company B, there was more fatalistic resignation: 'I think I'll be glad of a change. There's nothing we can do about it (Company B); 'relieved — I want to stop work for a bit' (Company B).

As the previous paragraph indicates, there was a range of reactions to the redundancies. However, the predominant feeling was one of shock, sadness, and loss. Such sentiments were especially strong in the garment factory, but also predominated in the other plants. Only in plant B could the fatalistic resignation mentioned as characteristic of female reactions to redundancy be discerned — but this reaction could hardly be attributed to a specifically feminine orientation, in view of the evident obsolescence of the product and the long-term run-down of the plant and its feeder factories.

The majority of respondents stated that their reactions to the redundancy had not changed between its original announcement and the interview. However, a minority had become more resigned to redundancy, and a smaller minority had become less resigned, as Table 3.6.4 shows. In the plants that had the most experience of union militancy respondents had become more resigned to redundancy, especially in plant C, as the failure of plant-level unionism to halt the redundancy, or to improve redundancy terms, became apparent. In plant A there was growing feeling that employees had been slow in reacting to the redundancy, showing itself in a growing feeling that 'something should be done'.

In all five cases management announced the redundancy at plant level meetings; only in Company B was there a formal warning from management.

Table 3.6.4
Change in reactions to redundancy between initial announcement and interview

	A (%)	B (%)	C (%)	D (%)	E (%)	Total (%)
No change	53	73.5	48.5	72	63	62
More resigned	12	13	23	19	18	17
Less resigned	27.5	3	11	7	16	12
Other	8	10	14	2	4	8
Missing data			4.5			
N	51	68	66	43	51	279

Since leaving dates for individuals differed according to production requirements, notices of individual dismissals were sent individually. Management's handling of the redundancy in plant B differed from management's handling in the remaining four plants: the company had extensive experience of handling labour reductions; there was the possibility of internal transfer and therefore the closure was not as dramatic; there was more flexibility in permitting time off to look for alternative jobs; and the whole process was relatively gradual. As is shown below, employees were relatively satisfied with management's handling of the process. The process was far less orderly and less predictable in the remaining four companies, especially in Company C. In Company A management had always adopted a flexible approach towards its employees, for example over hours of work: this did not change in the period between the announcement of the closure in May 1981 and the plant's closure in October, employees being able to take time off from work to look for alternative employment, and to leave on a mutually convenient date if jobs were found. In so far as it was possible, within the constraints of maintaining output and transferring capital equipment during a plant closure, management maintained its traditional paternalism — involving stringent opposition to collective demands, but sympathy for individual problems. In Company D local management's handling of the redundancy was flexible, for example over time off to find alternative work, and the use of company facilities, including telephone and stationery, to apply for jobs. But there was extensive criticism of headquarters management for the closure decision itself, and of the local Job Centre for the initial failure to provide an on-site service for redundant employees. In case study E the over-capacity in manufacturing capability in the group of which Company E was a part had been obvious for years. However, the implications of the over-capacity for plant E were unclear at plant level, and the closure decision was unexpected when it came. Management handled the redundancy clumsily, in allowing many workers to read about the closure in the newspapers before providing information themselves. Moreover, there was a feeling that the redundancy terms did not compensate adequately for length of service, especially among skilled craftsmen. The most rigorous handling of the redundancy process was in plant C, where management kept firmly to statutory commitments and the closure terms: no time off other than that statutorily required was provided, and no flexibility was shown over leaving dates, either for cases of ill health (of which respondents cited many examples) or where redundant employees had found alternative jobs.

In view of the differences in management's handling of the redundancy process it is not surprising that there were significant differences in employees' evaluations. Only in plant B was extensive satisfaction reported, as Table 3.6.5 shows.

Table 3.6.5
Responses to *How do you feel about the way management handled the process of redundancy?*

	A (%)	B (%)	C (%)	D (%)	E (%)	Total (%)
Satisfied	24	63	15	23	18	30
Mixed feelings	6	7	1.5	12	8	6.5
Resigned	23.5	10	12	14	14	14
Aggrieved	47	10	56	35	51	39
Other			11	2		3
Don't know		9	4.5	14	10	7
N	51	68	66	43	51	279

In the remaining plants the balance between a sense of grievance and resignation differed, the former prevailing in all cases. It is perhaps not surprising that workers in Company A, primarily part-time garment workers, were more likely to be resigned to management's handling than either clerical workers were, or, notably, manual employees in a Midlands engineering plant. The extent of mixed feelings in plant D is notable, reflecting the contrasting evaluations of the actions of central and plant management, with plant management able to make only a limited impact upon outcomes. In view of the importance of employees' reactions to management's handling of redundancy the major sources of criticism made in plants A, C, and E are worth investigating further, although the wide variety of responses makes the data unsuitable for quantitative analysis.

In all three plants the most common criticisms were of inadequate notice and inadequate information; in plants C and E there were also complaints about the impersonal and inconsiderate way in which the redundancy was handled. For example, for plant A:

I think it was terrible the way they told us – it was really sprung on us – we thought when we got the [————] that they would guarantee our jobs.

Not very well. Come out of the blue – those here a long time won't come out of it well money-wise. Not told anything – and that whitewash rumours. Not know where you are.

Rather underhand. Didn't tell us anything — should have warned you in advance — so it wouldn't have been such a let down.

On the other hand, it was recognized in plant A that local management were probably not very well informed themselves, and that headquarters was making the major decisions, but leaving local management to carry them out, without much assistance from headquarters: 'Own managers/supervisors explained it — to me — quite fair. Not seen any higher up — top management should have come down from [headquarters] to explain what's happened. They've left things very unsettled and no one really knows why the firm is closing down.' (The tactic of limited headquarters involvement caused resentment, but worked effectively: both local and headquarters management were insulated, and the resentment could be ignored, since the plant was closing completely.) Criticisms of management were more extensive in Company C:

Very bad. I think they should have told us more. They knew before they told us, and they haven't given us a finishing date — they don't seem to know what they're doing.

It's not done fair. It seems silly to me to take jobs off people who are working well and to take it to a factory where they're not coping with it. We'd already taken cuts in the work force and still do the same amount of work — and then they still make you redundant. Not hear much about the actual redundancy — keep changing dates. You build yourself up to a pitch to think you're going and then the date is changed and you feel the strain. Also can't plan to get another job because you can't give a definite date. Can't now get a job and ask for voluntary redundancy because can't necessarily let you go.

Disgusting, you're just a number, they don't seem to have any feelings towards you. Was made redundant before and they were quite different — they said they were sorry to see us go and tried to help us.

The clerical workers in Company E also criticized the lack of information, and the initial leak of the story of the redundancy to the newspapers:

It could have been done a lot better, very bad policy that we read about it in the newspaper and some of the instances of dismissal have been grim considering the service involved, no human contact no-one to say good-bye and sorry.

Not very well, we are all treated as if we were a number, they don't want to know, the ones at the top give you the impression that they think that it's just our hard luck, the way they've treated some of the men who've worked here for thirty years it's shocking, you'd think after all these years of service there'd be some personal touch, some recognition of long service.

The provision of full information, rigorous attempts to keep to schedules, and personal contact and expression of regret between management and employee, do not change the outcome of the redundancy process. But they do affect their evaluations of the process, and of the firm carrying it out, as Tables 3.6.5 and 3.6.6 show. (In the case of Company C many respondents commented that their views of company management had changed before the redundancy: these were coded as 'no change'.) There was thus a sharp contrast between the evaluation of Company B and of the remaining companies; although relatively

Table 3.6.6
Responses to *Have your feelings about the firm changed as a result of the way the redundancy was handled?*

	A (%)	B (%)	C (%)	D (%)	E (%)	Total (%)
For the better			4.5	5	2	2
For the worse	47		39	19	37	28
No change	53	100	54.5	70	59	68.5
Other			1.5	5	2	1
Missing data				2		
N	51	68	66	43	51	279

few respondents had changed their evaluation of Company D's management, 47 per cent of workers in Company A, 39 per cent in Company C, and 37 per cent in Company E had changed their opinions of the company for the worse. It might be thought that such views were irrelevant, since employees were being dismissed. However, production continued during the run-down even in the plants due for total closure, and managements often wished to secure extra co-operation from employees because of the disruption caused by a changing labour force and the inability to schedule production accurately, often requiring extended deadlines. Moreover, multi-plant companies may wish to transfer the more productive, skilled, or younger employees from the closing plant to other plants. Finally, even redundant employees may have future work careers in which favourable evaluations from past employers might be helpful, either to future managements or even, in view of the unpredictability of future labour requirements, to management in the present firm. Such considerations are of course additional to those of personal consideration.

One issue we were concerned with in evaluating company handling of the redundancy process was the extent to which redundant employees made use of professional advice provided by the company about pensions, use of redundancy money, and other financial matters. Unfortunately the provision of such assistance was limited, and awareness of the limited services provided even more so. Financial advice was offered only in Company C, where the advice included help in calculating precise entitlement to redundancy payments, and the implications for pensions. However, little use was made of the service, partly because uncertainty about leaving dates and bonus levels made precise calculation impossible. In general, respondents appeared to prefer to rely upon advice outside the company for what was regarded as private business — although in different circumstances competent professional advice might have been used more extensively. Company A was most active in helping redundant employees to find alternative work, perhaps because it operated in a relatively small industry, in a relatively small town, with good contacts with the limited number of firms that had jobs to offer similar to those provided by Company A. Even in the company where advice was available the majority of respondents stated that advice or counselling was not offered, underlining the difference between general availability and help offered to the individual.

The role of the unions in the redundancies studied was limited, especially at plant level: there was little scope for plant-level collective bargaining, and union actions were primarily concerned with securing sympathetic implementation of the redundancy agreements. However, although there was little difference in the level of ineffectiveness shown by the unions in the five cases, there were very substantial differences in respondents' reactions to what the unions had done. Moreover, there is no evidence to support a feminine 'fatalistic' response to redundancy — although respondents had few specific ideas of what the unions should have done differently.

There was a difference, but not a major one, in the evaluations by the women interviewed of plant-level and extra-plant-union officials, the women evaluating their plant-level representatives more positively, although with major differences between factories (as would be expected). A majority of women thought that their plant-level representatives had done everything possible to prevent the redundancies occurring, and a majority in every plant except A thought that extra-plant officials had done everything possible. Dissatisfaction was greatest with both plant-level representatives and paid officials at Company A, as would be expected in view of the events described above, pp. 124–5. Since the major responsibility for negotiations with management rested with the paid official it was inevitable that dissatisfaction with his activity should be more extensive, although it is significant that almost half of the respondents thought that their factory representatives had not done everything possible. (The plant-level representatives in the negotiations with management were male, although the majority of workers were female.) In the remaining four companies only small minorities felt that factory representatives had failed to do everything possible: in Company B some respondents felt that insufficient pressure had been exerted to secure the introduction of new products, and in Company E many felt that their steward had been generally incompetent; the level of satisfaction in Companies C and D was notably high. The women were less confident in evaluating the actions of full-time officials, 22 per cent not knowing whether the full-time official had done everything possible or not: only in plant C was the proportion of 'don't knows' below 10 per cent (8 per cent) — as one might have expected in a major Midlands engineering plant. Overall, 26 per cent thought that full-time officials had not done everything possible, the highest proportion being found in plant A (59 per cent), the lowest proportion in plant D (2 per cent). The reasons for the findings in plant A have been outlined above. In plant D the obvious decline of the company's product market, and the strenuous efforts to keep the plant open made by the full-time official meant that little blame was attached to her for her failure to influence the redundancy process. Significantly, 30 per cent of respondents in Company C thought that their paid officials had not done everything, reflecting the well-publicized failure of national officials to support Company C stewards, although local paid officials had done so.

Many women were conscious of the inadequacy of the actions taken by their representatives. But, not surprisingly, they had difficulty in making specific suggestions for additional action. When the women were asked what their factory representatives or full-time officials should have done, too few specific suggestions were made to permit quantitative analysis. Some women, especially in plant A, suggested that the unions should have tried harder to keep the plant open through negotiations (eight women, five in plant A); others suggested that alternative products ought to have been suggested (three women, all in plant B); others that the workers concerned ought to have been involved in discussions more. There was little spontaneous mention of strikes, sit-ins, or other forms of industrial action: six women suggested that a strike should have been organized. The most frequent comment was simply that the unions should have been more militant, made by 8 per cent of respondents.

Only a small minority of the women interviewed spontaneously suggested that the unions should have been more militant. However, a very substantial majority stated that they would have been prepared to take part in industrial action to halt the redundancy if their union had asked them to do so: those least willing to do so were clerical workers in plants D and E.

Table 3.6.7

Responses to *If the union had asked you to take part in industrial action to halt the redundancy would you have agreed to do so?*

	A (%)	B (%)	C (%)	D (%)	E (%)	Total (%)
Yes	88	78	80	30	65	71
No	12	18	15	42	29	22
If majority vote only		1.5	3	12	6	4
In some circumstances				2		0.4
No answer/non-TU		3	1.5	14		3
N	51	68	66	43	51	279

In plant D a number of women were unwilling to take part in industrial action because they did not think it would do any good: when asked if they would have been willing to take part in a strike or sit-in if they thought it would be any use, the proportion willing to do so increased from 30 to 46.5 per cent.

Where unions organized meetings and protests about the redundancy the women interviewed nearly all took part, as Table 3.6.8 shows. As we have seen, in Company A the redundancy agreement was not put to the vote, and in Company B the very gradual phasing out of the valve production unit meant that there was no call for a special meeting. In the other plants only four women,

Table 3.6.8

Responses to *Did you attend any meeting open to you to discuss or vote on matters concerning the redundancy?*

	A (%)	B (%)	C (%)	D (%)	E (%)	Total (%)
Yes	16	19	92	86	67	55
No	4	3	6	5	23.5	8
No meeting/did not know of meeting	80	76.5	1.5		9	35.5
Not answered		1.5		10		2
N	51	68	66	43	51	279

all in plant C, did not attend a meeting 'voluntarily', either because they did not think it would achieve anything (1), did not think they could contribute (1), or that it was not relevant to their situations (2) – all other non-attenders were either absent from work (5), could not leave their work posts (3), or did not know about the meeting (5). In short, involvement in the decision to accept or reject the redundancy was as complete as practically possible.

Only in plant C was there any active opposition to the redundancy, involving protest marches, lobbying of local councillors and MP's, and a brief one-day stoppage. A very substantial majority of women interviewed took part in the protest march (76 per cent), and a very small proportion reported that they had taken part in industrial action (9 per cent). Since no action apart from holding meetings occurred in the other plants, there was no involvement in any action: whether the unions would have organized any additional action if the workers involved had not been predominantly female, and whether the women would have taken part in such action if it had been organized, it is of course impossible to say. However, there is no evidence to suggest that the women involved would not have done so, except in plant D, and some evidence to suggest that they would have done so.

In view of these factors it might have been expected that workers in plant A would have been least satisfied with the redundancy terms negotiated, and workers in plant B the most satisfied. Expectations were confirmed about the least satisfied, but the most satisfied were workers in plant D, as Table 3.6.9 shows. Workers in plant A were right to be dissatisfied in comparison with well-publicized redundancy agreements in the public sector, although their impressions of the level of benefits provided by medium-sized firms in the private sector was mistaken. They were particularly dissatisfied with the provision made for long-service employees. It is also hardly surprising, in view of their general hostility to the handling of the redundancy by management and by union officials, that a very substantial minority of workers in Company C thought that the unions had not obtained the best terms possible. But the

Table 3.6.9
Responses to *Did the unions secure the best terms possible for employees in general?*

	A (%)	B (%)	C (%)	D (%)	E (%)	Total (%)
Yes	35	46	53	74	59	52
No	53	34	38	9	12	30.5
Don't know	10	19	8	7	29	15
Not answered	2	1.5	1.5	9		2.5
N	51	68	66	43	51	279

number of women in plant B feeling that the unions did not secure the best terms possible is higher than might have been expected, in view of the generosity of the redundancy agreement compared with those obtained elsewhere. Those who were dissatisfied simply felt that the unions should have obtained more money — there was no feeling that specific groups had been neglected. The explanation lies in the failure of paid union officials to publicize their role in obtaining such favourable terms (or at least, claiming such a role if they did not in fact play one): significantly, 25 per cent of respondents at plant B did not know whether their paid officials had done everything possible to prevent the redundancy or not, and few are likely to have had any knowledge of the role of the union in negotiating the agreement at company level. In such circumstances the GMWU's policy of concentrating responsibility outside the plant, and playing a limited role where employers were willing to follow progressive personnel policies, was an ineffective way of acquiring credit with rank-and-file members — the limitation of doing good by stealth.

In this section we have hitherto been concerned primarily with women's subjective reactions to redundancy and to management and union handling of the process. We have also shown the women's degree of involvement in collective responses. However, redundancies are unpropitious occasions for collective action: collective action can make little impact on the fact of the redundancy, and only limited impact on the process, especially in situations of total closure. In view of the limited utility of collective action and the inevitable ultimate dispersal of work-mates, reducing collective loyalty, there is an obvious pressure for individual action — towards the search for alternative employment as quickly as possible. The alternative is fatalistic resignation. In the five case-study plants, following the announcement of the redundancy, a substantial minority of women applied for other jobs where they could be secured without jeopardizing redundancy pay; where redundancy pay was jeopardized by the search for alternative work no effort was made to find it — an economically rational calculation made by mainly middle-aged working-class women who had little chance in any other circumstances of acquiring even the modest capital sum represented by the redundancy pay due to them.

The proportion of women applying for jobs following the announcement of the redundancy ranged from 27 per cent in Company C to 42 per cent among clerical workers in the North West engineering firm (plant D), as Table 3.6.10 shows.

Table 3.6.10
Responses to *After you realised that there would be a redundancy did you take any steps to get a different job before being made redundant?*

	A (%)	B (%)	C (%)	D (%)	E (%)	Total (%)
Applied for jobs	35	35	27	42	37	35
Sounded out job market only	2	12	9	5	8	7.5
No	63	51.5	64	51	55	57
Not answered		1.5		2		
N	51	68	66	43	51	279

($P = 0.469$)

There was thus very little variation in the proportion of women looking for jobs after the announcement of the redundancy, perhaps surprisingly so in view of the different occupations covered, and the different levels of labour demand in the five labour markets: one might have expected more job applications in a labour market with a relatively low level of unemployment, such as area A, than in an area with a high level of unemployment, such as area B, reflecting the relative chances of success.

The reason for inactivity was not primarily fatalism, as Table 3.6.11 shows.

Table 3.6.11
Responses to *Why did you not take any steps?*

	A (%)	B (%)	C (%)	D (%)	E (%)	Total (%)
Did not think of it	2	3		2		1
No jobs to apply for	10	10	9	7	18	11
Afraid of losing redundancy money	14	1.5	9	2	6	6.5
No point until leaving date		6	24	5	4	9
Seeing job through	4	7	3	12	2	5
Not in hurry for job	10	7	3		2	5
Pregnant	2		1.5			1
Giving up work	8	9		14	10	7.5
Other	16	13	14	9	14	13
Not applicable (did apply for jobs)/ no answer	35	43	36	49	45	41
N	51	68	66	43	51	279

($P = 0.001$)

The figures are only suggestive, since the numbers involved are small and there is a very large miscellaneous 'other' category. However, the most frequently mentioned reasons related either to the practical difficulties posed by the firm's conduct of the redundancy, or to the limited jobs available. Hence 14 per cent at Company A stated that they were afraid of jeopardizing their redundancy money (small though it was), and 9 per cent at Company C had the same fear. By far the most common reason cited in Company C was the impossibility of applying for alternative work until definite leaving dates had been fixed, a difficulty echoed in Company B. Company C's policy on leaving for manual workers was administered less flexibly than Company E's policy for clerical workers. Pessimism about the lack of alternative jobs was most pronounced in Company E, where the interviews were held latest, and where unemployment had risen above the levels of the other four labour markets (see below, pp. 218–19). The other group having a relatively pessimistic assessment of the alternative jobs available was at the feeder factory in Company B, again a realistic assessment. Significantly, relatively few women stated that they were intending to give up work – 7.5 per cent overall, mainly clerical workers and a few elderly operatives in Company B.

The substantial number applying for alternative jobs, and the firm-related and economically rational reasons frequently given for not applying for alternative jobs, do not indicate a picture of fatalistic resignation. The number of 'active' responses ranged from 57 per cent in the Company E to 73 per cent in Company C, 'active' including not applying for jobs because of fear of losing redundancy money, inability to take steps because of uncertainty over leaving dates, and the desire to see the job through. It is of course impossible to say whether the provision of 'firm-related' explanations for inactivity was a rationalization of a fundamental fatalism, the provision of a personally acceptable reason for lack of initiative. In default of evidence for alternative interpretations, we feel that explanations have to be taken at face value.

Very few of the respondents who applied for jobs had been successful at the time of interview, only 5 per cent or fifteen respondents. The findings on post-redundancy employment are presented in Chapter 4, on redundant women in the labour market.

In short, there was little evidence to indicate a fatalistic response to redundancy amongst our respondents. In four of the five cases the majority of respondents believed that the redundancy could have been avoided: only in Company B did a majority believe that redundancy was inevitable, reflecting the obvious technological obsolescence of the product and the gradual run-down of the plant. The major reasons given for the redundancies were the overall fortunes of the economy and bad management. Only in plant B was there advance warning of redundancy, and the most favourable evaluation of management handling of redundancy was also in plant B. There was considerable feeling that workers ought to have been kept better informed about the impending threats to their jobs. There was also some criticism of the handling of the redundancies by the trade unions. The majority of women interviewed felt that plant-level officials had done everything possible to prevent redundancy (except in plant A); a majority of women who expressed an opinion also believed that their paid officials had done everything, again with the exception of plant A. Although there was little the unions involved could do to prevent the closures, keeping the membership informed and showing an active interest made a difference to employees' evaluations of their unions. The majority of women would have been prepared to take part in industrial action to prevent closures if they had been asked. Finally, a majority of women either took steps to find another job before their redundancy, or were unable to do so because of management policies: few women intended to give up working.

3.7 Redundancy pay

The redundancy pay received by the respondents comprised two elements, statutory entitlement which employers were required to make under the Employment Protection (Consolidation) Act 1978, for which employers received a proportional reimbursement from the Redundancy Fund, and *ex gratia* payments. Under the 1978 Act employees' payments were calculated according to a formula based on age, length of service, and earnings. The amount was calculated on the basis of one and a half week's pay for each year of service between the age of 41 and normal retirement age, plus one week's pay for each year of service between the ages of 22 and 40 inclusive, and half a week's pay for each year of service up to the age of 21.[9] The principles governing the *ex gratia* payments varied from company to company, as explained above, pp. 128–31. The primary factor in Company A was length of service, age not being taken into account in *ex gratia* payments; in Company B age and length of service were both taken into account; in Companies C, D, and E the basic *ex gratia* payment depended on length of service, in addition to the closure terms.

There are at least two different reasons for making redundancy payments: compensation to employees for the loss of jobs, and financial assistance with the transitional costs of changing jobs or moving from employment to unemployment. These two types of reasons can be further subdivided. The compensation could be provided as a means of avoiding potential industrial-relations problems associated with the reduction of the labour force, or as socially just compensation for the loss of job property rights. The transitional costs could also be justified on grounds of utility (the avoidance of industrial conflict, easing the introduction of new processes), equity, or social welfare. At the time of the initial passage of the Redundancy Payments Act in 1965 the government's major interest was in facilitating labour mobility by helping with the transitional costs, and by providing some recompense for accumulated job property rights. With the emphasis upon payment linked to length of service, rather than anticipated transitional costs, the criterion of recompense was in practice paramount. The positive transitional role has been further eroded as unemployment has increased by the growing importance of the negative welfare role of providing a financial cushion during the initial period of unemployment, especially necessary with the ending of earnings-related unemployment benefit in 1981 and changes in the rules governing tax rebates in 1982.

As Table 3.7.1 shows, our respondents were aware of the range of reasons for making redundancy payments.

Table 3.7.1
Responses to *Why do you think redundancy payments are made?*

	A (%)	B (%)	C (%)	D (%)	E (%)	Total (%)
Compensation	24	29	54	33	62	41
To avoid trouble	10	1.5	9	7	6	6.5
Tide over/ease transition to new job	41	46	42.5	51	31	42
Other		1.5	1.5		4	1
Don't know	31	26.5	6	14	6	17
No answer				2		0.4
N	51	68	66	43	51	279

Percentage is that of respondents mentioning given type of reason.

The most commonly cited reasons for redundancy payments were 'compensatory' ones (41 per cent), although the precise terms used differed. But there were interesting contrasts between plants — over twice as many women in the two Midlands engineering firms mentioned 'compensatory' reasons as women in the South East garment factory or the North West electronics firm. In Company C this may have been due to the highly 'unionate' character of industrial relations in the plant, and in plant E to the relatively high level of awareness shown by Midlands clerical workers, as shown in replies to other questions. Similarly, very few women in either plant said that they did not know why redundancy payments were made. Almost an equal number of women mentioned 'utilitarian' reasons for redundancy payments, primarily as a means of tiding them over until a new job is found. The only difference found between the five plants was in the comparatively small number of Midland clerical workers mentioning such reasons, although even amongst that group 31 per cent mentioned utilitarian reasons. One issue of interest would be to examine the extent to which 'compensatory' explanations had increased in comparison with 'utilitarian' ones, with a consequential growth in industrial citizenship rights.

At the time of the first interview, not all respondents knew the amount of redundancy pay they would receive, a fact which is important in itself. However, Table 3.7.2 shows the amount of redundancy pay received by the women interviewed after the redundancies. There were marked differences in the level of redundancy payments received, women in Companies B, C, D, and E receiving substantially higher payments than women in Company A. The women from

Companies B, C, D, and E received payments averaging between £3000 and £4000, up to a maximum of £9300 (possibly higher, as the most senior woman from Company D did not reveal how much she received nor did some other senior women). In Companies C, D, and E no payment was lower than £1000 and in B only 5 per cent of payments were below £1000. In all four companies the great majority of payments were £2000 or over. In Company A, however, payments averaged only £847, 62 per cent of payments were under £1000, and the highest payment was of £2800. Only five women, two from Company A and three from B, received no redundancy payment at all.

Table 3.7.2
Size of redundancy payments (by firm)

£s	A (%)	B (%)	C (%)	D (%)	E (%)	Total (%)
0	5	7	–	–	–	1
1–999	62	5	–	–	3	15
1000–1999	26	17	2	19	7	14
2000–2999	7	24	36	13	38	24
3000–3999	–	17	13	29	14	14
4000–4999	–	15	15	10	7	10
5000–5999	–	–	13	10	–	5
6000–6999	–	2	1.5	6.5	24	7
7000–7999	–	–	6	3	–	2
8000–9300	–	5	4	3	–	3
Unwilling to say	–	7	4	6.5	7	6
N	42	41	53	31	29	196

Note: Data on size of redundancy payments were derived from the second questionnaire.

In Companies B, C, D, and E the average redundancy payment was equivalent to just over one year's net pay for the average worker in each company: in Company A the average redundancy payment was equivalent to only nineteen weeks' net pay for each worker.

Women are more likely than men to have interrupted service with the same employer. This is especially likely where employers follow a specific policy of recruiting women whom they have previously employed, for example on re-entry into the labour force after children had reached school age, as Companies A and B did. Hence redundancy payments do not always cover the whole period of service with a given employer, as Table 3.7.3 shows. The redundancy payments were far less than the total length of service for slightly more than a fifth of the women overall, but for as many as 41 per cent in the garment factory and 25 per cent in the electronics factory. Since plant C had been open for only a relatively brief period there had been less opportunity for interrupted service.

Opinions about the fairness of the amount received as redundancy pay also differed between plants, the highest level of satisfaction being reported in

Table 3.7.3
Responses to *Was your redundancy payment for your total service with the firm?*

	A (%)	B (%)	C (%)	D (%)	E (%)	Total (%)
Total service	51	69	77	86	82	73
Less than total service	41	25	18	14	14	23
Don't know	4	3	1.5			2
Missing data	4	3	3		4	3
N	51	68	66	43	51	279

$(P = 0.009)$

plant D, the lowest in plant A. In view of the relatively low level of payments in plant A the prevalence of a belief that the redundancy pay was not enough is hardly surprising. It is more surprising that 53.5 per cent of women in plant D thought that the level of payment was generous, compared with 23.5 per cent in plant E and 4.5 per cent in plant C, although the criteria for the payments were the same in all three plants. A majority of respondents thus thought that the payments received were either generous or fair: satisfaction was particularly evident amongst the clerical workers in plants D and E. However, a majority of respondents in plants A and C and a surprisingly large number of plant B (in view of the relative generosity of the terms) thought that the payments were insufficient.

3.8 Conclusion

The five redundancies examined comprised four plant closures, one clothing factory and three engineering plants, and one unit closure in the electronics industry. All five companies experienced major declines in their product markets, although the reasons for the decline, and its trajectory, differed. The clothing factory had survived the decline in the industry throughout the 1970s notably well, occupying a distinctive niche by producing high-quality garments: however, even its product market was seriously weakened in 1980. The electronics plant faced reduced demand because of the technological obsolescence of its product, and the reduced labour required for its replacement products. All three engineering companies suffered from increased competition in export markets, and increased import penetration, throughout the 1970s: recession in 1979 produced severe difficulties for all three companies already weakened by long-term decline and financial pressures.

Although redundancies are specific events, they are often the final stage in a long-term process, involving earlier and less drastic attempts to reduce the labour force, as in the five companies studied. The process of contraction was especially evident in the electronics company. The policies followed to achieve a reduced labour force resulted in a relatively ageing labour force.

Strategic decisions on redundancy are rarely taken at plant level. In all five companies major decisions were taken either at company, group, or international headquarters. The influence of trade unions upon the five redundancies was limited, the most extensive opposition being mounted in the Midlands engineering plant. Despite the limited impact of trade unions upon the redundancies, the majority of women were satisfied with the role of their plant-level representatives in the engineering and electronics plants, although many women were critical in the clothing factory. The redundancy agreements provided for enhancement in all five plants, although the terms of the agreement, and the average level of payment received, were significantly less generous in the clothing plant than in the other four closures. There was no evidence that women were discriminated against in the five closures, although no attempt was made to cater for the distinctive employment patterns of women workers (for example in the treatment of broken service).

There was no evidence of a distinctively feminine fatalism towards the redundancies. The majority of women did not believe that the redundancies were inevitable. Similarly, the majority of women said that they would have gone out on strike if there union had asked them, and a majority either took steps to find alternative work, or did not do so for economically rational reasons, following the announcement of the closures. Like men, the women found the experience of redundancies stressful, and had few definite proposals for countering management policies.

Notes

1. Massey and Meegan, *The Anatomy of Job Loss*, p. 41.
2. Ibid., p. 209.
3. Report to the National Economic Development Council by the Electronics Components Sector Working Party, 1981, p. 6.
4. William Brown (ed.), *The Changing Contours of British Industrial Relations* (Basil Blackwell, 1981), p. 118.
5. C. Airey and A. Potts, 'Workplace Industrial Relations', (Social & Community Planning Research, 1981), p. 28.
6. Report of the Committee of Inquiry on Industrial Democracy (Bullock), (HMSO, 1977, Cmnd. 6706), p. 44.
7. Institute of Manpower Studies, *Manpower Commentary No. 13: Redundancy Provisions Surveys*, Vol. I, Part 1: *Commentary*, pp. iv and 52, and Vol. 2, Table 103.
8. Ibid., Vol. 1, pp. iv–v.
9. Employment Protection (Consolidation) Act, Schedule 4, in B. A. Hepple *et al.*, *Labour Relations: Statutes and Materials* (Sweet & Maxwell, 1979), p. 502.

4

WOMEN IN THE LABOUR MARKET

In previous chapters we have documented women's work experiences and attitudes before redundancy. In this and the following chapter we are concerned with their experiences and attitudes following redundancy: this chapter focuses upon job search, re-employment, and retraining, home-working, and setting up in business, at least potentially money-making alternatives to conventional market employment; Chapter 5 focuses upon unemployment. The behaviour of redundant women in the labour market is important in its own right: they comprise an experienced and, in many instances, skilled group of workers. The extent to which they found future employment in jobs that matched their experience and skills, or at least were regarded by the women as being as good as their pre-redundancy jobs, is an indication of the extent to which the redundancies studied resulted in a more efficient allocation of labour: a more efficient allocation of labour would have resulted if women had moved from firms experiencing product-market difficulties (as the case-study firms were) to firms which were not doing so, whilst the women continued to make use of their skills and experience. The behaviour of the redundant women in the labour market is also important indirectly, as an indication of the extent to which women were committed to market employment, or regarded market employment as an ancillary activity, to be given up either out of pressure or out of choice in the face of difficulties in securing paid employment. Finally, the extent to which the women secured satisfactory jobs is an indication of the extent to which they were able to achieve work objectives which, as we showed in Chapter 2, were important to them.

This chapter is divided into five sections. The first section outlines briefly the overall experience of the redundant women in the labour market. The second section examines the process of job seeking, including the methods used, their relative effectiveness, and the extent to which the women regarded themselves as handicapped (by age, sex, disability, or other disadvantages) in the search for work. The third section presents data on post-redundancy employment experience, involving a comparison between pre-redundancy and post-redundancy

152 *Working Women in Recession*

jobs. In the fourth section we examine alternatives to going out to work, covering retraining, home-working, and independent business activity. In the final section we place the experience of the women we interviewed in the context of the overall labour-market situation in their travel to work areas. The major source of data for this chapter is the second personal interview, supplemented by data from the first interview and from the postal questionnaire where appropriate.

4.1 Post-redundancy experience in the labour market

The majority of women interviewed before the redundancy planned at that time to continue going out to work after the redundancy. Most intended continuing employment without a break if possible, but a substantial minority intended taking a break either for a holiday, to move house, or for a pregnancy. However, only a minority of the women interviewed in the first stage of the project were in employment at the time the second interviews were carried out, and only a small minority of those actually interviewed a second time were in employment. After the redundancy, the largest group of women were looking for work (36 per cent), a slightly smaller number had been re-deployed in the same firm or obtained further employment (28 per cent), some had retired temporarily (12 per cent), some had retired permanently (9 per cent), and no information was available on 15 per cent. Put simply, the major employment consequence of the redundancies was to increase the number of women who wanted to work out of work. There was no 'alternative' role of looking after a family available to the majority of the women — their families no longer needed full-time care.

When interviewed before the redundancy, the majority of women planned to continue working after the redundancy: 69 per cent said that they would be looking for another job immediately, 14 per cent that they would be looking for another job after an interval, and 17 per cent that they would not be looking for another job. Married women were, of course, less likely than single women to intend continuing to work. Marital status, however, was not decisive: the major difference between women intending to look for another job and women not intending to do so was in their breadwinner status: fewer women who described themselves as joint breadwinners intended to look for work than any other group, as Table 4.1.1 shows. Having additional sources(s) of income obviously made it possible to withdraw from the labour market or to delay looking for alternative work, although prolonged delay would lead to serious financial hardship in view of the substantial financial contribution made to household income by the women interviewed.

The reasons given for stopping work were primarily personal and domestic. The largest number were planning to retire early (6.5 per cent), whilst a further 2 per cent did not think that there was any point in looking for work because of their age. A further 1 per cent of women wanted a rest, one women (.4 per cent) intended to help in the family business, one women (.4 per cent) intended

Table 4.1.1
Intention of looking for another job (by breadwinner status)

	Earning own keep (%)	Sole breadwinner (%)	Main breadwinner (%)	Joint breadwinner (%)	Earning extras (%)	Missing (%)	Total (%)
Yes	82	81	50	62	65.5		69
Yes after break	6	5	50	18	17		17
No	12	14	–	20	17	.4	14
N	51	43	2	153	29	1	279

($p = 0.067$)

to retire because her husband was invalided, and 1 per cent of women intended to have children.

The majority of women intended to look for further employment, but not all intended to do so immediately: 62 per cent of the women who intended to seek work intended to do so immediately, 20 per cent after a holiday, 1 per cent after having a child, and 16 per cent after moving house. Women were less likely to intend looking for work immediately in plants A, C1, and B1 than in the other factories, the most common reasons for delay in A and C1 being to take a holiday, the most common reason in B1 being to move house.

Table 4.1.2
Responses to *When do you intend to start looking for work?* (by area)

	A (%)	B1 (%)	B2 (%)	C1 (%)	C2 (%)	D (%)	E (%)	Total (%)
Immediately	39	44	59	38	67	58	53	52
After a holiday	23.5	17	–	43	18	14	10	17
After pregnancy	2	2	–	–	2	–	–	1
After moving house	8	29	15	9.5	11	5	16	13
No intention of looking	27.5	7	26	9.5	2	23	22	17
N	51	41	27	21	45	43	51	279

($p = 0.017$)

The high proportion of women from C1 intending to take a holiday, contrasting sharply with the low proportion in C2, was probably due to the timing of the redundancy: women were due to leave C1 shortly before Christmas, and to leave C2 in the New Year. Not unexpectedly, women who described themselves as earning extras or as joint breadwinners were less likely to be looking for work immediately than other women: 41 per cent of women earning extras, 43 per cent of joint breadwinners, 50 per cent of main breadwinners, 69 per cent of women earning their own keep, and 70 per cent of sole breadwinners intending to look for work immediately.

The women who intended to have a break from employment intended to have only a short break: 13 per cent of women interviewed intended to have a break of six months or less, whilst a further 4 per cent said that the length of time they wanted to elapse before looking for work again depended upon circumstances: only 2 per cent of women interviewed envisaged a gap of over six months.

To summarize, before the redundancy 14 per cent of women intended to cease employment, 2 per cent intended to retire from the labour market for more than six months, and could thus be described as planning 'temporary retirement', 4 per cent said that the amount of time they would postpone looking for work depended upon circumstances, and 13 per cent said that they intended having a break in employment of six months or less. Hence 33 per cent of the women originally interviewed intended to have some interruption in their employment after the redundancy. However, a considerably smaller proportion never intended to look for work after redundancy, only 17 per cent. The range of potential withdrawals from the labour market ranged from 17 to 33 per cent, the latter figure including women who intended having a gap of up to six months in employment (the majority of whom were envisaging a gap of under three months).

Of the 279 women initially interviewed 101 (or 36 per cent) were in employment at the time of the second interview, of whom twenty-two (or 8 per cent) had had their redundancies postponed: 28 per cent had thus found new jobs. Table 4.1.3 summarizes the employment status of all initial respondents at the time of the second interview.

Table 4.1.3
Employment status of all respondents at time of second interview (by company)*

	A (%)	B (%)	C (%)	D (%)	E (%)	Total (%)	N (%)
Working	35	16	30	39	25	28	79
Looking for work	35	43	39	35	25	36	101
Temporarily retired	12	9	21	9	8	12	34
Permanently retired	12	13	3	7	8	9	24
No information/redundancy postponed	6	19	6	9	35	15	41
N	51	68	66	43	51		279

*Including those not re-interviewed.

Of the women who had been initially interviewed only 28 per cent had been declared redundant and had obtained subsequent employment: 36 per cent described themselves as looking for work, 12 per cent as temporarily retired, and 9 per cent as permanently retired.

Table 4.1.3 presents data on all women interviewed before the redundancy. However, it was not possible to re-interview all initial respondents. Before examining the data derived from the second interviews it is helpful to present data on the employment status of women whom we were unable to re-interview. Table 4.1.4 therefore summarizes data on the employment status of women not interviewed a second time. Of the original group 9 per cent were still working for or redeployed within the same company or group, 4 per cent were unwilling to be interviewed because they had permanently retired from the labour market, 4 per cent were unwilling to be interviewed because they were working full time and did not have the time available, and 4 per cent were unemployed, but refused to be interviewed. No information was available on 7 per cent of the original group, the largest number (12) from case study B: many respondents in this case study who had been intending to retire from employment at the time of the first interview said that they would not be willing to be interviewed a second time, and their addresses were not available for recontacting. A further

Table 4.1.4
Employment status of women not interviewed at second stage

	A N	B N	C N	D N	E N	Total N	Total (%)
Still working at original firm	–	–	8	2	15	25	9
Working	3	3	1	3	–	10	4
Unemployed	–	5	–	3	2	10	4
Permanently retired	3	6	–	1	–	10	4
Left district	3	1	–	3	2	9	3
No information	–	12	4	–	3	19	7
Interviewed	42	41	53	31	29	196	70
Total	51	68	66	43	51	279	100

3 per cent had left the district and could not be contacted. In short, we could not re-interview 30 per cent of the original respondents. Of this 30 per cent, 30 per cent were never declared redundant, or finally left too close to the date of the second interview to be eligible for re-interview, and 12 per cent were known to be in employment, making a total of 42 per cent of non-respondents in employment. On this basis, the sample interviewed in the second stage over-represents the unemployed. However, it is known that seventeen out of the twenty five women still with their original companies were about to lose their jobs, or had lost them in the days immediately preceding the second interviews: the overrepresentation of the unemployed in the group interviewed is thus a result of the particular timing of the second interviews, and does not present a substantively misleading picture of the post redundancy employment experience of the women first interviewed.

The primary source of data for the analysis of post-redundancy experience was the second-stage interview. As Table 4.1.5 shows, 17 per cent of the women interviewed in stage two were working full time at the time of the second interview, 12 per cent part time; 17 per cent described themselves as temporarily retired, 7 per cent permanently retired, and the largest group, 46 per cent were looking for work.

Women employed in Companies D and E, who were primarily clerical workers, were thus much more likely than other workers to have found alternative employment: 32 per cent of women in Company D and 28 per cent in Company E. Women employed in Company C had particularly severe difficulties in finding alternative employment, only 6 per cent having found full-time work. As many as 26 per cent of women formerly employed in Company C had retired temporarily from work, reflecting the difficulties experienced in finding work. (These findings are discussed below, pp. 202–4.)

The employment difficulties of workers in Company C were not the artefact of there being a relatively short period of time between their leaving Company C and their being interviewed: workers in Company C had been out of work longer than workers in any other company. As explained in Chapter 1, the women were not interviewed the same length of time after leaving their pre-redundancy employment: since leaving dates were staggered, and the interviewing process itself took several weeks in each case study, the time elapsing between leaving and being interviewed varied within and between case studies. Table 4.1.6 summarizes the length of time of unemployment experienced by all respondents interviewed at the second stage.

Table 4.1.5
Employment status of women interviewed at the second stage

	A (%)	B (%)	C (%)	D (%)	E (%)	Total (%)	N
Working full time	17	12	6	32	28	17	33
Working part time	17	7	15	10	7	12	23
Looking for work	43	58.5	49	39	38	46	91
Temporarily retired	14	15	26	13	14	17	34
Permanently retired	7	7	4	6.5	14	7	14
Own business	1					.5	
N	42	41	53	31	29		196

Table 4.1.6
Length of time of unemployment of all respondents re-interviewed (by company)

No. of weeks	A (%)	B (%)	C (%)	D (%)	E (%)	Total (%)	N
0	19	7	6	32	20	15	30
1– 3	2	–	2	–	2	1.5	3
4– 7	2	2	2	10	7	4	8
8–11	5	5	6	16	3	7	13
12–15	5	2	4	10	49	11	22
16–19	7	5	15	10	–	8	16
20–23	33	71	24.5	23	14	34	67
24–27	26	7	9	–	3	10	20
28–31			15			4	8
32–33			17			5	9
N	42	41	53	31	29		196

The majority of women were out of work for several months: 72 per cent of women interviewed were out of work for twelve weeks or more. Secondly, the majority of women out of work for under three months were not unemployed at all: 15 per cent of all respondents went directly from their pre-redundancy jobs to alternative work. Thirdly, differences in the length of time out of work for women in the different case studies were largely due to the pattern and phasing of the redundancies: once women had become unemployed there was little difference in the chances of finding re-employment – the differences in re-employment prospects for full-time work were largely due to differences in the number of women finding work before leaving pre-redundancy employment. The chances of finding full-time work before leaving pre-redundancy employment were heavily influenced by age, occupation, and the policies of the employing company.

As expected, there were important differences between age groups in employment status at the time of the second interview. In all age groups except the relatively small groups aged under 25 and over 55 the largest proportion of women described themselves as looking for work: 44 per cent of women aged 25–34, 55 per cent of women aged 35–44, and 50 per cent aged 45–54. Amongst the under 25s the largest group were working full time (60 per cent), and amongst the over 55s the largest group were temporarily or permanently retired (54 per cent). Table 4.1.7 summarizes the data on age and employment status.

Table 4.1.7
Age and employment status at second interview

	≤ 25 (%)	25–34 (%)	35–44 (%)	45–54 (%)	55 + (%)	Total (%)	N
Working full time	60	28	8	14	12.5	17	33
Working part time	–	–	18.5	14	12.5	12	23
Looking for work	40	44	55	50	21	46	91
Temporarily retired	–	26	14	14	29	17	34
Permanently retired	–	–	5	9	25	7	14
Own business	–	3	–	–	–	.5	1
N	10	39	65	58	24		196

Women aged under 25 were very substantially more likely than other women to have found re-employment in full-time work, 60 per cent having done so: the next-highest group was of women aged 25–34, 28 per cent of whom had secured full-time employment. Women aged under 25 constituted only 5 per cent of the women interviewed, but 18 per cent of women in full-time employment. The chances of women aged under 25 obtaining full-time employment, especially non-manual workers, were thus relatively good. Significantly, none of the women in this age group had taken part-time employment, or retired from the labour force (temporarily or permanently): if out of work, they were still intending to hold out for full-time work at the time of the second interview.

The largest group of women aged 25–34 were looking for work (44 per cent). However, a number of women had retired temporarily from the labour force (26 per cent), the majority to have a family. In addition, one women had decided to try to launch her own business. Twenty-eight per cent had succeeded in finding full-time employment. Again, no woman had taken part-time employment, and no woman had retired permanently from the labour force. In comparison with the under 25s, this group had alternative family roles which they were able and willing to assume. However, the alternatives appeared to be having a family or full-time employment, not attempting to combine the two roles through part-time employment.

Women aged 35–44 were much less successful than younger women in securing full-time work: only 8 per cent had obtained full-time work, and as many as 55 per cent were looking for work. Of the remainder, 14 per cent had retired from work temporarily, and 5 per cent permanently. Significantly, 18.5 per cent were in part-time employment, a higher proportion than in any other age group. The implications of these figures will be discussed fully below. However, it is for this and the next age group that the redundancy is likely to have the most serious impact. The economic burden of growing children and the need for work to maintain customary standards of living are likely to be greater than for other age groups.

The employment status of women aged 45–54 was not very different from that of women aged 35–44. As for the 35–44 age group, the largest number of women aged 45–54 were looking for work — 50 per cent. Slightly more were working full time (14 per cent compared with 8 per cent) and slightly fewer working part time (14 per cent compared with 18 per cent); slightly more were permanently retired (9 per cent compared with 5 per cent) and exactly the same proportion were temporarily retired (14 per cent). There were thus few differences between women aged 35–44 and women aged 45–54, possibly reflecting similar pressures for employment, and similar requirements from employers.

As expected, the position of women aged 55 or more was very different. Fewer women in this age group described themselves as looking for work than in any other age group — only 21 per cent, compared with 46 per cent overall. This was not because such women had been especially successful in finding work, only 12.5 per cent being in full-time work (more than women aged 35–44, but fewer than any other group) and 12.5 per cent having found part-time work. Instead, the majority had retired from the labour force, either permanently or temporarily. Hence 29 per cent described themselves as temporarily retired, and 25 per cent as permanently retired. Although the larger number described themselves as temporarily retired, for women aged 55 or more the distinction between temporary and permanent retirement may simply be one of perspective, some women recognizing that their chances of finding future employment are negligible more rapidly than others. (However, the difference in perspective is important, since temporarily retired women may appropriately be regarded as members of the labour force: see below, pp. 268–9.)

There were also differences in employment status between women in different occupational status groups. As Table 4.1.8 shows, women in non-manual occupations were substantially more likely than manual workers to have found full-time employment after the redundancy. Hence 25 per cent of women employed in professional administrative and supervisory jobs before the redundancy found full-time work after it, and 29.5 per cent of clerical workers: amongst manual workers the most successful group were semi-skilled workers, 16.5 per cent of whom obtained full-time employment. Expressed differently, non-manual

Table 4.1.8
Occupational status and employment status

	Prof./Admin. Supervisory (%)	Clerical (%)	Semi-skilled (%)	Slightly Skilled (%)	Unskilled (%)	Total (%)	N
Working full time	25	29.5	16.5	3	–	17	33
Working part time	6	4.5	11	23.5	18	12	23
Looking for work	50	32	52	47	54.5	46	91
Temporarily retired	19	25	13	15	27	17	34
Permanently retired	–	9	7	12	–	7	14
Own business	–		1			.5	1
N	16	44	91	34	11		196

($p = 0.119$)

workers comprised 31 per cent of respondents in the second interview, but 51.5 per cent of women in full-time employment. Despite this relative success, for all occupational statuses the largest group of women was of those who were looking for work.

Occupational status group 1 did not have the highest rate of success in securing re-employment, 25 per cent having found alternative full-time work, and 6 per cent part-time. However, the bulk of women in this group were employed in Companies D and E, where the last two case studies were carried out: there was thus a shorter period between leaving the pre-redundancy firm and the second interview. In addition, 19 per cent had retired temporarily from the labour force. Clerical workers were the most successful in finding alternative employment, 29.5 per cent having found full-time work, and 4.5 per cent part-time work; there were also significantly fewer clerical workers looking for jobs than any other group, 32 per cent looking for work. A substantial proportion, 25 per cent, had retired temporarily from the labour force, mainly young clerical workers planning pregnancies. However, it is significant that even in the most successful occupational-status group only slightly over a third (34 per cent) had found alternative work.

The employment experience of manual workers following redundancy was poor: 16.5 per cent of semi-skilled and 3 per cent of slightly skilled were in full-time employment, and no unskilled woman at all. In contrast with non-manual workers, more manual workers had found part-time work than had found full-time work: 56 per cent of manual workers in employment were in part-time work, compared with only 15 per cent of non-manual workers in employment. The highest proportion of part-time workers was found amongst the slightly skilled, primarily hand-sewing machinists from company A, although the largest number were found among the semi-skilled, primarily former engineering-assembly workers from Company C. Many more manual workers had withdrawn from the labour market, describing themselves as temporarily retired, than had found full-time employment: 13 per cent of semi-skilled,

15 per cent of slightly skilled, and 27 per cent of unskilled workers had temporarily retired from the labour force. Out of the 136 manual workers interviewed after the redundancy, 12 per cent had obtained full-time employment, 15 per cent had obtained part-time work, 22 per cent had retired from the labour force, and 51 per cent were still looking for work.

In this section we have outlined in general terms the experience of the redundant women in the labour market. Before the redundancy 86 per cent of respondents intended to look for another job, 69 per cent of respondents immediately and 17 per cent after a break. Women in case study B were more likely to be giving up employment than any other group (26 per cent), women in case study C less likely than in any other group (4 per cent). At the time of the second interviews, four to seven months after redundancy, 28 per cent of the initial sample were known to have found alternative work, and a further 9 per cent had not, after all, been declared redundant: 36 per cent were looking for work, 12 per cent had temporarily retired, and 9 per cent had permanently retired, no information being available about the employment status of the remainder. Seventy per cent of the initial sample were interviewed in the second stage, of whom 17 per cent were working full time and 12 per cent part time: 46 per cent were looking for work, 17 per cent were temporarily retired, and 7 per cent were permanently retired. Thus, instead of the 86 per cent who hoped to obtain a future job, 17 per cent had obtained a full-time job and 12 per cent a part-time job. Young women were much more successful in finding alternative work than older women, women aged under 25 being the most successful. Women in non-manual jobs were more likely to secure alternative jobs than women in manual jobs, although even amongst non-manual workers only a minority found work. Where women in manual jobs found alternative work it was more likely to be part time than full time, although of course a very large majority were in full-time employment before the redundancies.

4.2 Job search

This section is concerned with the process of job search; the outcome of the process is examined in section 4.3. The process of job search is important in its own right, and as a possible indicator of women's commitment to the labour market. The direct importance of job search is obvious: in labour-market terms, the process determines the extent to which workers find jobs that match their skills, experience, and preferences out of the range of jobs available — obviously, no job search can be effective if relevant jobs are not available. Moreover, considerable public expenditure is incurred in providing employment services, especially Job Centres, whose role is to facilitate the process of job search; it is obviously important to obtain information on the use women make of such services, and their evaluations of the services provided. In this context comparison between 'formal' and 'informal' methods of job search is especially relevant. The use of different methods of job search cannot be taken as a direct index of commitment to market employment; there are several reasons for using only a limited range of services, or for making only limited use of particular services, which have no implications for commitment to market employment. However, at a minimum, it is clearly relevant to understand how far commitment is associated with action.

The section is divided into three subsections. The first examines the timing of job-search activity. The second presents evidence on the methods used in looking for jobs, and the effectiveness of alternative methods in obtaining interviews and jobs. The same subsection includes an examination of respondents' evaluations of the effectiveness of alternative methods. In the third subsection we examine the extent to which the women interviewed regarded themselves as handicapped in the search for work, and the specific issue of discrimination.

4.2.1 The timing of job search

Slightly under a half of the women interviewed began looking for jobs before they left their pre-redundancy employment (43 per cent): the majority of the remainder began looking within the first month after leaving. Women in case studies B and C were less likely to have begun looking for work before leaving than women in the other three case studies: women in Company B, especially in the feeder factory, were notably pessimistic about their chances of finding alternative work, whilst women in Company C faced considerable practical difficulties in looking for work whilst working. Younger women were more likely to have begun to look before leaving than older women, and non-manual workers more than manual workers. Early search was associated with — although not necessarily the cause of — relative success: women who began to look for work before leaving were significantly more likely than others to find work. Detailed analysis of application rates for jobs showed that women aged under 25 submitted more job applications than women in any other age group, and women aged 55 or over substantially fewer. Clerical and semi-skilled women submitted more job applications than other occupational groups, and unskilled women substantially fewer. The number of women applying for jobs in the last month was fewer than in the first month, but more than in the intervening months: the average number of jobs applied for was lower. The following paragraphs document and explain these conclusions.

As Table 4.2.1.1 shows, 43 per cent of women asked said that they had begun to look for work before leaving their previous employment, 17 per cent began to look in the first week, and a further 16 per cent after the first week but within the first month. The data have been presented by area rather than by company, since, as explained in Chapter 1, research in Companies B and C covered two plants in each, a main site and a feeder factory. In Company B the two plants were in separate travel to work areas, although in Company C the two plants were in the same area. Since experience in the labour market is likely to be influenced by the travel to the work area within which the factory is located, it is appropriate to regard the unit of analysis as the area, rather than

Table 4.2.1.1
Time of beginning job search (by area)

	Area							Total (%)	N
	A (%)	B1 (%)	B2 (%)	C1 (%)	C2 (%)	D (%)	E (%)		
Before leaving	63	23	33	15	26	80	30	43	66
Within 1 week	17	9	–	38.5	22	8	25	17	26
1–4 weeks	6	50	25	–	18.5	8	10	16	25
5–12 weeks	3	9	25	31	15	–	25	12	19
Over 3 months	3	–	–	15	15	–	–	4	7
Offered job without looking	9	9	17	–	4	4	10	7	11
N	35	22	12	13	27	25	20		154

the company, although in many cases the differences between the plants in the same case study are likely to be small. For convenience, data on the two plants involved in Company C are presented separately, although there are unlikely to be sociologically significant differences in labour-market experience between the two factories.

There were major differences between companies in the timing of beginning job-search activity: women in case studies B and C were less likely to begin to look for work before leaving than women in the other case studies. However, the reasons for the delay were not the same. Overall, the most frequently mentioned reason for not looking for work before leaving was the desire for a rest, mentioned by 9 per cent of women. In Company B the most frequently mentioned reasons for not looking for work before leaving were that the leaving date was at Christmas holiday time, and therefore there was little point in looking, that the respondent needed time to get over the shock of redundancy, that there was little chance of work and therefore looking was pointless (especially in area B1), and that the women concerned wanted a rest. In Company C some of the reasons were personal (illness) and domestic (home decorating). However, most of the reasons related to the lack of time available for looking for work, and the danger of losing redundancy money.

In general, younger women were more likely to begin looking for work before leaving their pre-redundancy jobs than older women: 80 per cent of women aged 35–44, 33 per cent aged 45–54, and 33 per cent aged 55+ did so. However, the age differences were not due simply to an age effect: they were also influenced by family circumstances, and by the policies of the women's pre-redundancy employers. As expected, married women were more likely to delay looking for work until after they had left their pre-redundancy employment than single women: only 36 per cent of married women, compared with 78 per cent of single women (and 40 per cent of widows, and 53 per cent of divorced and separated women) began to look for another job before leaving. Similarly, 17 per cent of married women, but only 11 per cent of single women, had a gap of over a month before looking for work. For young single women the incentive to begin looking for work as soon as their impending redundancy was announced was obvious. For women aged 35–44 the pressures of combining market employment with domestic responsibilities were acute, owing to their responsibilities for children: although only 2.5 per cent of women had children under 5, 27 per cent had children under 16, who required time and energy. It is hardly surprising that women aged 35–54 were more likely to delay looking for work to have a rest than any other age group. Secondly, employers differed in their policies towards allowing women to have time off to look for work. In Company C many women did not apply for jobs before leaving because they did not have a definite leaving date, or could not find the time required to look for work. The age groups containing high proportions of women previously employed in Company C were therefore likely to have fewer women applying for work before leaving than other age groups; former employees of Company C were concentrated in the age range 35 upwards.

Women in non-manual occupations were more likely to apply for jobs before leaving than women in lower status groups, as table 4.2.1.2 indicates.

Table 4.2.1.2
Time of beginning job search (by occupational status)

	Prof./Admin. Supervisory (%)	Clerical (%)	Semi-skilled (%)	Slightly Skilled (%)	Unskilled (%)	Total (%)	N
Before leaving	58	63	37	36	22	43	66
Within 1 week	8	13	13	29	33	17	26
1–4 weeks	17	7	21	11	22	16	25
5–12 weeks	17	3	15	14	11	12	19
Over 3 months	–	3	8	–	–	4	7
Offered job without looking	–	10	5	11	11	7	11
N	12	30	75	28	9		154

The numbers involved in individual occupational groups are small, especially in groups 1 and 5. However, there is a clear contrast between non-manual and manual workers in the numbers looking for work before leaving previous employment. This was partly influenced by the age composition of the different groups. However, differences in the age composition were less important than differences in the policies of the firms involved: where companies limited opportunities for looking for work before the redundancy it was obviously difficult for the women involved to look for work. Moreover, it is perhaps unsurprising that women in manual jobs, especially unskilled manual jobs, were more likely to delay looking for work to have a rest than women in non-manual jobs.

In view of the foregoing, it is not surprising that women who applied for jobs before leaving their pre-redundancy jobs were more likely to be in employment at the time of the second interview than other women. As shown earlier, women were far more likely to obtain jobs between the announcement of the redundancy and their leaving their pre-redundancy job than at any other time. Table 4.2.1.3 summarizes the data on the timing of beginning search and on employment status at the time of the second interview.

Table 4.2.1.3
Timing of beginning job search (by employment status)

	Working full time (%)	Working part time (%)	Looking for work (%)	Temporarily retired (%)	Total (%)	N
Before leaving	70	52	31	37.5	43	66
Within 1 week	9	17	19	25	17	26
1–4 weeks	3	13	23	–	16	25
5–12 weeks	–	4	20	–	12	19
Over 3 months	6	–	5.5	–	4	7
Offered job without looking	12	13	1	37.5	7	11
N	33	23	90	8		154

$(p = 0.011)$

Hence 70 per cent of the women who were working full time had started looking for work before leaving, and 52 per cent of women working part time; only 31 per cent of women who started looking before the redundancy were still looking for work. Put differently, at the time of the second interview 35 per cent of the women who began looking for work before leaving were in full time employment, and 18 per cent in part time employment: 42 per cent were looking for work. However, at the same time only 11.5 per cent of women who started looking for work in the first week after leaving their pre-redundancy job were in full time employment, and 15 per cent working part time: 65 per cent were looking for work. There were similar differences in length of time out of work. Of course, it was difficult for women who did not apply for jobs until after the redundancy to have no experience of unemployment, although one woman did so, looking for work in the first week, finding it, and regarding the time out of work as a natural break: 38 per cent of women who started looking for work before the redundancy had no experience of unemployment. There were also differences in the length of time out of work between women who began applying for jobs at different times: hence 24 per cent of women who began looking before leaving were unemployed for fifteen weeks or less, compared with 15 per cent of women who began looking in the first week. The timing of job search was not, in itself, decisive: women who began looking before leaving were younger, and of higher occupational status, than women who did not: such women were likely to have better re-employment prospects, independently of the timing of job search (see above, pp. 158–61). However, the differences were not solely explicable by the differences in the age and occupational status of the two groups: the timing of job search made a difference.

Early job search did not guarantee employment, but delaying job search made it highly unlikely that jobs would be found. Hence only five women who did not start looking for work until three weeks or more after leaving subsequently obtained full time employment, and six found part time work: of the twenty-three women who delayed looking for work in order to have a rest, seventeen (or 74 per cent) were still looking for work at the time of the second interview, four to seven months later.

In previous paragraphs we have indicated differences in the timing of job-search activities between areas, occupational-status groups, age groups, and marital statuses. However, it would be misleading, for two major reasons, to use the timing of the beginning of job-search activity as an index of commitment to market employment. First, company personnel policies made a major difference to the ability of women to spend time in looking for work before leaving: women in Company C had the least time available for looking for work, but were more intent on continuing in market employment than women in any other company. Secondly, the timing of the redudancies made it impossible to make a meaningful comparison between different groups of women who only began to look for work after leaving: the women left Company B, and plant C1, directly before Christmas, making a delay in looking for work inevitable, since Christmas involves women in even heavier domestic responsibilities than other times of the year, and in any event employers were unlikely to be recruiting long-term employees immediately before the Christmas break.

Previous paragraphs have concentrated on the timing of the beginning of active job search. We now turn to job search after leaving previous employment. To provide basic data on this activity as a possible index of commitment to market employment and as a way of providing precise information on the possible process of discouragement amongst women in the labour market, we asked women how many jobs they had applied for during the first, second, most recent, and intervening months out of work. The data are not reliable in detail, since women who made many applications obviously could not be precise about specific numbers, and their recollection of the time of applications may have been faulty. Moreover, the number of applications is influenced by the number of suitable jobs of which the respondents were aware, as well as by the depth of the respondent's commitment to finding market employment. Nevertheless, Table 4.2.1.4 does provide relevant evidence on the amount and timing of job-search activity.

Three general conclusions emerge from changes in the number of job applications over the time out of work. First, the proportion of women applying for any job at all in any single month was low: the largest number of women applying for jobs in any month was seventy-four, in the first month of job search — only 59 per cent of women who were out of work for at least a week. Secondly, the number of women applying for jobs declined after the first month, but increased in the month immediately before the interview. The size of this increase may be

Table 4.2.1.4
Proportion of women applying for specific numbers of jobs (by month)

No. of job applications	First month (%)	Second month (%)	Intervening months (%)	Last month (%)
1	38	42	32.5	53
2– 5	45	40	47.5	33
6–10	14	13	10	9
11–20	1	2	7.5	5
21 +	3	2	2.5	–
N	74	45	40	57

Percentage is that of women who applied for jobs that month.

exaggerated, women not remembering precisely whether they applied for a specific job over a month ago or within the last month. Moreover, the 'last month' is an uneven length of time away from the date of leaving the pre-redundancy job: the length of time was between four and seven months, and it might have been expected that there would be fewer applications from women who had been out of work for seven rather than for four months. However, this was not a major factor: although there were differences in the number of job applications submitted in the last month between women with different periods of time out of work, the number of women making job applications did not decline significantly with length of time out of work. There is thus evidence that the major change in the likelihood of applying for jobs at all is after the first month: thereafter the likelihood of applying appears to change little, at least within the time period covered by our study, up to thirty-three weeks. However, thirdly, women were applying for fewer jobs in the last month than they had done in the first month. Although the number of women applying for jobs increased in the month before the interview over the level in preceding months, the number of jobs applied for was, on average, fewer than in previous months: the women applying for jobs applied for an average of 4.94 jobs in the first month, 4.47 jobs in the second month, 4.7 jobs in the months intervening between the second and last months, and three jobs in the last month. More women applied for jobs in the last month out of work before the interview than any month except the first, but they applied for fewer jobs.

Detailed interpretation of the data on application rates and their changes over time is difficult, for variations in application rates could be due to success, failure, or lack of interest. Obviously, women who secure jobs quickly are likely to submit fewer applications than women who have difficulty in finding work. Alternatively, women who have no success in obtaining interviews are likely to be discouraged, and are likely to reduce their level of application. Finally, women who are not greatly concerned about re-employment are unlikely to submit many job applications.

As a means of showing the effect of the experience of unemployment on application rates initial attention is focused only on those women who were unemployed at the time of the second interview: women who submitted few applications because of their rapid success are therefore excluded. Table 4.2.1.5 summarizes the distribution of application rates of women who were unemployed at the time of the second interview.

As Table 4.2.1.5 indicates, there was no evidence of discouragement amongst the relevant group of women: more women submitted applications in the last month than had submitted applications in any previous month. The data may not be wholly reliable: job applications made in the recent past are more likely to be remembered than job applications made several months earlier. However, there is no indication that, among women seeking work at the time of the second interview, the number of applications was declining. There is therefore no support for the view that women who were still looking for work were discouraged to the point of not submitting applications. This was so, regardless

Table 4.2.1.5
Changes in application rates (women looking for work at second interview only)

	First month N	Second month N	Intervening months N	Last month N
1	11	16	10	23
2– 5	18	11	13	15
6–10	4	3	2	5
11–20	–	1	2	1
21 +	–	–	–	–

of the number of months intervening between the second and last months, which ranged from 0 to 4. In short, the women who were looking for work at the time of the second interview were as energetic as they had been earlier: however, some women had dropped out of the labour market completely and were temporarily retired at the time of the second interview, despite having applied for jobs earlier.

We have shown earlier that there were differences between women in different companies, age groups, occupational statuses, and domestic circumstances in the likelihood of their beginning to look for work before leaving their previous firm. There were also differences in application rates between different social groupings. Since the numbers of women were so few, we do not present data on all the variations. Instead, we have concentrated on two which we examine in turn: age and occupational status.

Table 4.2.1.6 summarizes the data on application rates and age: in view of the small numbers, the detailed data have not been presented. By the presentation of average figures, the relative size of the different age groups is ignored: there were far fewer women looking for work in the extreme age categories, under 25 and over 55, than in the middle three categories. Moreover, the most frequent number of applications submitted, by every age group in every month, was one. Nevertheless, four general conclusions emerge. First, although the

Table 4.2.1.6
Age and job-application rate (by month)

	Age				
	≤ 25	25–34	34–44	45–54	55 +
Average no. of job applications					
First month	14.17	4.4	2.29	7.82	2.2
Second month	7.5	2.36	3.72	7.08	1
Intervening months	8.67	2.36	6.54	4.17	1
Last month	9.00	2.82	3.19	1.84	1

$N =$ Average number of jobs applied for.

number of women aged under 25 was small, their application rate was very high: their job prospects were relatively bright, as was shown in Section 1 (pp. 158–9), but those actively looking for work were looking very actively. Secondly, women aged 55 or more were relatively inactive in applying for jobs. Thirdly, women aged 25–34 applied for fewer jobs, on average, than women aged 35–44 and 45–54. Finally, there were few systematic differences in application rates between women aged 35–44 and women aged 45–54.

The evidence presented in Table 4.2.1.6 also shows variations in the impact of length of time out of work in application rates by different age groups. Women aged 55 + submitted fewer applications, on average, than women in the other age groups even in the first month after leaving their pre-redundancy employment. But they submitted even fewer in later months. Similarly, there is a significant drop in the application rates of women aged 45–54: whereas they applied on average for 7.82 jobs in the first month after leaving, they applied for only 1.84 jobs in the most recent months. Amongst women in the age groups 25–34 and 35–44 there is no similar trend downwards: in the former group women applied for more jobs, on average, in the last month than in the second and intervening months, whilst women in the latter group applied for more jobs, on average, in the last month than in the first month. There was also no decline in the average number of applications submitted by women in the youngest age group, the average number applied for being higher (9.00) than in the second and intervening months.

As Table 4.2.1.7 shows, clerical workers and semi-skilled manual workers made more job applications than other groups: unskilled manual workers had an especially low application rate. Differences in application rates reflected the number of vacant jobs for which the women thought they were eligible and which they would have been willing to do: clerical (group 2) and semi-skilled manual (group 3) workers thought that there were more vacancies for which they were eligible (as shown below, pp. 196–7, they were not more catholic in the jobs they were prepared to consider than other groups, clerical workers being especially restricted in the type of jobs they were looking for). The ap-

Table 4.2.1.7
Occupational status and job-application rate (by month)

	Occupational status				
	Prof./Admin./ Supervisory	Clerical	Semi-skilled	Slightly skilled	Unskilled
First month	4.40	7.89	4.85	2.43	2.00
Second month	2.14	3.30	6.63	4.20	1.50
Intervening months	3.00	4.70	6.50	2.30	3.50
Last month	2.50	4.14	3.08	2.0	1.60

N = Average number of jobs applied for by women applying for jobs.

plication rates for professional, administrative, and supervisory (group 1) workers were lower than for clerical or semi-skilled workers, reflecting the limited range of vacancies for which they thought they were eligible. The low number of applications made by unskilled manual workers (group 5) is also notable, reflecting the limited openings available to them: they submitted fewer job applications than any other occupational status group in every time period except 'intervening months', where their application rate was higher than that of professional, administrative, and supervisory, and semi-skilled workers.

All groups of women submitted fewer job applications, on average, in the last month before the interview than in the first month, the rank order of occupational-status groups being the same on both occasions. The decline in the number of applications was especially marked amongst groups who had submitted relatively large numbers of applications in the first month: the application rate for occupational group 1 dropped from 4.40 to 2.50, for group 2 from 7.89 to 4.14, and for group 3 4.85 to 3.08, compared with a decline from 2.43 to 2.00 for slightly skilled workers and 2.00 to 1.60 for unskilled workers. Although the numbers involved in all groups, especially groups 1 and 5, are small, and thus averages are liable to distortion by single examples of women making large numbers of applications, the trend is clear: with lengthening periods out of work the women were submitting fewer job applications on average, with a particular decline in the number of women submitting very large numbers of job applications.

In this subsection we have been concerned solely with the limited subject of the timing of the process of job search. This has shown substantial variations in the timing of beginning the process of job search, and in the number and timing of job applications. However, timing is only one limited aspect of the process of job search. Moreover, timing was only partially determined by the women themselves: the policies of their previous employers, and the scheduling of their leaving dates, exercised a major influence upon the commencement of job search. Furthermore, the extent and timing of job applications was influenced by the availability of suitable jobs, as well as by the women's actions in looking:

they cannot therefore be used as a direct measure of commitment to the labour market. Nevertheless, the data on the timing of job search provided initial evidence on commitment: 76 per cent of women interviewed began to look for work before leaving their pre-redundancy job or within four weeks of leaving, and a further 7 per cent were offered jobs without looking. The commitment did not lead to great success, even measured by the number of job applications: more women applied for jobs in the first month after leaving their pre-redundancy employment than in any other month, but they comprised only 59 per cent of women with experience of unemployment.

We now turn to the methods used in looking for work, and the women's views on the effectiveness of different methods.

4.2.2 Methods used in job search

The search for work can be undertaken through the formal institutions set up to facilitate the process or informally, by asking amongst friends and family, and by calling on potential employers on chance. The most frequently used methods of job search were formal: 78 per cent of women sought jobs through the newspapers, and 77 per cent used the Job Centre; 56 per cent asked around among friends, and 27 per cent amongst family members. The newspapers were thought to be the most effective means of finding a job, although by only a minority — 20 per cent; few women could mention three effective methods of looking for work, and 14 per cent said that no method was effective. The Job Centre was mentioned by more women as the least effective means of finding work than any other method, 24.5 per cent. As measured by the number of applications the women made as a result of the different methods used, newspapers were the most effective method: 62 per cent of women who used newspapers applied for jobs advertised, and 37 per cent obtained interviews. Only 6 per cent successfully obtained jobs through that method. Comparable figures for women using Job Centres were: 43 per cent applied for jobs through the Job Centre and 25 per cent obtained interviews. Eleven per cent were successful through using the Job Centre.

The data on methods of job search used are summarized in Table 4.2.2.1, showing the proportion of women using specific methods. Each woman used, on average, 3.23 methods of looking for work. As we have shown, newspapers and the Job Centre were by far the most frequently used methods of looking for work, with asking friends as the third most popular: no other method was used by even a third of women. No woman used her union at all, although almost all women had been union members in their previous employment.

The popularity of different methods of job search varied from group to group. A distinction can be drawn between formal, market mechanisms (newspapers, Job Centre, secretarial and private employment agencies, and shop-window advertisements) and informal methods (asking family, friends, and applying to firms on spec whether in person, by telephone or by writing). It might be expected, on general grounds, that reliance upon one type of method or another

Table 4.2.2.1
Methods of job search used

	Percentage	N
Newspapers	78	120
Job Centre	77	118
Asked friends	56.5	87
Asked family	27	42
Writing to firms on spec	22	34
Telephoning firms on spec	21	33
Visiting firms on spec	13	20
Shop window ads	11	17
Secretarial/private employment agencies	8	13
Recruited from previous firm directly	5	8
Factory-gate advertisements	3	5
Trade union	–	–
Other	1	1

Percentage is that of women who looked for work: multiple response permitted.

would be determined by two factors, of unequal weight: the local labour market, and the type of occupation involved. Women in major metropolitan areas, as in case study C, might be expected to rely upon formal methods more than women living in smaller communities, as in case study A and factory B1. Similarly, women in occupational-status group 1 (professional, administrative, and supervisory) and in group 2 (clerical) might be expected to be part of a wider labour market, reached primarily through impersonal methods, than women in manual jobs. To explore this issue we have examined formal and informal methods separately, showing the differences between areas and between occupational status groups.

As Table 4.2.2.2 indicates, there were differences between areas in the use made of different methods of job search, but the differences do not indicate any close connection between local labour markets and reliance upon formal methods of job search; the differences were less systematic. The use made of secretarial and private employment agencies was confined to cases with large numbers of clerical workers, case studies D and E; following up factory-gate advertisements was only done in the case of manual workers, in the South East market town and the Midlands engineering case study. More significantly, women living in the major metropolitan areas did make more use of newspapers than women in other areas. But there was no link between type of labour market and use made of the Job Centre: women in case studies E and A made less use of the Job Centres than women in other areas did, but this was not because of the nature of the local labour market.

Much less use was made of informal methods than formal methods, but there was no general contrast between smaller communities and major metropolitan areas. Women were more likely to ask around amongst their family and friends in areas A and B1 than elsewhere, as is shown in Table 4.2.2.3, but the differences were small: 31 per cent of women in area A and 36 per cent of women in area B1 asked members of their family, compared with 28 per cent in area D, 26 per cent in area C2, 25 per cent in each of areas B2 and E, and only 8 per cent in area C1. Women in case study A were more likely to ask their friends about jobs than in any other area, 66 per cent, but again the differences were relatively small.

Table 4.2.2.2
Use of formal methods of job search (by area)

	A (%)	B1 (%)	B2 (%)	C1 (%)	C2 (%)	D (%)	E (%)	p
Newspapers	69	73	50	92	81.5	88	90	0.053
Job Centre	66	91	83	92	74	84	60	0.094
Secretarial/private agencies	3	–	–	8	–	28	20	0.001
Factory ads	6	–	–	15	4	–	–	0.151
Shop-window ads	11	14	–	38.5	11	8	–	0.027
N	35	22	12	13	27	25	20	

Percentage is that of women mentioning given method.

Table 4.2.2.3
Use of informal methods of job search (by area)

	A (%)	B1 (%)	B2 (%)	C1 (%)	C2 (%)	D (%)	E (%)	p
Asking family	31	36	25	8	26	28	25	0.697
Asking friends	66	59	58	61.5	48	48	55	0.816
Recruited from previous firm directly	9	–	42	–	–	–	–	0.000
Applying on spec by phone	31	18	8	31	26	4	25	0.169
Applying on spec in person	17	18	25	38	4	–	5	0.010
Applying on spec in writing	26	18	–	23	11	28	40	0.126

Percentage is that of women mentioning given method.

There were few differences in the use made of different methods of job search by women in different occupational status groups, and no confirmation for the suggestion that formal methods would be more likely to be used by women in non-manual occupations than women in manual occupations: indeed, women in professional, administrative, and supervisory jobs were more likely to ask members of their family about jobs than women in any other occupational-status group, 42 per cent doing so, compared with 27 per cent overall. Table 4.2.2.4 summarizes the data on the use made of different methods of job search by occupational status.

Table 4.2.2.4
Methods of job search (by occupational-status group)

	Occupational status					
	Prof./Admin./ Supervisory	Clerical	Semi-skilled	Slightly skilled	Unskilled	p
Formal						
Newspapers	100	87	72	70	100	0.034
Job Centre	83	73	77	75	78	0.968
Secretarial/employment agency	33	27	1	–	–	0.000
Ads outside factory	–	7	3	4	–	0.752
Shop window ads	8	7	15	11	–	0.592
Informal						
Asked family	42	23	28	21	33	0.707
Asked friends	67	43	57	61	67	0.522
Recruited from previous firm	–	–	11	–	–	0.065
Applied on spec by phone	8	–	28	25	22	0.124
Applied on spec in person	–	3	16	25	–	0.045
Applied on spec in writing	42	33	13	32	–	0.015

There were thus few differences between occupational-status groups in the relative use of the most popular methods: the three most popular methods with professional, administrative, and supervisory staff, newspapers, Job Centre, and asking friends, were the three most popular with all other occupational-status groups, the only variation in ranking being a slightly greater use of Job Centres than newspapers by semi-skilled and slightly skilled manual workers.

There was thus only slight evidence to indicate a connection between the character of the community and the use of particular methods of job search, or between occupational statuses and the use made of different methods of job search. The most common methods used were newspapers, Job Centres, and asking amongst friends. Nor were there systematic differences linked with age or marital status. Younger workers were more likely to ask other members of their family than older workers (40 per cent of women aged under 25, 35.5 per cent of women aged 25–34, 31 per cent of women aged 35–44, 20 per cent of women aged 45–54, and 8 per cent of women aged 55 +), probably reflecting the degree of contact between the women interviewed and relatives likely to be knowledgeable about possible jobs. Older women were more likely to ask their friends than younger women were, under 25, 40 per cent, 25–34, 55 per cent, 35–44 64 per cent, 45–54 50 per cent, and over 55 67 per cent – although the relationship was not statistically significant.

In addition to general questions about the use made of different methods of job search we examined two specific issues in greater detail: the use of newspapers, and the extent to which the women came into contact with people able to provide information about jobs. A large number of women said that they used newspapers in looking for work (78 per cent); an even larger majority said they looked at job advertisements in newspapers — 95 per cent, with little difference between area, occupational status, age, or marital status. The newspapers used were overwhelmingly local ones — 99 per cent used local ones, compared with only 10 per cent looking in national newspapers (counting the (*Manchester*) *Guardian* as a national newspaper), and 7 per cent using other printed media.

Access to formal methods of job search is in principle unrestricted (although buying several newspapers can be expensive, and transport costs to Job Centres could be substantial). However, informal methods depend upon local contacts. We therefore asked women whether they had opportunity to meet people able to tell them about jobs where they worked. Table 4.2.2.5 summarizes the data by area.

Table 4.2.2.5
Contact with people able to tell about jobs (by area)

	Area							Total
	A (%)	B1 (%)	B2 (%)	C1 (%)	C2 (%)	D (%)	E (%)	(%)
Contact	80	59	45.5	38.5	52	43.5	53	57
No contact	20	41	54.5	61.5	48	56.5	47	43

Women in case study A, carried out in a medium-sized market town, had more contacts with others who could tell them about jobs than women in the other areas; women in area C1 were especially likely to feel isolated from others who could tell them about jobs. Women in the youngest (under 25) and the oldest (55 +) age categories were less likely than others to believe that they came into contact with possible sources of information about jobs. Similarly, women in slightly skilled and unskilled jobs were more likely to feel isolated than women in other occupational-status groups.

To the question of how they came to meet people able to tell them about jobs, the most common answer was simply through friends, mentioned by 38 per cent of women who said that they had such contacts. Social clubs, pubs, social outings, keep-fit classes, and the Church were also mentioned. We were especially interested in the role of ex-work mates: 34 per cent of women who had such contacts said that they were through ex-work mates. This was especially important in case studies A and B1, where contacts were maintained with former work colleagues, in case study A on a regular basis through informal Friday morning gatherings. The contrast is especially marked with C2; women in C2 comprised 18 per cent of respondents, but only 4 per cent of those who felt that they heard about possible jobs through former work mates. There were two major reasons for not having relevant contacts: either that their friends were out of work like themselves, mentioned by 33 per cent, or that they had few friends and did not go out very much, mentioned by 35 per cent.

The three most frequently used methods of job search were newspapers, Job Centres, and asking amongst friends. We were, of course, interested in establishing the most effective methods of looking for work. Effectiveness was examined in four ways: the methods the women said were the most, and the least, effective; the methods that led to the most job applications, the methods that led to the most interviews, and the methods that led to the most jobs.

As Table 4.2.2.6 indicates, there was considerable difference of view on which were the most effective ways of finding suitable jobs.

Table 4.2.2.6
Responses to *Which methods did/do you find most effective in producing suitable jobs for you to apply for?*

	N	Percentage
Newspapers	39	25
Job Centre	34	22
None	28	18
Asking friends	24	16
Don't know	11	7
On spec in person	9	6
On spec by phone	7	5
On spec in writing	5	3
Asking family	3	2
	(N = 154)	

Percentage is that of women answering job-search questions.

The most frequently mentioned way was through newspaper advertisements, mentioned by 25 per cent of women who actively sought jobs; it was also the method used most frequently. The second most frequently mentioned method was the Job Centres, mentioned by 22 per cent, and the third asking friends, mentioned by 16 per cent. However, there was little conviction or enthusiasm: 18 per cent said that no method was effective, whilst a further 7 per cent said that they did not know. All other methods were mentioned as being particularly effective by fewer than ten women. It is hardly surprising that the most widely used methods of job search were also thought to be the most effective. However, very few respondents who used such methods also thought that they were the most effective. Although 78 per cent of women said that they used newspapers as a means of looking for work, only 25 per cent said that they found them the most effective method; although 77 per cent said that they used the Job Centre, only 22 per cent said that it was the most effective method; and although 56.5 per cent asked friends about jobs, only 16 per cent said that it was the most effective method.

Although there were no differences between areas in the likelihood of asking friends for jobs, there were differences in evaluations of the effectiveness of the method. Women in case study A, and in area C1, were more likely to refer to asking friends as the most effective way of looking for work. Also, women aged 45–54 were more likely to see asking friends as the most effective way of looking for work than any other method. Finally, manual workers were more likely than non-manual workers to regard asking friends as the most effective method: manual workers comprised 69 per cent of respondents, but 92 per cent of those who thought that asking friends was the most effective means of finding work. In short, the third most popular effective method was asking friends, but its popularity as an effective means was confined almost exclusively to manual workers.

More women thought that formal methods of job search were more effective than informal methods, amongst both manual and non-manual workers. Amongst manual workers, there were no systematic differences between different occupational groups in the perceived effectiveness of newspapers and the Job Centre: amongst non-manual workers women in professional, supervisory, and administrative jobs were far more likely to see newspapers as the most effective, whilst there was little difference in perceptions of their relative effectiveness amongst clerical workers.

Although the numbers involved are small, there are indications that the perceived effectiveness of different methods changes with length of time out of work. It is hardly surprising that pessimism about the effectiveness of any method of job search tended to increase as the length of time out of work increased: women out of work for sixteen weeks or more comprised 61 per cent of the relevant group, and 68 per cent of those who did not think any method of looking for work was effective. The perceived effectiveness of newspapers also declined: women who were out of work only a relatively brief period were more likely to regard newspapers as the most effective, informal methods being perceived as more effective by women out of work for longer periods. However, there were major differences in occupational status and age between women experiencing short and long periods out of work, and it is impossible to disentangle the effects of occupational status and age from the effects of length of time out of work.

The reasons for believing that particular methods were effective were very varied, and responses too few to analyse statistically. In explaining why newspapers were the best method, the women mentioned that the jobs advertised were new and more numerous than elsewhere. Also, it was possible to ring immediately for application forms. The Job Centre was seen as being effective because it put all the jobs it had available on display, and was therefore convenient to consult; the Job Centre was in a better position than anyone else to match skills and experience to the jobs available; and the Job Centre would take the initiative and telephone if a suitable job was available. Asking around amongst friends was stated as being the best because friends gave early notification of jobs, and could give useful recommendations to future employers. Finally, calling on firms on spec was seen as the most effective because it enabled the women to see what the job really involved, and also showed employers that the applicants were really interested.

The women were also asked about the methods they had found least effective. By far the most frequently mentioned were the Job Centre, mentioned by 31 per cent of the relevant group, and the newspapers, mentioned by 16 per cent. Although a significant number of women had asked friends, very few thought that it was the least effective method. In view of the limited use made of other methods, figures on their perceived ineffectiveness are unhelpful. Evaluations of the Job Centres varied from area to area: whereas 23 per cent of women in area A, and 14 per cent in area B1, thought that the Job Centre was the least effective in their experience, 46 per cent in area C1 and 44 per cent in area C2 thought that the Job Centre the least effective method. There were no general differences in evaluation by age, occupational status, or marital status. The major reason for the ineffectiveness of methods used was simply the paucity of jobs available, specifically mentioned by 20 per cent of women looking for work, whilst other women commented that they were often too late in applying. Small numbers of women made specific comments. Job Centres were criticized for failing to remove cards once jobs had gone, for having only low-paid jobs, and for being badly organized. Newspapers were seen as ineffective because jobs had often gone before the women were able to submit applications, or because they advertised jobs requiring skills or experience that the women did not have. Telephoning on spec was ineffective because it always resulted in a negative answer, whilst writing on spec was ineffective because firms had more enquiries than they could cope with, and therefore did not bother to reply. Visiting firms on spec was ineffective because any disadvantages (especially age) were obvious. Finally, shop-window ads were ineffective because they were primarily directed at school leavers.

The effectiveness of job-search methods is not simply a matter of subjective assessment: applications submitted, interviews obtained, and jobs found are more precise measures. These are examined in turn.

As Table 4.2.2.7 indicates, more women submitted applications for jobs seen in newspapers than for those heard of through any other means: seventy-four women, or 62 per cent of women who said that they used newspapers in looking for work actually applied for jobs they had seen there; fifty-one women, or 43 per cent of women who reported using the Job Centre, applied for jobs heard of through the Job Centre; and thirty-seven women, or 43 per cent of women who reported asking friends, applied for jobs heard of through friends. Newspapers were thus the most widely used source of information on jobs for which applications were submitted, followed by the Job Centre and then friends — as would be expected from the relative frequency of usage of the different methods.

Table 4.2.2.7
Source of information on jobs applied for

	N	Percentage
Family	11	26
Friends	37	43
Newspapers	74	62
Job Centre	51	43
Secretarial/private employment agencies	5	38
On spec by phone	11	33
On spec in person	8	40
On spec in writing	12	34

N = Women submitting applications (any number) for jobs via method.
Percentage is that of women reporting using method (see p. 000).

Newspapers were more effective as a means of generating applications than the Job Centre, with an 'application-generating' rate of 62 per cent, compared with 43 per cent for the Job Centre: the contrast between the two would be greater if the number of applications submitted by each woman was taken into account: individual women submitted a larger number of applications in response to newspaper advertisements than in response to information acquired at Job Centres. Since replying to newspaper advertisements required less effort than visiting the Job Centre, this is hardly surprising. Asking one's family about jobs was a relatively ineffective way of acquiring information about jobs for which applications could be submitted.

Submitting applications was of course at the initiative of the respondent: being called for interview depended upon the assessment of the potential suitability of the applicant for the post by the prospective employer. Table 4.2.2.8 summarizes the data on the source of information on jobs for which interviews were obtained, together with the proportion of women who used a given method being successful in obtaining an interview by that method. Newspapers remained the most 'successful' method, a higher proportion of women obtaining interviews from replying to newspaper advertisements than by any other method. Not surprisingly, telephoning firms on spec was a particularly unsuccessful way of obtaining interviews, although asking members of the family was only slightly more successful. Asking friends was slightly more successful than the Job Centre in generating interviews.

The most important criterion for evaluating the effectiveness of alternative methods of job search is the extent to which they lead to jobs. As indicated earlier, the women obtained seventy-eight jobs: seventy-two women obtained one job, and six had two jobs following the redundancies. On this criterion the most successful method was asking friends: twenty-three jobs, or 29 per cent, were obtained by this method. The Job Centre was the second-most effective, thirteen jobs, or 17 per cent, being obtained through the Job Centre. Replying

Table 4.2.2.8
Source of information on jobs for which interviews were obtained

	N	Percentage
Family	9	21
Friends	27	31
Newspapers	44	37
Job Centre	29	25
Secretarial/private employment agencies	3	23
On spec by phone	5	15
On spec in person	6	30
On spec in writing	5	26

to newspaper advertisements led to only eight jobs, or 10 per cent of the jobs obtained. Asking one's family, applying on spec by telephone, or applying on spec by writing each produced five jobs; applying on spec in person led to three jobs. In addition, nine jobs were obtained through former employers, either directly or as a result of employer action with other firms. No other method led to more than two jobs. Hence some methods of job search were more effective at generating interviews than in generating jobs. Although 37 per cent of women who used newspapers obtained interviews by replying to advertisement, only 10 per cent of the jobs obtained were obtained through that method; although only 31 per cent of women who asked friends obtained interviews by doing so, the same proportion obtained jobs through that method; although only 25 per cent of women who reported using the Job Centre obtained interviews for jobs through that method, 17 per cent of the jobs obtained were obtained through that method. In short, asking friends was not the most common method of looking for work, nor the most effective in producing jobs for which applications could be submitted, nor the most effective in producing interviews; but it was the most effective, absolutely and compared with other methods, in producing jobs.

Although statistics on application, interview, and job-finding rates provide a basis for comparing the effectiveness of alternative methods of job search, they are profoundly misleading in themselves. The demand for women with different skills and experience (and ages) differed between and within areas: the value of crude 'placement' rates as indices of effectiveness is therefore limited. In particular, it was more difficult for manual workers, especially manual workers aged 45 or more, to get jobs than for non-manual workers, especially young clerical workers: methods resulting in the placement of more 'difficult' workers might thus be more effective than the overall figures indicate. We have therefore examined differences in 'interview-generating' rate and in success rate by area and by occupational-status group: Table 4.2.2.9 summarizes the data on interviews by area, and Table 4.2.2.10 by occupational status.

Women in the Labour Market 181

Table 4.2.2.9
Number of women obtaining interviews in each area (by method)

	Area							Total N	Total using method
	A N	B1 N	B2 N	C1 N	C2 N	D N	E N		
Family	–	1	–	–	3	3	2	9	42
Friends	10	1	1	4	3	4	4	27	87
Newspapers	5	4	1	3	7	14	10	44	120
Job Centre	7	4	1	2	2	12	1	29	118
Secretarial/private employment agency	–	–	–	–	–	2	1	3	13
On spec by phone	2	–	1	1	1	–	–	5	33
On spec in person	3	–	1	1	1	–	–	6	20
On spec in writing	1	–	–	–	1	2	1	5	34
Total N of women in area	35	22	12	13	27	25	20		

Table 4.2.2.10
Number of women obtaining interviews in each occupational status (by method)

	Occupational-status group					Total N	Total using method
	Prof./Admin./ Supervisory N	Clerical N	Semi-skilled N	Slightly skilled N	Unskilled N		
Family	–	3	4	1	1	9	42
Friends	1	4	13	8	1	27	87
Newspapers	5	16	12	7	4	44	120
Job Centre	3	8	12	4	2	29	118
Secretarial/private agency	1	2	–	–	–	3	13
On spec by phone	–	–	5	–	–	5	33
On spec in person	–	–	4	2	–	6	20
On spec in writing	2	1	2	–	–	5	34
No. of women in occupational status	12	30	75	28	9		

Because of the small numbers involved, and the differences in proportions made by using different denominators, the data have been presented in absolute rather than in proportional numerical terms. As Table 4.2.2.9 shows, there were marked differences between areas in the relative effectiveness of different methods in generating interviews: newspapers were more effective than Job Centres in generating interviews in the Midlands and in case study D, but not more so elsewhere. The difference was largely due to differences in the ability to generate interviews for clerical workers: replying to newspaper advertisements led to interviews for sixteen clerical workers, but the Job Centres involved obtained interviews for only eight clerical workers. Whether the difference in the relative performance of newspapers and Job Centres was due to their being concerned with different clerical workers, or to the failure of potential employers to notify Job Centres, it is impossible to say on the data available: it was probably due to the failure of potential employers to notify Job Centres of vacancies.

Although newspapers were more effective in obtaining interviews than the Job Centres, Job Centres were more effective in producing jobs. Overall, thirteen women obtained jobs through Job Centres, compared with seven through newspapers. The most effective Job Centres in this respect were in areas D, A, and B1: eight women obtained jobs through Job Centres in area D, three in area A, and two in B1 — all the jobs obtained through Job Centres. Newspaper advertisement led to jobs for four women in area D, and one in each of areas A, C2, and E: no woman obtained jobs through replying to newspapers advertisements in areas B1, B2, and C1. The most effective method of obtaining jobs was through asking friends in all areas except B2 and D; hence eight women in area A, five women in area E, four women in area C1, three women in area D, and one woman in each of areas B1 and C1 obtained jobs through friends. In area B2 the only women who obtained jobs obtained them with their former employer; in area D the Job Centre was the most effective method. There was thus no indication that the relative effectiveness of formal and informal methods differed between different types of community or different types of labour market: informal methods were the most effective in a medium sized market town, area A, and in a major conurbation, areas C1, C2, and E.

There was some evidence to suggest that formal methods of job search were more effective for non-manual workers in producing jobs than informal methods, although informal methods were important for both groups. Table 4.2.2.11 presents evidence on the relationship between job status and the method successfully used to obtain post-redundancy jobs. As Table 4.2.2.11 shows, for women in occupational status groups 1 and 2, non-manual workers, the Job Centres were the single most successful means of obtaining jobs; a third of the professional, administrative, and supervisory women who obtained jobs obtained them through Job Centres, and 29 per cent of clerical workers, compared with 17 and 19 per cent respectively who obtained them through friends. On the other hand, only 13 per cent of semi-skilled manual workers, 9 per cent of slightly skilled manual workers, and no unskilled manual worker obtained her job via Job Centres, compared with 26, 64, and 67 per cent who obtained them through friends. (The figure for semi-skilled workers is distorted by the number who obtained jobs with or through their former employer.) Replying to newspaper advertisements was not a very successful method of obtaining jobs, especially for manual workers: only three manual workers obtained jobs through replying to newspaper advertisements, and even for clerical workers newspaper advertisements were less successful than the Job Centres.

In this section we have presented evidence on the methods used in job search,

Table 4.2.2.11
Method of obtaining job (by occupational status)

	Prof./Admin./ Supervisory (%)	Clerical (%)	Semi-skilled (%)	Slightly skilled (%)	Unskilled (%)	Total (%)	N
Family	–	5	10	9	–	7	5
Friends	17	19	26	64	67	31	22
Newspapers	–	19	3	9	33	10	7
Job Centre	33	29	13	9	–	18	13
Secretarial/private employment agency	17	5	–	–	–	3	2
Previous employer	17	5	23	–	–	12.5	9
On spec by phone	–	–	13	–	–	6	4
On spec in person	–	5	3	–	–	3	2
On spec in writing	17	5	6.5	–	–	6	4
Factory-gate ad	–	–	–	9	–	1	1
Shop-window ad	–	–	3	–	–	1	1
Other	–	9.5	–	–	–	3	2
N	6	21	31	11	3		72

($p = 0.314$)

Note: For convenience of comparison with previous data the table ignores the six jobs obtained between the redundancies and the second interview by the women who had two jobs: the inclusion of the six jobs would not change the table substantively.

and the effectiveness of different methods. The three most widely used methods of job search were consulting newspapers, visiting Job Centres, and asking around amongst friends. More women mentioned newspapers as the most effective means of finding out about jobs than mentioned any other method, but the method was named as the most effective by only a minority of women. The second method most frequently mentioned as being the most effective was using the Job Centre, followed by asking friends. The Job Centre and the newspapers were also most frequently mentioned as the least effective, largely because they were the methods of which women had the most experience. Newspapers were the most widely used source of information on jobs for which applications were submitted, and also the most effective means of obtaining interviews — although even newspapers only led to interviews for a minority of the women who used them. The most effective method of obtaining a job was by asking around amongst friends, although Job Centres were moderately effective for non-manual workers.

4.2.3 Female handicaps

Workers are not a homogeneous group, and the demand for different kinds of workers differs: we were concerned to see what difficulties the women felt themselves to be under, whether deriving from the economic situation in general, or from their own characteristics in particular. It is hardly surprising that the majority of women interviewed said that they experienced difficulty in finding a job after the redundancy — 61 per cent. The degree of difficulty differed from area to area, and from job to job: difficulties were greater in the North West and the Midlands than in the South East, and more difficult for manual workers, except hand sewing machinists in the South East, than for non-manual workers. The major difficulties were due to the lack of jobs, but a minority of women also felt that they were handicapped by their age, lack of formal qualifications, or, amongst manual workers, sex. Very few women were inhibited from taking jobs by their family commitments. Although a minority of women felt they were handicapped in looking for jobs by their sex, there was no evidence of discrimination experienced on grounds of sex at the interview stage. There were few suggestions on how either government or private organizations should help women experiencing employment difficulties specifically, suggestions being the same as for men in the same situation.

As Table 4.2.3.1 shows, the majority of women interviewed experienced difficulty in finding a job, the difficulties being especially great in case studies B and C.

Table 4.2.3.1
Difficulty in finding jobs (by area)

	A (%)	B1 (%)	B2 (%)	C1 (%)	C2 (%)	D (%)	E (%)	Total (%)	N
Difficulty	44	82	58	85	67	56	50	61	92
No difficulty	37.5	18	17	15	30	32	50	30.5	46
Don't know/Not thought about it	19	–	17	–	4	8	–	7	11
Other	–	–	8	–	–	4	–	1	2
N	32	22	12	13	27	25	20		151

$(p = 0.041)$

The proportion reporting difficulty thus ranged from 85 per cent in C1 to 44 per cent in A. The contrasting experiences were not due solely to regional differences in themselves, but also to differences in the occupational composition of the groups in the different areas. In both the Midlands and the North West manual workers experienced more difficulty in finding work than non-manual workers. Hence the proportion of women reporting difficulty ranged from 82 per cent, in the North West area B1, manual workers, to 50 per cent in the Midlands area E, primarily clerical workers. (Only 58 per cent of former electronics-assembly workers in plant B2 reported difficulty, the relatively low proportion being due to a relatively large number of women retiring permanently from the labour force and therefore not looking for work.)

The importance of occupation is indicated clearly in more detailed analysis. As Table 4.2.3.2 indicates, under half of the women in administrative, clerical, and hand-sewing reported difficulty in finding work.

Table 4.2.3.2
Difficulty in finding jobs (by occupation)

	Occupation										Total
	Nurse (%)	Catering (%)	Administration (%)	Clerical (%)	Computing (%)	Machine sewing (%)	Hand sewing (%)	Electrical assembly (%)	Engineering assembly (%)	General service (%)	(%)
Difficulty	100	64	33	44	100	58	42	74	68	80	61
No difficulty	–	27	33	47	–	37.5	25	15	32	20	30.5
Don't know	–	9	–	9	–	4	33	7	–	–	7
Other	–	–	33	–	–	–	–	4	–	–	1
N	2	11	3	34	1	24	12	27	22	15	

($p = 0.002$)

The small numbers in some of the occupations renders detailed statistical analysis inappropriate. However, the overall pattern is clear. In general, manual workers were more likely to report difficulty than non-manual workers. But within each group there were important differences. Amongst manual workers sewing machinists were less likely to report difficulty than assembly workers or workers in general services (cleaning). Amongst non-manual workers clerical and administrative workers were less likely to report difficulty than women in more specialized — if sometimes more qualified and higher-paid — occupations, where the number of vacancies was likely to be few. When women were asked about their difficulty in finding a job that suited them there was a small overall increase in the number of women reporting difficulty (from 61 to 65 per cent), due largely to a jump in the number of hand-sewing machinists reporting difficulty: jobs were there but they were not seen as suitable (because of low pay and poor working conditions and lack of transport).

Overall differences in the reported difficulty of securing re-employment between occupations were not due to age: there was relatively little difference in age between clerical workers and engineering assembly workers. However, age was a relevant factor for specific occupations, notably electronic assembly and general services, where the women were handicapped by age as well as, in the former case, by a decline in demand for electronics assembly workers. As in previous studies, older workers were more likely to report employment difficulties than younger workers, although the small numbers in extreme age categories reduces the significance of the findings: the data are summarized in Table 4.2.3.3.

Table 4.2.3.3
Difficulty in securing jobs (by age)

	Age					
	≤ 25 (%)	25–34 (%)	35–44 (%)	45–54 (%)	55 + (%)	
Difficulty	50	55	63	61	75	
No difficulty	50	29	30	32	17	
Don't know	–	16	4	7	8	
Other	–	–	4	–	–	
N	10	31	54	44	12	151

($p = 0.487$)

Women under 25 were less likely to report difficulty, women over 55 more likely, than women in intervening years.

It is hardly surprising that the likelihood of reporting difficulty in finding work increased with length of time out of work: the proportion reporting difficulty ranged from 17 per cent of women with no experience of unemployment to 100 per cent of women out of work for thirty-two weeks or more.

Table 4.2.3.4
Difficulty in finding jobs (by weeks out of work)

	0 (%)	1–3 (%)	4–7 (%)	8–11 (%)	12–15 (%)	16–19 (%)	20–3 (%)	24–7 (%)	28–31 (%)	32+ (%)	Total (%)
Difficulty	17	33	50	58	67	70	78	57	100	100	61
No difficulty	79	67	50	33	20	10	16	14	–	–	30.5
Don't know	3	–	–	–	13	20	4	29	–	–	7
Other	–	–	–	8	–	–	2	–	–	–	1
N	29	3	6	12	15	10	50	14	6	6	151

The women believed that they were experiencing difficulty for two major reasons, the recession and their age. By far the most common reason for believing they were experiencing difficulty was the recession, and the lack of jobs available. However, a minority of women believed that they were experiencing difficulty because of their age. Table 4.2.3.5 summarizes the data on reasons for experiencing difficulty by age.

Table 4.2.3.5
Reasons for difficulty in finding jobs (by age)

	Age					Total
	≤ 25 (%)	25–34 (%)	35–44 (%)	45–54 (%)	55+ (%)	(%)
Recession	60	71	53	71	44	61
Age	–	12	15	44	67	27
Lack of qualifications	40	6	29	11	–	17
Not trying hard	–	–	12	7	–	7
Jobs not well enough paid	–	12	15	4	11	10
Other	–	24	15	11	33	16
N	5	17	34	27	9	92

Percentage is that of women answering question giving particular answer: two explanations were permitted.
N = Women who were experiencing difficulties.

Of course, for many women both the recession and their age were reasons for their experiencing difficulty in finding jobs.

When asked directly whether they felt handicapped in finding work by the fact that too many people were looking for too few jobs, a majority of women agreed: 78 per cent. There were, however, differences between areas: 65 per cent of women in area A thought that they were handicapped in this way, compared with 82 per cent in area B1, 92 per cent in area B2, 100 per cent in area C1, 89 per cent in area C2, 72 per cent in area D, and 70 per cent in area E. The women felt that they were handicapped, but not that their position was

Table 4.2.3.6
Responses to *Are there jobs available for women with your skills?* (by area)

	Area							Total (%)
	A (%)	B1 (%)	B2 (%)	C1 (%)	C2 (%)	D (%)	E (%)	
Yes	64	27	25	31	59	64	55	51
No	28	64	67	69	41	28	35	43
Don't know	8	9	8	–	–	8	10	6.5
N	36	32	12	13	27	25	20	155

($p = 0.059$)

hopeless. Hence 51 per cent of women thought that there were jobs available within reasonable travelling distance for people with their skills. The most pessimistic group were women in area B2, where only 25 per cent thought that there were such jobs, and area B1, where only 27 per cent thought that there were suitable jobs; the most optimistic were in area D (64 per cent) and area A (64 per cent). The data are summarized in Table 4.2.3.6.

Younger women were more optimistic than older women and, hardly surprisingly, women in full-time employment more optimistic than women looking for work (or in part-time employment). Significantly, clerical workers were more optimistic than any other occupational-status group, by a very considerable margin, as Table 4.2.3.7 shows.

Table 4.2.3.7
Responses to *Are there jobs available for women with your skills* (*by occupational status*)

	Prof./Admin./ Supervisory (%)	Clerical (%)	Semi-skilled (%)	Slightly skilled (%)	Unskilled (%)	Total (%)
Yes	58	81	45	36	33	51
No	33	10	51	57	57	43
Don't know	8	10	4	7	11	6.5
N	12	31	75	28	9	155

($p = 0.009$)

Although many women thought that jobs were available, they were very aware that there was considerable competition for them: 72 per cent of women thought that there were many women with the same skills as them competing for the jobs available, and only 14 per cent that there were not – the remaining 15 per cent not knowing.

Of the women who explained their difficulties in finding employment 27 per cent mentioned age disabilities. However, when specifically asked, a larger number of women said that they felt that they were handicapped by their age in competing for jobs for which they were otherwise qualified. Table 4.2.3.8 summarizes data on age and employment handicap by area: the percentage believing that they were handicapped by age varied from 77 per cent in C1 to 35 per cent in E (the same rank order, although at a higher level, as revealed in the analysis of spontaneous explanations for employment difficulties). More women felt that they were handicapped by age than did not do so: 50 per cent felt that they were regarded by potential employers as too old, 3 per cent too young, and 2 per cent as both too old for some jobs and too young for others. It is hardly surprising that the proportion of women thinking that they were handicapped by age increased with age, the proportion believing themselves to be too old ranging from 10 per cent of women aged under 25 to 92 per cent of women aged 55+. The women correctly appreciated that age was a handicap in finding re-employment – although the effects of age would of course have

Table 4.2.3.8
Percentage of women believing that they were handicapped by age (by area)

	Area							Total
	A (%)	B1 (%)	B2 (%)	C1 (%)	C3 (%)	D (%)	E (%)	(%)
Too old	47	54.5	50	77	41	56	35	50
Too young	6	–	8	–	4	–	–	3
Both	–	–	–	8	–	4	5	2
Don't know	3	4.5	17	–	4	–	–	1
Not handicapped	44	41	25	15	52	40	60	42.5
N	34	22	12	13	27	25	20	153

($p = 0.178$)

been less if the level of unemployment had been lower; during periods of high unemployment employers could be more selective in their recruitment.

Although a majority of women answered that they were experiencing difficulty in obtaining a job, a minority were nevertheless successful in obtaining jobs. We asked this group why they were able to obtain jobs when other people were experiencing difficulties. Since only forty-six women said that they were not experiencing, or had not experienced, difficulty in finding a job, and no single reason was mentioned by more than ten women, statistical analysis is inappropriate. The most frequently mentioned reason was that the women concerned had good contacts amongst potential employers (ten). Personal characteristics were also mentioned — determination (by seven women), personality (by three), attitude (by three), drive (by one), being young and attractive (by one). Luck was mentioned by seven women, and willingness to do anything by four. Reference to being in the right place at the right time was made by seven women. The women who obtained jobs thus saw a wide variety of reasons responsible for their relative success. The reasons why mainly related to luck, good fortune, and personal characteristics; only a very few references were made to possessing relevant experience, or to there being a demand for women with their particular skills.

The major difficulties mentioned by the women themselves as encountered in looking for jobs were the recession and, for the elderly, age. However, women have been seen as suffering from a number of disadvantages, especially family commitments and inability to work normal hours, lack of formal qualifications and lack of experience, which may make their prospects of re-employment especially difficult. Finally, there is the issue of the extent to which women felt themselves to be handicapped by their sex.

The women were not seriously handicapped by family commitments: 86.5 per cent of women were not restricted in their choice of jobs by family commitments, the only significant number of 'restricted' women being found amongst clothing-industry workers in area A, 28 per cent of whom were restricted by family commitments. When asked specifically about difficulties involved in working specific hours, only 8 per cent (nearly all of whom were in area A) felt that they were handicapped in this way. More substantial handicaps were the lack of formal qualifications and the lack of experience.

A substantial 42.5 per cent of women interviewed said that they felt that they were handicapped by a lack of formal qualifications. The lack of formal qualifications was felt especially by women in areas C1 (69 per cent), B2 (67 per cent), and C2 (56 per cent), where over half of the women felt that they were handicapped by a lack of formal qualifications. The lack of qualifications was felt especially by semi-skilled workers (engineering-assembly workers), 53 per cent of whom felt that they were handicapped by lack of formal qualifications. Slightly skilled workers (hand-sewers, catering workers, and storewomen) were less likely to feel that they were handicapped in this way, only 22 per cent feeling so, and clerical workers, 35.5 per cent. As would be expected, fewer women felt that they were handicapped by lack of experience than felt handicapped by lack of formal qualification, although only slightly fewer, 40 per cent compared with 42.5 per cent. As before, women in case studies B and C felt more handicapped than either the clothing-industry workers in A or the clerical workers in D and E.

Table 4.2.3.9
Percentage of women believing that they were handicapped by lack of formal qualifications (by area)

	Area							Total
	A (%)	B1 (%)	B2 (%)	C1 (%)	C2 (%)	D (%)	E (%)	(%)
Handicapped	21	45.5	67	69	56	44	25	42.5
Not handicapped	71	50	33	31	44	56	75	55
Don't know	9	4.5	–	–	–	–	–	3
N	34	22	12	13	27	25	20	153

($p = 0.020$)

There was relatively little feeling amongst the women interviewed that they were handicapped by their sex: only 16 per cent. The women were asked whether they were handicapped in obtaining jobs by 'sex, that is men are competing for and more likely to get the jobs you apply for': the distribution of replies between areas is shown in Table 4.2.3.10. As Table 4.2.3.10 shows, there were large differences between areas. Women in manual jobs in the Midlands engineering industry were much more likely than any other group to believe that they were handicapped by their sex: 38.5 per cent in C1 and 30 per cent in C2, compared with 17 per cent in the next-highest area, B2. Very few clothing-industry workers, and very few clerical workers, felt that they were handicapped by their sex. The explanation lies in the different patterns of job segregation, discussed in detail above, pp. 36–9. Midlands engineering workers had been employed in a fully desegregated factory, working alongside men: the jobs for

Table 4.2.3.10

Percentage of women believing that they were handicapped by being female (by area)

	Area							Total
	A (%)	B1 (%)	B2 (%)	C1 (%)	C2 (%)	D (%)	E (%)	(%)
Yes	9	14	17	38.5	30	4	15	16
No	85	86	67	61.5	70	88	85	80
Don't know	6	–	17	–	–	8	–	4
N	34	22	12	13	27	25	20	153

($p = 0.043$)

which they were best qualified by experience were jobs for which men were in direct competition. Since their earnings had been high, their earnings aspirations were also high, rendering them reluctant to confine themselves to competing for relatively low-paid women's jobs. On the other hand, there was little competition from men for clerical jobs, and in the clothing industry the machinists did not feel themselves in competition from men, since men in the plant (and in neighbouring plants) were employed as cutters rather than as machinists. In short, the more effectively desegregated the occupational experience, the more women felt handicapped by their sex.

The women interviewed felt that their employment difficulties were due to there being too few jobs and, on a personal basis, to age: there was little feeling of being handicapped by their sex, because women and men were not competing for the same jobs.

There are obviously different stages at which discrimination could be made against women, only some of which would be known to the women involved. Discrimination could be shown in calling for references (where relevant), selecting for interview, and finally in appointing. The women would have direct experience of the interview, and of course of the actual outcome of the process. There was little feeling that the women had been discriminated against at interviews, and none at all that they had been discriminated against on grounds of gender. (Two women said that they had been refused interviews on grounds of their sex: for the jobs of chef and bingo caller.) Hence thirteen women reported that they had experienced discrimination at interview (compared with eighty who reported no discrimination and fifty-nine who reported no interviews). Of the thirteen cases of discrimination claimed, with varying degrees of bitterness, seven were on grounds of age, two on grounds of race, one on religious grounds, one on trade-union grounds, one because the woman concerned was pregnant, and one because the job had already been promised to someone else. The only instance of claimed direct discrimination on sexual grounds involved the non-appointment of a pregnant woman.

The women interviewed believed that they were handicapped in obtaining re-employment, but the handicaps were those which affected men as well as women: lack of jobs, old age, lack of formal qualifications, and lack of relevant experience. That the women suffered from these disadvantages may have been influenced by their being female; but the fact of being female was not seen as a major source of difficulty in itself. When asked whether they had any suggestions on how the Government could help women to find suitable jobs, the most numerous suggestions made were similar to suggestions made for finding suitable jobs for men – providing money to help industry to expand, job sharing, reductions in the retirement age, lower wages, higher wages, fewer immigrants, less overtime, more retraining. Specific suggestions relating to women, made by individual respondents, were for more female MPs, the provision of a Job Centre for women only, retraining programmes for women who were unable to train when younger because of children, and educating managers to make better use of women. It was also suggested that fewer married women should work, to provide opportunities for single women. In general, such suggestions as were made related to policies relevant to men as well as to women, but the most frequent answer to the request for suggestions was that they had no suggestion to make: some respondents were surprised at a question concerned with government policy towards women specifically. The most frequently mentioned suggestion on how other organizations could help women find suitable jobs was by not giving preference to men in jobs, mentioned by four women.

In short, the majority of women said that they experienced difficulty in finding a job after redundancy: as sections 4.1 and 4.3 indicate, their perceptions were accurate. The difficulties were especially great in the North West and the Midlands, although even in such areas clerical workers were relatively optimistic about the availability of jobs. The major difficulties the women saw were the lack of jobs and, for the old, their age, although when asked directly, a substantial number said that they were also handicapped by lack of formal qualifications and by lack of relevant experience. There was no feeling that women were losing out to men in competition for jobs because men and women were not seen as competing for the same jobs.

4.3 Post-redundancy employment experience

In this section we are concerned with the outcomes of the process of job seeking, the jobs obtained by the minority of women who succeeded in obtaining work. The section begins with a brief discussion of the importance of continuing in work. We then discuss the types of jobs the women were looking for, and were not looking for, the hours wanted, and the minimum level of earnings acceptable. Thirdly, we discuss the jobs obtained, the reasons for taking them, and compare post-redundancy and pre-redundancy jobs.

For the majority of women having a jobs was regarded as either very important or important. A substantial minority of women were prepared to take any job, the remainder looking for work broadly similar to the work they had been doing before the redundancy. The majority of women wanted full-time work, although a number of previously full-time workers were prepared to consider, or actually expressed a preference for, part-time work. Earnings aspirations were modest, indicating a willingness to accept lower pay than in their pre-redundancy jobs.

Only a minority of the women obtained jobs following the redundancy; only 24 per cent were in what they regarded as permanent employment. Previously non-manual workers were primarily in non-manual jobs: manual workers were likely to have had to accept low-grade service jobs, except for electronic-assembly workers re-employed by their former employer, and sewing machinists. All women lost the benefits of employment in large-scale industry — pensions, fringe benefits, and effective trade-union representation. However, the financial impact upon previously manual workers was greater than upon non-manual workers: a third of women previously employed in professional, administrative, and supervisory jobs reported that their rate of pay was less, and 48 per cent of clerical workers, compared with 75 per cent of manual workers. Only a minority of non-manual or manual workers reported that their post-redundancy jobs were less interesting. The following section documents and elaborates upon these general comments.

Following the redundancy the majority of women interviewed regarded having a job as either very important or important: 69 per cent. Having a job was regarded as either very important or important by more women interviewed in the two Midlands case studies, C and E, than in the other case studies; women in case study B were less likely to regard having a job as very important or important, as shown in Table 4.3.1.

Table 4.3.1
Responses to *How important is it for you to have a job?* (*by area*)

	Area							Total
	A (%)	B1 (%)	B2 (%)	C1 (%)	C2 (%)	D (%)	E (%)	(%)
Very important	43	23	33	54	63	48	65	47
Important	26	27	17	38.5	11	20	15	21
Fairly important	14	32	33	8	22	20	5	19
Not important	17	18	17	–	4	12	15	12
N	35	22	12	13	27	25	20	154

($p = 0.229$)

Since women who had retired permanently from the labour market have been excluded it is unsurprising that only 12 per cent regarded having a job as unimportant. More significant are the differences in the degree of importance attached to having a job between the different case studies. The degree of importance attached to having a job did not determine whether a job was obtained or not: jobs could only be found if they were available. However, the greater the importance of having a job, the greater the effort in finding one is likely to be. More particularly, where having a job is either not important or only fairly important the effort spent in looking, and therefore, other things being equal, the degree of success in finding, is likely to be less.

There were few differences between age groups in the proportion of women regarding having a job as important or very important, although women 55+ were slightly more likely than younger women to see having a job as important or very important. However, there was a predictable tendency for married women to attach less importance to having a job, as Table 4.3.2 shows.

Table 4.3.2
Importance of having a job (by marital status)

	Married (%)	Widowed (%)	Divorced/Separated (%)	Single (%)	Total (%)
Very important	39	40	76.5	74	47
Important	22	40	18	16	21
Fairly important	23	–	6	10.5	19
Not important	16	20	–	–	12
N	113	5	17	19	

($p = 0.028$)

None of the single or divorced and separated women regarded having a job as unimportant, and only one widow: however, 16 per cent of married women did so. Similarly, only 10.5 per cent of single women, 6 per cent of divorced women, and no widows regarded having a job as fairly important, compared with 23 per cent of married women.

Less predictable was the association between the women's stress on the importance of having a job and actually having one at the time of the second interview: 33 per cent of the women who regarded having a job as very important were in full-time employment at the time of the second interview, and 18 per cent in part-time employment, compared with overall figures of 21 per cent in full-time employment and 15 per cent in part-time employment. Table 4.3.3 summarizes data on the relationship between attitudes to the importance of work and employment status at the time of the second interview. As Table 4.3.3 shows, 45 per cent of women for whom having a job was very important,

Table 4.3.3
Employment status (by importance of having a job)

	Very important (%)	Important (%)	Fairly important (%)	Not important (%)	Total (%)
Full-time work	33	18	7	5	21
Part-time work	18	15	14	5	15
Temporarily retired	4	6	7	5	5
Looking for work	45	61	72	84	58
N	73	33	29	19	154

($p = 0.048$)

compared with 84 per cent for whom having a job was not important, and 72 per cent for whom it was only fairly important, were looking for work at the time of the second interview. Expressed differently, 73 per cent of women in full-time employment, and 56.5 per cent of women in part-time employment, compared with 37 per cent of women looking for work regarded having a job as very important.

The chances of the women obtaining work were obviously influenced by the type of work they were looking for, or willing to accept. Twenty-six per cent of women were willing to take any job at the time of their redundancy; a further 12 per cent were willing to do so by the time of the second interview. As was expected, in general women were primarily looking for the type of work with which they were familiar, although women in professional, administrative, and supervisory jobs (except nurses) before the redundancy were willing to take clerical jobs. Table 4.3.4 summarizes the data on the jobs looked for, classified into ten groups. Table 4.3.4 clearly indicates that non-manual workers were looking for jobs in non-manual occupations, and manual workers primarily for jobs in the manual sector (although a small number of unskilled manual workers were also looking for clerical jobs). There was little positive interest in sales jobs.

Table 4.3.4
Job preferences (by occupational status)

	Occupational status				
	Prof./Admin./ Supervisory (%)	Clerical (%)	Semi-skilled (%)	Slightly skilled (%)	Unskilled (%)
Professional	12	3	3	–	7
Supervisors	12	3	–	3	–
Self-employed	–	–	3	–	–
Clerical	59	65	5	–	40
Skilled manual/ higher-grade service	–	5	4	9	–
Manual semi-skilled	6	–	27	12	7
Sales	–	8	13	6	7
Service (lower grade)	6	–	9	24	–
Manual (unskilled)	–	3	10	18	20
Miscellaneous	–	3	7	–	–
Any job	6	11	21	29	20
N	17	37	107	34	13

N = Number of jobs mentioned.
Percentage is that of total mentions falling in specific categories.
'Any job' is classified as a single job; the percentage of mentions of 'any job' seriously understates the relative significance of a willingness to undertake any job in the population, since it is expressed as a percentage of mentions, not as a percentage of women. Women could mention up to four jobs.

The women were also asked if there was any type of job they would not take. The replies indicate both those factors in work that are salient to women, and those that they do not like: failure to mention an item could indicate that it was not salient, or that it was not disliked. Thirty-eight per cent said that there was no job they would not be prepared to take, and a further 4 per cent that they did not know. Statistical analysis of the remaining replies would be misleading, since the replies were open ended, and varied widely — some women mentioned specific jobs, others types of jobs. However, indistinct patterns emerged. Women in professional, administrative, and supervisory positions were likely to rule out jobs below their qualifications, or at factory level: there was also some hostility to cleaning work, domestic or industrial. They were not concerned about physically exhausting or stressful work — presumably because physical exhaustion was not perceived as a major problem. Clerical workers were also concerned to avoid factory work, although a small number also specifically mentioned physically tiring work. Amongst the semi-skilled manual workers there was considerable concern to avoid physically tiring work, linked to the pressures of assembly work and piece-rates. Some were also concerned to avoid cleaning work, eight women saying that they were not willing to do domestic cleaning, and seven that they were not prepared to do industrial or office cleaning. Slightly skilled workers had similar concerns: physical tiredness, and cleaning. Unskilled workers made no mention of tiredness, but four specifically mentioned that they would not do cleaning. Although the quantitative evidence is not strong, three conclusions are suggested. First, non-manual workers are concerned to avoid factory work. Secondly, manual workers are concerned to avoid physically tiring work. And thirdly, cleaning, especially domestic cleaning, is an occupation of last resort.

The range of jobs that the women were prepared to consider was influenced by two further factors, additional to the characteristics of the jobs themselves: hours and earnings. We asked the women whether they wanted full- or part-time employment, and also whether they would be willing to work evenings or night shifts. Before the redundancy the majority of women worked full time (78 per cent of the women interviewed twice). A majority of women were either willing to work only full time or preferred to work full time — 55 per cent. As we expected, preference for full-time work was related to marital status: 74 per cent of single women were willing to work full time only, and a further 21 per cent preferred to work full time, compared with 18 per cent of

Table 4.3.5
Attitudes to full- or part-time work (by marital status)

	Married (%)	Widowed (%)	Separated/Divorced (%)	Single (%)	Total (%)
Full-time only	18	40	59	74	30
Full-time by preference	25	20	23.5	21	24.5
Part-time only	20	–	12	5	17
Part-time by preference	18	40	6	–	15.5
Don't mind	17.5	–	–	–	13
N	114	5	17	19	155

married women willing to work only full time and 25 per cent preferring to work full time. The full data are summarized in Table 4.3.5.

The preference for, or at least indifference towards, part-time employment was greater than would have been expected on the basis of experience before the redundancy: many women who worked full time before the redundancy said that they would, in future, prefer part-time work following the redundancy. The change was mainly amongst women in case studies C and D. Before the redundancy all the women in case studies C and D were employed full time, the part-time workers being found in case studies A and B. However, following the redudancy 15 per cent of women in Company C, and 20 per cent of women in Company D said that they would prefer part-time work, whilst 15 per cent in Company C and 16 per cent in Company D said that they did not mind whether they worked full or part time. Many married women who had previously been at work full time either preferred part-time work or did not mind whether they worked full time or part time.

Non-manual workers were more committed to full-time employment than manual workers, as Table 4.3.6 shows: 75 per cent of women in professional, administrative, or supervisory jobs were willing to work full time only, or preferred to work full time only, and 68 per cent of clerical workers, compared with 55 per cent of semi-skilled workers, 39 per cent of slightly skilled workers, and 11 per cent of unskilled workers.

Table 4.3.6
Attitudes to full- or part-time work (by occupational status)

	Prof./Admin./ Supervisory (%)	Clerical (%)	Semi skilled (%)	Slightly (%)	Unskilled (%)	Total (%)
Full-time only	42	42	32	14	11	30
Full-time by preference	33	26	25	25	–	24.5
Part-time only	–	10	13	32	44	17
Part-time by preference	17	16	12	18	33	15.5
Don't mind	8	6.5	17	11	11	13
N	12	31	75	28	9	155

($p = 0.080$)

Many married manual workers who had been working full time would thus in future prefer to work part time, or did not mind whether they worked part time or full time.

Attitudes towards full- or part-time employment were linked to experience of re-employment. At the time of the second interview the majority of women were still seeking work. However, 47 per cent of those willing to work only full time were in full-time employment, and 6 per cent in part-time employment; none of the women prepared to work only part time were in full-time employment, and 38.5 per cent were in part-time employment. Of those who would have preferred full-time work, 10.5 per cent were in full-time employment and 10.5 per cent in part-time employment; of those who would have preferred part-time employment 17 per cent were in full-time employment and 12.5 per cent in part-time employment. Where the women were strongly committed to full- or part-time employment they appeared to be willing to remain unemployed rather than take the alternative choice (apart from 6 per cent of the women willing to take full-time employment only); where only preferences were involved, they were willing to take up the type of work they did not prefer. Table 4.3.7 summarizes the data. Since non-manual workers were more likely than manual workers to be willing to accept full-time work only, and non-manual workers were more likely to secure re-employment than manual workers, it is not possible to infer any causal link between preferences for full-time or part-time work *per se* and re-employment chances.

Table 4.3.7
Employment status at second interview (by attitudes to full- or part-time work)

	Full-time only (%)	Full-time preferred (%)	Part-time only (%)	Part-time preferred (%)	Don't mind (%)	Total (%)
Looking for work	45	74	54	62.5	60	58
Temporarily retired	2	5	7	8	10	6
Working full time	47	10.5	–	17	15	21
Working part time	6	10.5	38.5	12.5	15	15
N	47	38	26	24	20	155

A majority of women were prepared to work evenings, 35 per cent saying that they would be willing to do so without qualification, 5 per cent saying that they did not mind, and 14 per cent saying that they would be willing to, but would prefer not to. As expected, married women were less willing to work evenings (51 per cent being willing to do so) than single women (63 per cent). There were also differences between areas, women in the Midlands case studies being more willing to work evenings than women in either the South East or North West case studies: the proportions being willing (if in some cases reluctantly) to work evenings ranged from 85 per cent in area E, 69 per cent in C1, 65.5 per cent in C2, 62 per cent in D, 45 per cent in B1, to 42 per cent in B2 and 42 per cent in A. In general, younger women were less willing to work evenings than older women, reflecting their desire to retain evenings for their families or for entertainment, although the difference between age groups were slight. Amongst occupational-status groups, clerical workers were markedly less willing to work evenings than other women were, 61 per cent being unwilling to do so. Since clerical jobs were easier to find than other jobs, and they rarely involved evening work, this unwillingness had little influence on their chances of re-employment.

As expected, women were less willing to work night shifts than to work evenings: 23 per cent were willing to do so without conditions, 11 per cent preferred not to, but would do so if necessary, and 3 per cent said that they did not mind. Married women were less willing to work nights than single women, 18 per cent being willing to do so without conditions, compared with

32 per cent of single women. Again, women in the Midlands engineering industry were more willing to work nights than other women, the proportions willing to do so (whether reluctantly or not) ranging from 60 per cent in area E, 48 per cent in C2, 46 per cent in C1, 36 per cent in D, 33 per cent in A, to 18 per cent in B1 and 8 per cent in B2. The difference was not due to differences in the occupational composition of the areas, since there was surprisingly little difference between occupational-status groups in the willingness to work nights (except that unskilled women were more willing to than others). The most frequently mentioned reason for not being willing to work nights was the desire to spend time with the family, mentioned by 55 per cent of women being unwilling to work nights: all other reasons were mentioned by fewer than 10 per cent of women answering.

Finally, in establishing the women's views on their job aspirations, we asked the women the minimum take-home pay they would accept for full-time and part-time work. As expected, the minimum acceptable take-home pay was not high; also, as expected, it varied between areas. Table 4.3.8 summarizes the data on the minimum earnings the women were willing to accept for full-time work by area, and Table 4.3.9 for part-time work, also by area.

Table 4.3.8
Minimum earnings willing to accept (by area: full-time)

(£s)	Area A (%)	B1 (%)	B2 (%)	C1 (%)	C2 (%)	D (%)	E (%)	Total (%)	N (%)
≤ 40	10	–	–	–	–	–	–	2	2
40–49	40	6	–	–	8	4.5	18	12	15
50–59	50	56	78	8	15	50	29	39	48
60–69	–	33	–	42	35	33	23.5	25	31
70–79	–	6	22	17	35	9	6	14	17
80+	–	–	–	33	7	4.5	24	9	11
N	20	18	9	12	26	22	17		124

($p = 0.028$)

Table 4.3.9
Minimum earnings willing to accept (by area: part-time)

(£s)	Area A (%)	B1 (%)	B2 (%)	C1 (%)	C2 (%)	D (%)	E (%)	Total (%)	N (%)
≤ 30	48	25	33	12.5	20	31	18	30	31
30–39	32	40	33	37.5	53	44	73	43	45
40–49	8	30	33	25	20	25	9	20	21
50+	8	5	–	25	7	–	–	6	6
Depends	4	–	–	–	–	–	–	1	1
N	25	20	9	8	15	16	11		104

($p = 0.094$)

As Tables 4.3.8 and 4.3.9 show, women in case study A were willing to accept lower pay than women in the other case studies: 50 per cent were willing to work full time for take-home pay of under £50, compared with 14 per cent overall, and 80 per cent for under £40 for part-time work, compared with 73 per cent overall. Women in case study C would work only for higher wages than women in other case studies, for full-time work, although not for part-time work.

As would be expected, the minimum earnings the women were prepared to accept were influenced by the level of earnings before the redundancy: women in low-earnings plants were willing to work for lower levels of earnings in the future than women in the high-earnings plants. However, there was an important contrast between attitudes to full- and part-time work: the dispersal of minimum-earnings aspirations was higher for full-time work than for part-time work (SD = 10.2644 for full-time work, 7.616 for part-time). This reflected the expectation of women who had previously been employed full time in jobs with relatively high wages for women that, if they were to work part time in the future, they would be obliged to work in jobs with a lower hourly rate, as well as a lower level of take-home pay overall. This was especially likely for women previously employed in Company C.

There was little overall difference in minimum-earnings levels between women in different occupational-status groups, except that women previously employed in professional, administrative, and supervisory jobs would work only for higher earnings than other women: as shown above, pp. 40–1, there was no overall association between occupational status and earnings before the redundancy. However, there were slight differences between age groups in minimum acceptable earnings for full-time work: there was little difference in minimum earnings for part-time work. As shown in Table 4.3.10, women aged under 25, or aged 25–34, were willing to work for lower earnings than older women, although the differences were not great. Because of the small numbers involved, and the smallness of the differences, it is impossible to say whether the effect is a genuine age-effect or due to differences in the age structures of the earnings groups before the redundancies.

Table 4.3.10
Minimum earning acceptable to full-time work (by age)

	Age					Total
	≤ 25 (%)	25–34 (%)	35–44 (%)	45–55 (%)	55 + (%)	(%)
> 40	–	–	–	3	11	2
40–49	22	26	9	3	11	12
50–59	44	22	45	40	33	39
60–69	22	26	19.5	34	11	25
70–79	11	18.5	14	12	11	14
80 +	–	7	9	9	22	9
N	9	27	44	35	9	124

($p = 0.087$)

Minimum-earnings levels are unlikely to be major influences on re-employment prospects in themselves. However, women with high-earnings aspirations were more likely to be still looking for work at the time of the second interview than women with lower aspirations, as Table 4.3.11 indicates. The differences between groups are not large: however, 66 per cent of the women in work at the time of the second interview regarded take-home pay of under £60 as acceptable, compared with only 51 per cent of women still looking for work.

Table 4.3.11
Earning aspirations for full-time work (by employment status)

(£s)	Employment status				Total
	Full-time employment (%)	Part-time employment (%)	Temporarily retired (%)	Looking for work (%)	(%)
≤ 40	3	–	14	–	2
40–49	20	–	14	11	12
50–59	43	33	14	40	39
60–69	17	33	29	27	25
70–79	7	8	29	16	14
80 +	10	25	–	7	9
N	30	12	7	75	124

($p = 0.016$)

To summarize the women's job aspirations: following the redundancy the majority of women were looking for jobs similar to their previous jobs – non-manual workers were looking for non-manual jobs, and manual workers were looking for manual jobs. However, women in professional, administrative, and supervisory jobs were also looking for clerical jobs, as were a small minority of manual workers: as is shown below, a minority of manual workers wanted to re-train for clerical jobs (p. 214). There was little interest in sales jobs, and some dislike expressed for cleaning jobs. Minimum earnings aspirations were not high – and were below previous earnings levels, indicating an accurate perception that it would be difficult to obtain jobs as well paid as their previous jobs. The minimum level of earnings acceptable for part-time work was lower, in hourly terms, than the minimum level acceptable for full-time work, a number of previously full-time women preferred, or were willing to consider, part-time work. A majority of women were prepared to take evening work, but only a minority to work night shifts.

As indicated in section 4.1, at the time of the second interview fifty-six women were in employment, thirty-three full time and twenty-three part time. However, a larger number had had at least one job following the redundancy, seventy-two. In addition, six women had had two jobs. The overall employment experience has been discussed above in section 4.1: here we are concerned with a more detailed analysis of the jobs obtained, and a comparison between

Women in the Labour Market 203

post- and pre-redundancy jobs. The analysis is concerned with the fifty-six jobs held by the women at the time of the second interview and the sixteen temporary jobs held following the redundancy. The intermediate jobs held by the six women who had two jobs following the redundancy are discussed separately (p. 212).

Table 4.3.12 summarizes the data on the jobs obtained by the women after the redundancy by occupational-status group.

Table 4.3.12
Jobs obtained (by occupational status)

	Prof./Admin./ Supervisory (%)	Clerical (%)	Semi-skilled (%)	Slightly skilled (%)	Unskilled (%)	Total (%)	N
Professional	17	–	–	–	–	1	1
Supervisory	33	–	–	–	–	3	2
Self-employed	–	5	3	–	–	3	2
Clerical	33	81	–	–	33	28	20
Skilled manual and service (higher grade)	–	–	3	9	–	3	2
Manual semi-skilled	–	–	62	18	–	25	18
Sales	–	10	6	9	–	7	5
Service (lower grade)	17	5	13	18	–	11	8
Manual (unskilled)	–	–	23	45.5	67	20	14
N	6	21	31	11	3		72

In view of the small number of women finding work, detailed quantitative analysis of the jobs obtained is impossible. However, three general comments are appropriate. First, women in professional administrative and supervisory jobs were able to obtain work in similar jobs or in clerical work, if they obtained work at all. (There was a single exception — one woman took a job in a canteen.) Secondly, nearly all clerical workers were able to obtain work as clerical workers, only two women taking up jobs in sales (one of whom became a shop manageress) and one in entertainment. Thirdly, manual workers were obliged to take service jobs of different kinds (cleaning, industrial and domestic, catering, including hospitals, school meals, and as barmaids, and packing), with two significant exceptions. The two groups of manual workers who were able to remain outside this type of work were electronic-assembly workers who were re-employed by their old company on a short-term basis (six women) and sewing-machinists who were able to find work using their existing skills, although in less-established firms than their previous employment. Women in manual jobs declared redundant were thus likely to find themselves out of work, or, if in employment, in low-paid service occupations.

A substantial minority of the jobs obtained after the redundancy were explicitly temporary jobs, according to the understanding with the employer: twenty-one jobs, or 29 per cent of the jobs held. Since the numbers involved are small detailed statistical analysis would be inappropriate. However, one professional job was temporary (training officer), one catering job, eight clerical jobs, four semi-skilled manual jobs, two sales assistant jobs, one service job, and four unskilled manual jobs. Slightly more jobs were stated as being temporary by the women themselves, twenty-five or 35 per cent. There were marked differences in the proportion of temporary jobs between areas. The highest proportion of stop-gap jobs was in North West electronics (B2), where 80 per cent of the jobs were temporary – including jobs with previous employer. Area B2 was thus exceptional. However, there were also high proportions of temporary jobs in the Midlands: 67 per cent of jobs in area C1 were temporary, 45 per cent in area E, and 44 per cent in area C2. In contrast 33 per cent of the jobs in area D, 20 per cent in area A, and none in area B1 were regarded as stop-gap jobs. There is thus considerable evidence that post-redundancy jobs were only stop-gap jobs. The total number of even potentially permanent jobs obtained by the 196 redundant women interviewed twice was thus fifty-one. At the time of the second interview fifty-six women were in employment, nine of whom regarded their jobs as stop-gap jobs. Hence only forty-seven women (or 24 per cent) had jobs which they regarded as permanent at the time of the second interview, up to seven months after the redundancies.

For the majority of women with post-redundancy jobs the reasons given for taking the job taken was that it was the first or the only job offered: 58 per cent. The only other types of reason for taking a job mentioned by ten or more women were intrinsic reasons (mentioned by nineteen women, or 26 per cent of women who had jobs) and convenient travel arrangements (mentioned by ten women, or 14 per cent). Women in areas B1, D, B2, and E were more likely to give 'no alternative' as the reason for taking a job, women in C1 and C2 much less likely; the women in areas C1 and C2 also had higher earnings aspirations than women in other areas, as indicated above, helping to confirm the impression that women in the area may well have been more selective than women elsewhere. As expected, professional, administrative, and supervisory women, and clerical workers, were more likely to give intrinsic reasons for taking their jobs than were other occupational-status groups: three out of six in status group 1, and eight out of twenty-one in status group 2, compared with seven out of thirty-one in group 3, one out of eleven in group 4, and none out of three in group 5. Women in the clothing-industry case study A, were more likely to mention convenient hours or convenient travel arrangements than any other group: nine out of twenty, the next-highest number being two in each of areas D and E. Default reasons for taking particular jobs were thus very much more frequently mentioned following the redundancy than in explanations for choice of pre-redundancy job, or for choice of job on initial entry into employment (see above, pp. 69–72).

A majority of the women preferred their pre-redundancy jobs (53 per cent), 29 per cent preferred their post-redundancy job, the remainder having mixed feelings, believing that the jobs were about the same, or that they were not comparable. The proportion of women preferring their previous jobs was highest in area C2, and lowest in E, 78 per cent in area C2 preferring previous job, and only 27 per cent in E: the women employed in C2 were of course manual workers, the women employed in E clerical workers. Of the small number of women who preferred their post-redundancy jobs (twenty-one), six were clerical workers, four were sewing-machinists, and four were electronics-assembly workers who had been re-employed by their previous employer on inspection work: the remaining six were dispersed across a variety of occupations. The most common reasons for preferring post-redundancy job were that it was more interesting, mentioned by nine women and that the people were nicer, mentioned by eight women: no other reason was mentioned by more than two women. No woman mentioned better pay as a reason for preferring her post-redundancy job. The most frequently mentioned reason for preferring pre-redundancy job was a preference for the people, mentioned by fifteen women; ten referred to its being more interesting, nine to better money, seven to familiarity, and five to a sense of achievement in producing something: no other reason was mentioned by more than two women. From an analysis of the women's spontaneous comparisons between post- and pre-redundancy jobs, it could be inferred that the jobs were not much less interesting, but that they were much less well paid. This inference is confirmed by more detailed analysis.

The majority of women preferred their previous jobs in general terms. To investigate their experience more fully we asked the women to compare their post-redundancy jobs with their pre-redundancy jobs on a number of criteria. Table 4.3.14 presents the overall distribution of replies for each occupational group: the percentage is that of women saying that their post-redundancy job was less good.

There were three areas in which the majority of women saw a deterioration: rate of pay (62.5 per cent), pensions (64 per cent), and effective trade-union representation (60 per cent). Deterioration in these areas would be expected with movement from large-scale manufacturing industry, in which the women had previously been employed, into a wide variety of occupations and industries, very few of which were involved in manufacturing. There was also an extensive decline in the level of fringe benefits provided, 44 per cent reporting that the level of fringe benefits was worse. However, it is noteworthy that only a minority reported a worsening of conditions in two areas: the degree of friendliness of their colleagues, and the intrinsic interest of their work. Hence 36 per cent of women reported that they had less friendly people to work with than before, 43 per cent about the same, and 19 per cent that they had friendlier work-mates at their post-redundancy job. Only 22 per cent reported that their work was less interesting than in their previous job, 36 per cent saying that it was the same, and 40 per cent that their post-redundancy jobs were more interesting. Overall, the women thus experienced a deterioration in the type of rewards characteristic of large scale manufacturing industry in the 1970s, even for women: relatively high rates of pay, pensions, and fringe benefits, and effective trade-union representation. They did not, however, experience a

Table 4.3.13
Comparison between post- and pre-redundancy jobs

	Prof./Admin./ Supervisory (%)	Clerical (%)	Semi- skilled (%)	Slightly skilled (%)	Unskilled (%)	Total (%)	(p)
Rate of pay	33	48	81	54.5	67	62.5	0.009
Security	50	38	26	27	33	32	0.631
Convenient travel	50	43	26	18	33	32	0.101
Cost of journey to work	50	50	22	33	37.5	35	0.720
Convenient hours	33	33	23	27	33	28	0.558
Promotion prospects	33	43	29	50	33	37	0.327
Working conditions	33	48	35.5	30	33	38	0.537
Pensions	60	75	56	75	50	64	0.001
Fringe benefits	60	61	29	50	50	44	0.364
Interest	–	24	23	18	68	22	0.008
Friendly work-mates	17	33	45	27	33	36	0.254
Effective trade union	80	69	50	71	50	60	0.532
Efficient management	17	17	23	11	50	20	0.457
Considerate management	17	42	20	11	67	27	0.172
Opportunity to use skills	–	29	29	30	67	28	0.040
Variety	–	14	32	30	33	24	0.192
Responsibility	17	24	20	20	–	20	0.629
Being left alone to get on with job	17	9.5	10	–	–	8	0.558
Sick pay	25	37	35	20	33	33	0.501

Percentage is that of women saying that the post-redundancy job was worse.

major deterioration in the interest of the work performed, or in the warmth of social relations at work.

There were differences between occupational-status groups which it is important to explore briefly.

As only six women from occupational status group 1 were re-employed, quantitative analysis of their comparisons would be inappropriate. However, in general they appeared to lose little by the redundancy, provided that they secured re-employment. No one reported that their work was less interesting, or less varied or provided fewer opportunities to use their skills. Only one woman said that her work-mates were less friendly and only two reported that their rate of pay was worse. Three women reported that their travel arrangements were less convenient, and more costly. A majority in this group reported that their jobs were less secure, their fringe benefits and pensions were worse, and that they did not have as effective a trade union: but these were not major concerns for the women. In short, the women may have had to be satisfied with awkward travel arrangement or hours, but the jobs they obtained were otherwise satisfactory.

Clerical workers were relatively successful in securing re-employment, as shown above (pp. 159–60). The jobs they obtained were similar in character to the jobs they had had previously: the women were also likely to regard them as equally interesting – 52 per cent of clerical workers said that their jobs were equally interesting, 24 per cent that their pre-redundancy jobs had been more interesting, and 24 per cent that their present jobs were more interesting. Similarly, 52 per cent said that they had the same opportunity to use their skills and training, 14 per cent that they had more, and 29 per cent that they had less; 48 per cent said that they had the same amount of variety, 38 per cent that they had more, and 14 per cent that they had less. Their relations with their colleagues at work were also likely to be similar: 52 per cent reported that the people were as friendly to work with, 14 per cent that they were more friendly, and 33 per cent that they were less friendly. Like the professional, administrative, and supervisory women, the main loss was in the rewards associated with large-scale manufacturing industry – pensions (75 per cent reported worse), fringe benefits (61 per cent worse off), and effective trade-union representation (69 per cent worse off). On pay, 48 per cent were worse off, 38 per cent the same, and 14 per cent better off. There was also an indication that the women had to go to greater efforts to travel to work – as did professional, administrative, and supervisory workers: 33 per cent said that their travel arrangements were equally convenient, 24 per cent more convenient, and 43 per cent less convenient.

The pattern amongst manual workers was, in some respects, different, partly because the rewards of their pre-redundancy jobs had been different. (In view of the small number of slightly skilled and unskilled women in jobs – only eleven of the former and three of the latter – and the similarity in post-redundancy jobs amongst all manual workers, manual workers have been treated as a group in this analysis.) Like clerical workers, they had lost any pension rights or fringe benefits they may have possessed. Also like clerical workers, their jobs were no less interesting, nor less varied, than their previous jobs: 43 per cent reported that their jobs were more interesting, 32 per cent that they were equally interesting, and 25 per cent that they were less interesting. On variety, 41 per cent reported more variety, 25 per cent the same, and 32 per cent less variety. However, manual workers were less likely to have found equally friendly people to work with than clerical workers: 18 per cent said that they had more friendly people to work with, 41 per cent equally friendly, and 41 per cent less friendly. They were also substantially more likely than clerical workers to have a lower rate of pay: 16 per cent said that their rate of pay was better, 9 per cent that it was the same, and 75 per cent that it was worse. Finally, a lower proportion of manual workers than of clerical workers reported that their journeys to work were less convenient: 30 per cent reported that travel arragement were more convenient, 45 per cent the same, and 25 per cent that they were less convenient. (Comparable figures for clerical workers were 24, 33 and 43 per cent respectively.) This suggests that travel arrangements constituted a more significant disincentive to taking a job for manual workers than for clerical workers — as would be expected, in view of the less convenient hours, and lower earnings, of the jobs the redundant manual workers were able to obtain. (The contrast is even greater for the costs of travel: 27 per cent of manual workers reported that their journey to work was less expensive, 45 per cent the same, and 27 per cent more expensive; 14 per cent of clerical workers reported that their journey to work was less expensive, 33 per cent the same, and 52 per cent that it was more expensive.)

Since the major reason for the women working was financial, it is important to examine the economic impact of the redundancy. The economic impact of unemployment is examined below, in Chapter 5, section 2: here we are concerned with the economic rewards of work for the minority of women who obtained jobs. As shown in Table 4.3.13, 62.5 per cent of women reported that their rate of pay (including bonuses) was lower in their post-redundancy job than in their pre-redundancy jobs. This decline was especially extensive amongst manual workers: clerical workers were more successful financially. Table 4.3.14 shows the comparison between clerical and manual workers: the small number of women in occupational-status group 1 did even better financially.

Table 4.3.14
Comparison between earnings before and after redundancy

	Clerical workers (%)	Manual workers (%)
Better	14	16
Same	38	9
Worse	48	75
N	21	31

($p = 0.009$)

The decline was of course especially marked amongst women in previously relatively well-paid jobs: all of the engineering assembly workers who obtained jobs were paid less, as were 75 per cent of machine-sewers. Amongst the hand-sewers (in case study A) and the electronic assembly workers re-employed by their old firm, the extent of the decline was less, since in the former case their level of earnings was low anyway, and in the latter they were returning to very similar jobs with their previous employer. Table 4.3.15 presents the data on earnings changes by occupation: although the numbers are small, the table indicates the differential economic impact of redundancy upon the minority of women who obtained re-employment.

Table 4.3.15
Comparison of earnings before and after redundancy (by occupation)

	Nursing (%)	Catering (%)	Administrative (%)	Clerical (%)	Machine-sewing (%)	Hand-sewing (%)	Electrical assembly (%)	Engineering assembly (%)	General service (%)	Total (%)
Better	–	14	100	21	17	29	22	–	33	20
Same	–	14	–	33	8	–	22	–	–	17
Worse	100	71	–	46	75	57	57	100	67	62.5
N	1	7	1	24	12	7	9	8	3	72

($p = 0.289$)

Although there were very few single women, they were more likely to obtain jobs either as well paid as, or better paid than, their pre-redundancy jobs than either married or divorced and separated women. This was partly because single women were more likely to be employed in clerical jobs than married, divorced or separated women (and likely to be younger, although there was no statistically significant overall age effect). But there may also have been a greater willingness amongst married women to accept jobs that involved lower levels of earnings (provided that the job did not involve significant inconvenience in travelling to work). Table 4.3.16 summarizes the data on the relationship between marital status and change in earnings levels.

Table 4.3.16
Comparison of earnings before and after redundancy (by marital status)

	Married (%)	Divorced/Separated (%)	Single (%)
Better	18	12.5	33
Same	16	–	33
Worse	65.5	75.5*	33
N	55	8	9

($p = 0.037$)

*12.5 per cent = other.

The majority of women reported that their rates of pay in their post-redundancy jobs were lower than in their pre-redundancy jobs. This decline was true for both full and part-time employment. Before the redundancies the average net pay of the women was £63.90 for full-time work and £40.40 for part-time work; following the redundancies the average net pay was £56.40 for full time work and £30.23 for part-time work. Table 4.3.17 summarizes the distribution of earnings for full- and part-time employment.

Before the redundancy, as indicated in Table 1.3.5.2, there was little difference in the level of earnings between occupational-status groups, for full-time workers. As Table 4.3.17 indicates, there were substantial differences after the redundancy: 84 per cent of professional, administrative, and supervisory staff earned £50 or more in their post-redundancy employment, and 69 per cent of clerical workers. However, only 20 per cent of semi-skilled manual workers, and not a single slightly skilled or unskilled manual worker in employment earned £50 or more. Table. 4.3.18 summarizes the level of earnings following the redundancy by occupational status.

There was thus a very substantial drop in the average level of earnings of the women following the redundancy. This drop occurred in all occupational-status groups, but it was very much more marked amongst women who had been employed in manual jobs than amongst women who had been employed in non-manual jobs.

Table 4.3.17
Post-redundancy earnings, full- and part-time

£s	Full-time (%)	Average earnings (%)	Part-time (%)	Average earnings (%)
≤ 30	5	28.00	61	25.63
31–39	10.5	37.50	32	35.30
40–49	24	43.00	3	45.00
50–59	21	54.00	3	52.00
60–69	13	63.00	–	–
70–79	18	73.00	–	–
80 +	8	95.00	–	–
		Average £56.40		Average £30.23

Table 4.3.18
Post-redundancy earnings (by occupational status)

£s	Prof./Admin./Supervisory (%)	Clerical (%)	Semi-skilled (%)	Slightly skilled (%)	Unskilled (%)	Total (%)
≤ 30	–	5	33	45.5	33	24
30–39	17	21	27.5	36	33	26
40–49	–	11	17	18	33	16
50–59	–	21	14	–	–	13
60–69	17	16	3	–	–	7
70–79	50	16	3	–	–	10
80 +	17	16	–	–	–	4
N	6	19	29	11	3	68

($p = 0.243$)

Note: The occupational-status groups are based on jobs held before the redundancies.

As was indicated earlier, the chances of obtaining work were better before leaving pre-redundancy employment than at any particular time later: in addition, the jobs obtained by women who did not have any period out of work were better paid than the jobs obtained by women after a period of unemployment, as Table 4.3.19 shows. Hence 60 per cent of the jobs obtained by women before leaving their pre-redundancy job resulted in £50 per week or more take-home pay, compared with only 17.5 per cent of jobs obtained by women with a period out of work. The length of time they were unemployed was not, in itself, the reason for association between the length of time out of work and the level of earnings: non-manual workers were more likely to obtain higher-paid jobs and less likely to have a period out of work than manual workers were. However, it is significant that the impact of the redundancies upon manual workers should be two-fold: the chances of obtaining a job were worse than for non-manual workers, and the wages of the jobs which were obtained were markedly worse.

Table 4.3.19
Post-redundancy earnings (by length of time unemployed)

£s	Time out of work (weeks)							Total
	0 (%)	1–3 (%)	4–7 (%)	8–11 (%)	12–15 (%)	16–19 (%)	20+ (%)	(%)
≤ 30	11	33	33	25	33	20	45	24
30–39	14	–	33	25	50	60	36	26
40–49	14	33	–	25	17	–	9	16
50–59	18	–	33	17	–	20	–	13
60–69	14	–	–	–	–	–	9	7
70–79	21	33	–	–	–	–	–	10
80+	7	–	–	8	–	–	–	4
N	28	3	3	12	6	5	11	68

($p = 0.324$)

Although only a minority obtained work following redundancy, six women had two jobs, three in area C2, two in area D, and one in area A. Two of the jobs held between the redundancy and the job held at the second interview were part time – serving as barmaid: one of the women gave this up on obtaining a permanent job, the other continued after she had obtained a full-time job, because she enjoyed the work. A third job was serving as a casual silver-service waitress: the woman concerned obtained a permanent job after only a week. Two jobs were those of temporary secretary, one with an agency: both women left when they obtained permanent clerical jobs. Finally, one sewing-machinist in the South East case study left a sewing-machinist job because she was able to obtain a better-paid job elsewhere. These six women thus obtained stop-gap jobs, leaving when they had been able to obtain permanent, or better-paid jobs. The jobs they had are additional to the seventy-two analysed in the previous pages.

In this section we have presented data on the types of jobs the women were looking for following the redundancies, and the jobs obtained. The majority of women regarded finding a job as either very important or important: 69 per cent. In general the women were looking for jobs similar to the ones they had been doing before the redundancies, although a substantial minority, 39 per cent, said that they were willing to take any job. The majority of women wanted full-time work, but a substantial minority of married women, especially married women manual workers, were prepared to consider, or actually preferred, part-time work. A majority of women were prepared to take evening work, and a substantial minority (37 per cent) were prepared to work nights. The level of earnings looked for varied substantially between case studies: women in previously low-paid jobs were willing to take jobs with lower pay than women in higher-paid jobs.

Only a minority of women obtained jobs following the redundancy. Seventy-two women (or 37 per cent) had at least one job following the redundancy, and six (3 per cent) had two. However, many of the jobs were temporary, and at the time of the second interview only fifty-six women were in employment (29 per cent); a further nine jobs were regarded by the women as stop-gap jobs, leaving forty-seven women (24 per cent) in permanent employment. Previously non-manual workers were primarily employed in jobs similar to their previous jobs, only four non-manual workers taking jobs in either sales or lower service jobs. Manual workers were unlikely to have obtained jobs similar to their previous jobs, taking primarily lower-grade service jobs: the major exceptions were electronic-assembly workers re-employed by their former employer, and sewing-machinists. The majority of workers lost the benefits of working in large-scale industry — pensions, fringe benefits, and effective trade-union representation. However, the financial impact of the redundancies was greater upon manual workers than upon non-manual workers. Whereas the majority of non-manual workers obtained jobs paying either the same or higher wages than before the redundancy, the majority of manual workers earned less: the drop was especially marked amongst former employees of Company C. Manual workers were also less likely to report that their work-mates were at least as friendly as in their pre-redundancy jobs. There was less contrast in the degree of interest in the jobs themselves: only a minority of women in both non-manual and manual jobs reported that their jobs were less interesting.

4.4 Retraining, homeworking, and own business

For the women who did not obtain jobs following the redundancies there were three (not mutually exclusive) ways of earning or potentially earning money: retraining, home-working, and setting up own business. A majority of women said that they would like to retrain (57 per cent), primarily for jobs in clerical work or the caring professions. However, only a minority of women had taken any steps to undertake retraining. Of those who had not the most frequently mentioned reason for not doing so was simply that they had not seriously considered it, although a small number mentioned their age. In general, the women were receptive to the conception of retraining, but not very knowledgeable about how to proceed in entering training courses: a small number of comments on the Job Centres mentioned that they could play a more active role in providing information about training courses. There was little interest in homeworking: seventeen women had done homeworking before, but only six had tried to find paid work that could be done at home following the redundancy, and only one actually did it. Two women were involved in running their own businesses following the redundancy, one running an antiques business and one assisting her husband in a small garage.

A majority of women, 57 per cent, said that they would like to retrain. Women looking for work (68 per cent) or temporarily retired (64 per cent) were significantly more likely than women in part-time work (48 per cent), or in full-time work (30 per cent), to wish to retrain. The wish to retrain appeared to increase with length of time out of work; only 35 per cent of women who were, or had been, out of work for under two months (eight weeks) wished to retrain, compared with 63 per cent of women out of work for longer. There was no difference in the proportions wishing to retrain between non-manual and manual workers, nor between married and single workers, and the only difference between age groups was that fewer women aged 55+ wished to retrain than others (37 per cent, compared with 57 per cent overall) — hardly surprisingly.

The comparatively small number of women wishing to retrain, but in employment, were interested in a comparatively narrow range of courses (three in commercial subjects, three in catering, three in computing/word processing, one in an IPM course, and two did not know). But the women looking for work were interested in a very wide range of possible courses, falling into six groups: (1) thirty-four women would have liked clerical training; (2) thirteen women were interested in catering; (3) fifteen women were interested in one of the female caring professions (nursing, social work); (4) three women mentioned an interest in public exams in general — O level, A level, or degree; (5) individual women mentioned specific interests which they would like to develop further — flowers, electronics, dress-making; and (6) two women mentioned specific professional training, one in accountancy and a second in personnel management. As expected, women in non-manual occupations were interested in enhancing their qualifications through further professional and clerical training: women formerly employed in professional, administrative, and supervisory jobs mentioned courses in clerical skills (5), IPM (1), accounting (1), computing (1), and catering (1). The most frequently mentioned courses by clerical workers were: clerical (9), foreign languages (1), HNC in Business Studies (1), IPM (1), catering (2), computers (3), tailoring (1), anything interesting (1) and unknown (4). Semi-skilled manual workers mentioned a much wider range of courses — as expected, since there were more of them than any other group and they were unemployed for longer. Sixteen women would have liked to undertake training in secretarial work, ten in female caring professions, seven in catering, four in computers, three in hairdressing, two in flowers, one in each of painting and decorating, electronics, dress-making, O levels (unspecified), English, hobbies, six in anything interesting, four in anything leading to a job, and two did not know. Amongst women in occupational-status group 4, three mentioned catering, three nursing, two mentioned machining, two clerical, one computers, and three did not know. Amongst unskilled manual workers, three women mentioned clerical training, two nursing, one A levels, and two did not know. Not surprisingly, the courses the women wished to follow were linked closely to traditional women's jobs, although the relative frequency of mention of courses involving computers indicated that some women were aware of new opportunities for women in new technology areas. In general, women in employment, and women previously in non-manual jobs, whether in employment following the redundancy or not, wished to follow courses directly linked to their existing work experience; unemployed manual workers were interested in a very wide range of courses, including clerical courses, often not directly linked to their previous work experience.

The number of women who had considered retraining in the last twelve months was lower than the number of women who said that they would have liked to retrain when specifically asked: 24 per cent compared with 57 per cent. The major reason given by the women for not considering retraining was simply that they had not got around to it, although a small number, sixteen, said that they thought they were too old. Of the forty-three women who had considered retraining, twenty-six were still considering it and making enquiries at the time of the second interview, two had dropped the idea, and fifteen had made definite arrangements to attend courses, or had actually begun to attend.

By far the most popular courses were in clerical and typing: seven of the fifteen women were planning to undertake clerical courses. In addition, two women planned to undertake courses in catering (one in cordon bleu cooking), two women in geriatric social work, and one in each of computing, business management, being a nanny, and floristry. Two of the women were in employment — the women planning to undertake courses in cordon bleu cooking and in computing — and a third was involved in running her own business — the woman intending to do business management. The remaining twelve women regarded themselves as either temporarily retired from employment (two) or looking for work (ten). It is difficult to assess the depth of the commitment of the women to retraining. For some women the commitment to retraining was limited, their knowledge of the proposed courses shadowy, and the likely impact of retraining on their subsequent employment prospects probably small. However, the majority of the women proposing to retrain appeared to have obtained advice from the Job Centre on appropriate courses, primarily funded through TOPS, and knew what they hoped to achieve. Fourteen of the fifteen women had not yet embarked upon their proposed retraining: the one woman who had had completed a one day course in word-processing, which she had paid for herself.

Retraining was designed to enhance earning potential in the future. The second alternative to going out to work was homeworking. However, there was little interest in homeworking, only six women saying that they tried to obtain paid work that could be done at home following the redundancy, and only one actually doing it. All of the women involved in homeworking were married, aged 25–44; five had previously been manual workers, and one in occupational status group 1. Fewer women were looking for paid home-work than had previously done such work, six compared with seventeen. This is not surprising, since the women either did not like homeworking, or knew little about it. The most frequently mentioned reason for not seeking homeworking was that it was too badly paid, some women using the term 'exploitation': 27 per cent said that it was too badly paid. The other reason for not doing homeworking, mentioned frequently, was that it would confine them to the house when a major reason for working was to get out of the house (27 per cent). A smaller number, 16 per cent, did not know what homeworking involved. A small number of women either did not like the type of work that was done at home (eight women), or thought that homeworking would spill over into family life and disrupt it (seven women). Only five women who were not looking for homeworking thought that they would like it, either because it was convenient or because they thought that it paid well.

Two women were involved in their own businesses following the redundancy, one running an antiques business, the second sharing in the running of a garage with her husband. For the first woman the redundancy provided a stimulus, without which she would probably not have taken up the job full time: her redundancy money also made a contribution to the capital required to establish the business. The income from the business was irregular, and below her previous earnings. She very much preferred running her own business because of the independence it gave her, as well as the responsibility and inherent interest of the antiques themselves. The only disadvantages were irregular income and 'exhaustion' from working irregular hours. The second woman was involved in what was originally her husband's garage; before the redundancy she helped with the paper-work, on a part-time basis, beginning to work full time after the redundancy. She also very much preferred working in her own business, because of the freedom, variety, and the more congenial work-mates. The major disadvantage was the pay: since she was in a partnership with her husband she was not paid at all.

Very few of the women actively pursued other ways of making money than market employment following the redundancy. A majority of women expressed a general interest in retraining. However, only a minority of women took active steps to find out information about retraining, and only fifteen women either attended courses or made specific arrangements for doing so. There was very little interest in homeworking, only six women looking for work that could be done at home, and only one woman actually doing it. The most common reason given for not doing homeworking was that it was too badly paid (27 per cent) — an opinion confirmed by the experience of the one woman who was doing it. In addition, many women said that they worked for the company (27 per cent) and homeworking would be too isolated. Finally, two women were involved in running their own businesses, one independently and one in partnership with her husband; both very much preferred their present jobs to their previous jobs.

4.5 Conclusion: Women in the labour market

If the five redundancies studied had never occurred, it is highly likely that all the women we initially interviewed would have still been working with the same employer: none had specific plans to leave, or to cease going out to work. After the announcement of the redundancies, but before their implementation, 86 per cent of the women first interviewed said that they intended to look for another job, including 17 per cent after a break. At the time of the second interviews, between four and seven months after the redundancies had occurred, 17 per cent of the women interviewed were in full-time employment, 12 per cent were in part-time employment, 46 per cent were looking for work, 17 per cent were temporarily retired, and 7 per cent were permanently retired from employment (and one woman had started her own business). The major effect of the redundancies upon women's employment was thus to reduce it substantially. The reduction was substantial for all types of women workers, but was especially marked for manual workers: 31 per cent of professional, administrative, and supervisory women were in employment, 34 per cent of clerical workers, 27.5 per cent of the semi-skilled, 26.5 per cent of the slightly skilled, and 18 per cent of the unskilled manual workers. When in employment, manual workers were more likely to be in part-time than in full-time work.

In general terms, this reduction in employment was due to two sets of factors, of unequal importance: the attitudes and actions of the women themselves, and the number of jobs available. Since the overall concern of this study is with women's experience of redundancy and unemployment, not with the factors determining the demand for labour, we have naturally concentrated upon the women's attitudes and actions. However, the women's experience, and especially their chances of re-employment, were influenced by the level of demand for labour with the skills and experience they possessed: if there was little demand, their attitudes and actions could have little impact. Moreover, their attitudes and actions were likely to be more generally, and less perceptibly, influenced by their chances of re-employment: reactions to unemployment are likely to be conditioned by whether it is regarded as a transient or as a more or less permanent state. This could be expected to have a major effect on women's commitment to the labour market. In this concluding section we examine in general terms the interaction between the women's own attitudes and actions and the level of labour demand on their experience in the labour market. The discussion is necessarily speculative, since we do not have the evidence on labour demand to match the evidence we have gathered on the women themselves.

As we have shown, the majority of redundant women did not find jobs after their redundancies, and even fewer were in employment at the time of the second interview. This reduction in employment was not because the women had intended ceasing employment: only 14 per cent of the women initially interviewed did not intend to look for another job. Nor was it because the women had limited or unrealistic aspirations for their future jobs. Thirty-eight per cent of women said that they would be prepared to consider any job, a view especially common amongst manual workers, and the more defined aspirations of the non-manual workers did not prevent them from having a higher re-employment rate. Earnings aspirations were modest, many women, especially manual workers, recognizing that they would probably have to accept a drop in earnings if they were to get work. Nor was it because the women were limited in their choice of jobs by family commitments: over 85 per cent of women said that they were not restricted by family commitments, and the group of women who were most restricted, the South East clothing workers, were more successful in obtaining jobs after the redundancies than other women were. Finally, it was not because the women did not make serious efforts to find work: nearly all the women visited Job Centres and looked in local newspapers, although the intensity of use of the employment services differed substantially. Like men, women experienced employment difficulties in 1981—2 because there was limited demand for the skills and experience they offered.

It is impossible to establish satisfactorily the level of demand for the skills and experience of the women interviewed; even establishing it unsatisfactorily would require a specific research project, separate from, and complementary to, the present one. However, there were major differences between areas in the perceived difficulty of finding jobs: women in the South East were more optimistic than women elsewhere about their employment prospects. In the Midlands and North West, differences in assessment were conditioned by the occupational composition of the groups concerned: in both areas non-manual workers were more optimistic than manual workers. Hence the proportion of women reporting difficulty in finding jobs was 61 per cent overall, the proportions ranging from 44 per cent amongst South East clothing workers to 73.5 per cent amongst North West electronics workers: comparable figures were 72.5 per cent in case study C, 56 per cent in case study D, and 50 per cent in case study E. There is no reason to suppose, on general grounds, that the women's assessments would be inaccurate: they had a major interest in obtaining accurate information on the jobs available to them. However, it is worth considering two 'external' indicators of the level of labour demand in addition: unemployment rates, and job-vacancy rates.

The unemployment rates in the five travel-to-work areas in which the redundancies occurred are summarized in Table 4.5.1.

Table 4.5.1

Unemployment rate in travel-to-work areas (female and total) September 1981 and September 1982

	1981		1982	
	Female (%)	Total (%)	Female (%)	Total (%)
South East		10.1		12.3
North West (manual)	10.8	14.4	11.8	15.5
Midlands (manual)	11.2	16.2	12.4	18.2
North West (clerical)	13.9	14.7	14.3	15.9
Midlands (clerical)	14.4	16.7	14.6	17.7

Note: Case study B was carried out in two factories: data are presented on the travel to work area in which the major plant was located.

During the period in which the women were being declared redundant, the level of unemployment rose in all five travel-to-work areas, partly of course because of the women's own redundancies. In only one area, South East, was the level of unemployment below the national average. Two of the case studies were carried out in what was, at the time the research design was formulated, a high-unemployment region — the North West — and two in a region of rising unemployment: by the time the research was carried out, unemployment levels in the rapidly changing region, the West Midlands, and in the two travel-to-work areas in that region, Birmingham and Coventry, were higher than in the previously original 'high'-unemployment region. By the time of the second interviews, the overall unemployment rate was 18.2 per cent in Birmingham, and 17.7 per cent in Coventry, the official rates for women being 12.4 and 14.6 per cent respectively: the official female rate significantly understates the level of unemployment amongst women. The women's assessment of their employment situation accurately reflected the evidence as shown in official unemployment statistics.

Their views are also confirmed by data on job vacancies in the relevant labour markets. Table 4.5.2 provides an indication of labour demand at regional level by showing the notified vacancy: unemployed ratio for the three regions in September 1981 and September 1982: the notified vacancy rate is approximately a third of all vacancies.

Table 4.5.2
Ratio of notified vacancies to unemployed (male and female), September 1981 and September 1982 (by region)

	1981	1982
South East	5.99:100	5.49:100
Midlands	1.97:100	1.86:100
North West	2.03:100	2.09:100

Source: *Department of employment Gazette*, October 1981 and October 1982.

As Table 4.5.2 shows, for every 100 unemployed in the South East there were 5.99 notified vacancies in September 1981, and 5.49 in September 1982, in the Midlands 1.97 in 1981 and 1.86 in 1982, and in the North West 2.03 in 1981 and 2.09 in 1982. Since the Department of Employment itself estimates that approximately one third of vacancies are notified the overall vacancy ratio for the three regions was: South East 17.97 in 1981, 16.47 in 1982; Midlands, 5.91 in 1981 and 5.58 in 1982; North West 6.09 in 1981 and 6.27 in 1982.

With the help of data provided by Manpower Service Commission officials in the regions concerned it is possible to calculate the vacancy: unemployed ratio for the travel to work areas in which the redundancies occurred. Table 4.5.3 presents the data for the five relevant travel-to-work areas.

Table 4.5.3
Ratio of notified vacancies to unemployed (male and female), September 1981 and September 1982 (by travel-to-work area)

	1981 (%)	1982 (%)
South East	7.43	5.17
North West	3.08	3.41
Midlands (manual)	1.75	1.76
North West (manual)	3.25	3.02
Midlands (clerical)	2.2	1.50

Hence for every 100 unemployed people there were 7.43 notified vacancies in the South East market town in 1981 and 5.17 in 1982; in the North West area (B) 3.08 in September 1981 and 3.41 in 1982, in Birmingham 1.75 in 1981 and 1.76 in 1982; in North West area D 3.25 in 1981 and 3.02 in 1982; and in Coventry 2.2 in 1981 and 1.50 in 1982. To establish a more adequate index of labour demand the number of notified vacancies should be multiplied by 3, resulting in figures for September 1982 of 15.51 per hundred in the South East market town, 10.23 in the North West area B, 5.28 in Birmingham, 9.06 in the North West area D, and 4.50 in Coventry. There were thus only 15.51 jobs for every 100 unemployed in the most favoured area: in the least favoured area there were only 4.50 per hundred. (Since discrimination in employment is illegal there is of course no separate information on vacancies for women.)

The vacancy:unemployment ratio provides a useful, if crude, basis for comparing the level of labour demand between areas, and indicates the magnitude of the task the women faced in finding work. Nevertheless, ratios in themselves can be misleading: the same ratio has rather different implications for the chances of finding a job for a specific woman with specific skills depending upon whether the relevant labour market is small or large. The opportunities for finding work might be expected to be greater in large travel-to-work areas than in small ones. Table 4.5.4 therefore presents data on the total number of unemployed, the number of vacancies, and the number of women unemployed, for each area. Hence, in the most favoured travel-to-work area in the North West and Midlands in September 1981, area D, there were 387 vacancies notified, and 11 900 unemployed, including 3907 women; in the most-favoured area in the two regions in 1982, area B, there were 367 notified vacancies and 10 752 unemployed, including 3300 women. In the least-favoured area in 1981, Birmingham, there were 1974 notified vacancies and 112 853 unemployed, including 30 840 women; in the least-favoured area in September 1982, Coventry, there were 642 vacancies and 42 946 unemployed, including 12 668 women.

The evidence presented in the preceding paragraphs does not make it possible to assess precisely whether the women's perceptions of the labour markets in

Table 4.5.4
Job vacancies and unemployment levels, September 1981 and September 1982

	1981			1982		
	Notified vacancies	Total unemployed	Female unemployed	Notified vacancies	Total unemployed	Female unemployed
South East	452	6 081	1 966	381	7 374	2 538
North West (B)	308	10 014	3 027	367	10 752	3 300
Birmingham	1974	112 853	30 840	2234	127 281	33 941
North West (D)	387	11 900	3 907	388	12 868	4 023
Coventry	893	40 500	12 500	642	42 946	12 668

which they were involved were accurate or not: the local level data are not disaggregated by occupation. However, the data do indicate the limited number of vacancies which existed overall, and the competition for those vacancies the women could expect from both men and other women. In general there were substantially more vacancies in the South East, although the growth in unemployment, especially in female unemployment, in the local labour market in which the women from case study A were involved indicated that even in the South East openings in specific areas could be limited. The ratio of vacancies to unemployed was much lower in the remaining labour markets, in only one area in one year exceeding ten vacancies per 100 unemployed workers.

The majority of women thus perceived considerable difficulties in finding work following the redundancies: the overall data indicates an even less favourable situation than the women perceived. The women, especially in the Midlands and North West, did not think that there were many jobs for them, and they were right. Their attitudes and behaviour therefore had only slight impact upon their prospects of re-employment. However, their attitudes and behaviour are important, for they indicate the significance they attached to market employment: for the majority of women the difficulties they encountered in finding work had neither changed their preferences, inhibited their search for jobs, nor undermined their commitment to market employment at the time of the second interviews, four to seven months after leaving their jobs. Whether the extended period of unemployment they were likely to experience would eventually do so only time, and further research, will tell.

5

WOMEN AND UNEMPLOYMENT

In the previous chapter we examined the experience of the redundant women in the labour market; in this we examine the women's experience of, and attitudes towards, unemployment. We have attempted to provide a comprehensive picture of the effect of unemployment on the women concerned, covering their economic, domestic, and personal circumstances. The chapter is divided into eight sections. The first section presents basic data about the length of time unemployed of the women interviewed. In the second section we discuss the economic impact of unemployment. The third is concerned with women's activities during unemployment: how do women spend the time previously spent in paid employment? In the fourth section we discuss the effect of unemployment on family life and relationships. The fifth section covers the effect of unemployment on the women's relations with friends and with the wider community: does unemployment lead to social isolation? The sixth section is concerned with the effect of unemployment upon health, both physical and psychological. In section seven we examine the impact of redundancy and unemployment on the women's attitudes to government and employment. The chapter ends with a brief summarizing conclusion.

5.1 Length of time of unemployment

We have defined as unemployed all women who were out of work for at least a week and who did not have a job arranged before leaving their pre-redundancy employment; we have therefore excluded those women who had a job arranged before leaving their pre-redundancy job, even if they had a short break before taking up their jobs, and those women who were out of work for under a week; on this criterion 164 or 83 per cent of the women interviewed a second time had experienced unemployment.

The length of time between the women leaving their pre-redundancy employment and their second interviews, and hence the potential length of time out of work recorded at the time of the second interviews, differed between case studies. The majority of women from Company A were interviewed five to seven months after leaving, the majority from Company B five or six months after leaving, and the majority from Company E two to four months. Women in Companies C and D had widely staggered leaving dates, and hence a wider variation in length of time between interviews. Only twenty-five of the 164 women interviewed on experience of unemployment were working when interviewed, although a further sixteen had had jobs in the interim. Table 5.1.1 summarizes the length of time unemployed of the women interviewed.

Table 5.1.1
Length of time unemployed of all respondents interviewed at second stage

Length of time (weeks)	Company					Total	N
	A (%)	B (%)	C (%)	D (%)	E (%)	(%)	
0	19	7	6	32	21	15	32
1– 3	2		2		2	1.5	1
4– 7	2	2	2	10	7	4	8
8–11	5	5	6	16	3	7	13
12–15	5	2	4	10	49	11	22
16–19	7	5	15	10		8	16
20–23	33	71	24.5	23	14	34	67
24–27	26	7	9		3	10	20
28–31			15			4	8
32–33			17			5	9
N	42	41	53	31	29		196

The women who answered the questions on unemployment could not be considered as long-term unemployed; no woman had been out of work for more than thirty-three weeks, and the average length of time out of work was twenty weeks. However, the unemployment was not simply frictional unemployment: the majority of unemployed women (63 per cent) had been out of work for

Table 5.1.2
Average length of unemployment at time of interview

Company	Average no. of weeks	Standard deviation
A	20.3	6.0
B	20.5	4.5
C	22.8	7.6
D	14.2	6.0
E	15.5	4.9
Total average	19.6	7.0

($N = 164$)

twenty weeks or more, many women in the three earlier case studies being out of work for substantially longer periods of time. Moreover, since the rate of re-employment was low (see above, pp. 156–8), it was likely that women out of work at the time of the second interview would remain out of work in the future. We were therefore examining the early stages of the unemployment career of the long-term unemployed, but the full effects of long-term unemployment upon economic circumstances, activities, relationships, and attitudes had not yet begun to reveal themselves.

5.2 The economic impact of redundancy and unemployment

For most women money was a major incentive for going out to work. It would therefore be expected that the loss of income from work would be a major feature in their experience of unemployment, and that financial problems and the discomfort of having to adjust to a lower standard of living would be two of the women's chief concerns. However, although this was likely to be so in the long term, it was unfortunately not possible to study the likely major long-term effects of loss of income within the scope of this project because of the cushioning effect of redundancy payments, payments in lieu of notice, tax rebates, and unemployment benefit. As described above, the women were interviewed on their post-redundancy experience at varying lengths of time ranging from two to eight months after their redundancy and the average redundancy payment was sufficiently large to replace their net wages for at least eight months. It was possible therefore to collect fairly detailed data on the women's present financial position, but we could make only a broad assessment of the long-term effect of the loss of employment income on their standard of living.

5.2.1 *Women's post-redundancy financial status*

The women received widely varying amounts of redundancy money depending upon the terms of the redundancy agreement and their individual length of service. Details of the redundancy settlement in each company and the payments the women received are given in Chapter 3 (pp. 128–31, 147–8 above) and are not repeated here. As was shown there, there were marked differences in the level of redundancy payments received, women in Companies B, C, D, and E receiving substantially higher payments than women in Company A: the women from Companies B, C, D, and E received payments averaging between £3000 and £4000, the women in Company A receiving payments averaging only £847. In addition to the statutory and *ex gratia* redundancy payments, women who had paid full National Insurance contributions were eligible for unemployment benefit for one year dating from the end of the period during which wages in lieu of notice were paid. For women who had worked for twelve years or more without a break for the company, payment in lieu of notice continued for three months after leaving the company. Only a few women were interviewed under three months after leaving and all women who were eligible for unemployment benefit were receiving it when interviewed. All those women who had paid full National Insurance contributions had applied for unemployment benefit, and in total seventy-five women, 54 per cent of those unemployed when interviewed, were receiving unemployment benefit.

Whether the women had paid full insurance contributions or not was influenced by age, with older women less likely than younger women to have started work after contributions became compulsory, and possibly also less likely to have transferred when full insurance became more generally accepted, being compulsory for women starting a new job. There was thus a slight inverse correlation between age and eligibility for unemployment benefit with eligibility decreasing with age.

Table 5.2.1.1
Proportion of women receiving unemployment benefit (by age)

Age	Percentage	N
18–24	75	4
25–34	67	27
35–44	54	48
45–54	50	42
55–60	39	18
Total	54	139

N = women unemployed at the time of the second interview.

However, there was also a significant difference between companies, with women in Company B, where the average age was high, being the most likely to be fully insured. As the eligibility rate was also higher in C than in D and E the differences may also reflect different attitudes to benefits between clerical and manual workers, with manual workers more likely to be insured: the relatively low eligibility rate among the manual workers in Company A would be expected because of the high proportion of part-time workers in that company, only thirteen out of the thirty-seven formerly part-time workers unemployed when interviewed receiving benefit.

The different proportions of women paying full insurance may have been due to differences in company policy. However, the differences may also reflect differences in attitudes between manual and non-manual workers, manual workers, especially semi-skilled manual workers, being more likely to pay full insurance than non-manual workers: 58.5 per cent of semi-skilled manual workers were receiving unemployment benefit, compared with 41 per cent of unemployed clerical workers, although the former tended to be older than

Table 5.2.1.2
Proportion of women receiving unemployment benefit (by company)

Company	Percentage	N
A	44	27
B	73	33
C	59.5	42
D	39	18
E	37	19
Total	54	139

($p = 0.040$)
N = women unemployed at the time of the second interview.

the latter, and therefore contained a lower proportion of women legally required to pay the full rate.

5.2.2 *Uses made of redundancy money*

There are several potential ways of using redundancy money, a major factor influencing potential use being the availability of alternative sources of income, including spouse's wage. Unemployed married women with wage-earning husbands were likely to bank their redundancy money, to use gradually as a long-term income supplement and insurance against the difficulties likely to be encountered in adjusting to a reduced standard of living. However, not all married women had wage-earning husbands: fourteen women who were unemployed longer than three months also had husbands who were also unemployed, and in addition three had retired husbands and two husbands who were invalid pensioners. Four of these husbands had no income, and were presumably living upon their own and their wife's capital until eligible for social-security benefits.

Women who had no husband or whose husbands were unemployed were likely to be dependent upon social security benefits. However, they were eligible for that benefit only when their capital was reduced to £2000 (since increased to £2500). Alternatives for this group were therefore to use their redundancy payment for day-to-day expenditure until it was reduced to that amount, or to spend it on needed durables and in paying off mortgage and hire-purchase commitments in order to reduce future financial obligations. The latter course of action would result in the greatest financial advantage, especially if redundancy payments were small and home improvements or the purchase of domestic consumer durables were seen as major priorities, or if outstanding debts existed attracting substantial interest payments. Only if redundancy payments were substantially higher than the amount of capital legally permitted for recipients of supplementary benefit, and the family was already equipped with all the consumer durables considered necessary for comfort, was it expedient to use redundancy money for day-to-day expenditure. However, some women did not wish to rely on social-security benefits whilst they still had money of their own.

For women who were able to find work immediately, redundancy payments came as a windfall, although in many cases their new jobs paid less. This last group could use their redundancy money to purchase 'treats', holidays, or consumer goods they could not have bought with their normal salary, or the money could be banked as insurance against future job loss. Since many women who found work obtained only temporary jobs, financial caution was likely.

The use made of redundancy money therefore varied from individual to individual, depending upon a number of factors including the size of the redundancy payment, size of husband's income, current debts, current perceived need for home improvements and home durables, and anticipated future income. The use of redundancy money as a temporary substitute for employment income (income replacement) was uncommon, since most of the women who did not find work immediately were pessimistic about getting a job in the near future. In the event only ten (5.5 per cent) of women used their money as a substitute for wages, of whom only four had employed husbands.

Table 5.2.2.1
Uses of redundancy money

Use	Percentage	N
Income replacement only	5.5	10
Income supplement only (savings and some current expenditure)	5.5	10
Income replacement or income supplement and specific expenditure	23	42
Saved only	29	52
Specific expenditure only	17	31
Savings and specific expenditure	20	36
Total		181

N = no. of respondents who received and declared redundancy money.

The women were asked to list the specific uses made of redundancy money and were allowed to list up to six different uses, only seven women listing that number. Sixty-three per cent of women had put some aside for savings, although only 29 per cent gave savings as their only use. Forty-one per cent of women used some redundancy money for current expenditure, although only 5.5 per cent gave current expenditure as their only use. Twenty-five per cent spent at least some of their money on home improvements; 21 per cent on home furnishings or other consumer durables; 17 per cent on a holiday; and 14 per cent on outstanding bills.

A small number of women, thirty-one, or 17 per cent, used all their redundancy money for specific expenditures. In most cases expenditure was designed to improve the family's financial position through paying off debts and mortgages, or investment through home improvements, as Table 5.2.2.3 shows.

Table 5.2.2.2
Specific uses made of redundancy money

Uses	Percentage
Savings	63
To live on	41
Home improvements	25
Home furnishings/durables	21
Holiday	17
Outstanding bills	14
Pay off or purchase car	10
Give to or spend on children	7
Pay off house mortgage	4
Invest in business	4
Recreation/hobby	3
Knitting machine purchase	0.5(1)
Caravan purchase	0.5(1)
Undecided	0.5(1)
No redundancy money	1
Unwilling to say	5

Number of uses: 410
Number of respondents: 196.
Percentage is that of respondents.

Table 5.2.2.3
Uses redundancy money for specific items only

Use	N
Pay off house	2
Invest in business	2
Home improvements	12
Pay off outstanding bills	6
Purchase or pay off car	5
Home furnishings/durables	14
Holiday	3
Recreation/hobby	2
Spend on children	4
Clothes	1
Undecided	1

Number of uses: 52.
Number of respondents: 31.

Of the sixty-two women who used their redundancy money to replace or to supplement income, sixteen had exhausted it by the time they were interviewed. The length of time taken to use up their redundancy money varied widely. One had used up her money in three weeks, two in four weeks. Eight women had used up their money in three to five months, and a further five between five and seven months. Forty-six women were still using it as a regular income supplement when interviewed. As women were interviewed at periods varying from three to eight months after redundancy, all that can be said of this remaining group is that their money lasted longer than three months.

In general, the cushioning effects of extra payments, including redundancy money and unemployment benefit, meant that few women found themselves in serious financial difficulties by the time of the second interview. Only 12 per cent of those who had been unemployed for three months or more said that they found it very difficult to manage, and a further 1 per cent could not manage at all. Women from company A, where redundancy payments were relatively small, were no more likely to say that they found it difficult to manage than women from other companies, although all were interviewed six months after leaving: the two women who found it impossible to manage were from the Midlands Companies C and E. It is apparent that redundancy money, payment in lieu of notice, tax rebates, and unemployment benefit were sufficient even among company A women to maintain their standard of living for six months. Moreover, in Company A employment was available for sewing-machinists, if at inferior rates of pay and working conditions. Length of time out of work up to the maximum period of eight months made no difference in the degree of difficulty in managing. In reply to questions on the financial difficulties faced, the most commonly chosen response out of the four possible, was 'manage, but with not much money to spare.'

Table 5.2.2.4
Women's overall assessment of their financial situation

	Percentage
Manage without difficulty	34.5
Manage but with not much money to spare	49
Find it very difficult to manage	12
Really not manage at all	1
Missing	3.5
N	142

N = women unemployed for three months or longer.

5.2.3 Predicted long-term financial situation

Redundancy benefits and related payments, if used as a supplement to other sources of income, could be expected to forestall serious financial difficulties for one or two years, depending upon the size of the payment and upon other financial resources available to the women. However, the long-term prognosis for the women and their families was less promising. The results of a short postal questionnaire sent to the women approximately one year after the redundancies showed that, among women who were still unemployed, 64 per cent were then finding it difficult to manage financially.

In the long term, for married women loss of wages meant a decline in net joint income from an average £147 to an average £88.5 (see pp. 39–44). For single householders with children the financial consequences of a change from wages to social-security benefits were generally small, since the women's wages were low and employment usually involved additional expenses in fares, additional clothes, and use of convenience foods. The supplementary benefit for women with children often nearly matched what they could earn. However, at these very low levels of income small sums assume a major significance, and the little extra gained by employment could make a significant difference by adding some variety and scope to lives otherwise restricted by poverty. For young women living at home with their parents, board and lodging payments were usually small and would be easily covered by social-security payments, leaving some money for pocket money. This group may not suffer a much lower standard of living, but will no longer be able to save towards future independence in the form of their own or their marital home. Single women living on their own without children may suffer a drop in income to about half their normal income or less by going on social-security benefit, a drop which would mean a drastic change in their living circumstances.

The relative proportions of single and married women among our initial respondents was given in chapter 1 (pp. 21–2). However, these proportions were slightly different among those unemployed for three months or more. A slightly higher proportion of single women found work following redundancy, so that the proportion of married women among the unemployed was 79 per cent rather than the 74 per cent of initial respondents. There were thirty women who were supporting themselves (or were living with their parents) among the 142 women unemployed for three months or more. The remaining 112 were married, including fourteen whose husbands were unemployed, three whose husbands were retired, and two whose husbands were on invalide pensions. The proportion of unemployed married women who had unemployed husbands remained approximately the same as the proportion had been for the whole original sample of 279, changing from 12 to 13 per cent.

In the original sample the average net wage of all husbands was £88.5, although this figure was somewhat tentative (see above, p. 000). However, the average net income of the husbands of unemployed women was substantially lower: £78.50 (response rate was still only 68 per cent). In more detail, of those who declared their husband's income, 5 per cent had husbands with no income, a further 11 per cent of husbands had incomes of under £46, 23 per cent of under £66, 64 per cent of under £96, and only 30 per cent of £96 or over. The lower average income for husbands of unemployed women than for the whole sample was probably a result of a general tendency for more highly qualified women (such as industrial nurses and secretaries) to be both more likely to be re-employed and also more likely to have husbands earning higher incomes.

232 *Working Women in Recession*

Table 5.2.3.1
Incomes of husbands of unemployed women

Husband's net weekly income (£s)	Women who declared husband's income (%)
0	5
1– 45	11
46– 65	11
66– 95	42
96–115	25
116–205	5

($N = 79$)

5.2.4 *Economies*

Since few women had come to the end of the extra payments received on redundancy, the economies being made were marginal and 54 per cent of unemployed women said they had not had to economize at all. As Table 5.2.4.1 shows, the most common economy made was in clothes and shoes: although their replacement cannot be postponed indefinitely, it is not difficult to make clothes and shoes last longer. Seventy six women mentioned one economy, forty-five mentioned two, and twenty-eight mentioned three. Since only three responses were allowed, it is possible that more economies were made than were mentioned.

Because most of the women still had redundancy money in their savings

Table 5.2.4.1
Specific economies made by unemployed women

	No. of women mentioning specific economies
Clothes, shoes	29
Generally cutting back, no extras	24
Going out for meals, drinks	16
Less food	13
Holidays	8
Cuts in heating, power	8
Going out in car/petrol	6
Given up car completely	6
Smoking	5
Cuts in food variety	5
Family outings	4
Hairdressers	3
Savings	2
Present giving	2
Other	10
Total	141

Number of women making economies = 76.
Number of women with experience of unemployment = 164.

accounts the economies made by the women were generally in the areas in which economies might be anticipated when reduced expenditure is the result of careful budgeting rather than of immediate necessity. However, a minority of women (twenty-two) were already experiencing serious financial problems: four were cutting back on food and were unable to meet service bills, a further nine were cutting back on food, and a further nine were unable to meet service bills. All married women in this group (eighteen) had husbands with net incomes of £100 a week or under, and most had incomes of under £70. Four of the twenty-two were not married.

To summarize: as all unemployed redundant women were either eligible for unemployment benefit or married, redundancy money was generally used as an income supplement, saved for emergencies, or used to purchase needed goods, rather than used as income replacement. Most women had sufficient redundancy money to supplement their income to a reasonable level for at least one year. Under half the unemployed women had had to reduce their normal expenditure, and only a small minority had had serious financial difficulties. However, the long-term prognosis was less favourable. The women who had been unable to find jobs tended to have husbands with low incomes: the average income of the husbands of unemployed women being £78.5, compared to £88.5 for all husbands. When the redundancy money runs out families will probably find it difficult to manage on the husband's income alone, so that for many married, as well as single, women unemployment will result in serious economic hardship.

5.3 Activities

Before the redundancy the women had established a pattern of life, in many cases for several years, which they had expected to continue: 70 per cent were intending to work without a break until their retirement, and 65 per cent had already worked for ten years or more with their pre-redundancy employer. The redundancies initiated a change in routine, which was unanticipated in four of the case studies and in the fifth (B) the individual women were not certain that they themselves would be declared redundant, although it was known that the production facility was being phased out. The redundancies also initiated a major change in social environment; all the women had been working in plants employing over 100 workers, but 66 per cent lived in households of three or under. Unemployment therefore resulted in an inevitable constriction in social horizons. The contrast between the directed activity and companionship of the work-place and the freedom, comparative isolation, and quiet of home and neighbourhood, was sharp.

A sudden change of this nature in the pattern of daily routine has a number of possible consequences. In the following sections we investigate whether or not the women had time on their hands and difficulty in finding things to do, whether or not they found their non-work activities pleasanter and more interesting than their work tasks, whether their ceasing to work with a number of other people resulted in their feeling isolated or whether they preferred the relative autonomy of their domestic lives, and finally whether the termination of a role that had occupied a major part of their life resulted in feelings of loss of identity, leading to depression, stress, and feelings of worthlessness. This section is concerned with whether the women missed the activity of their work.

The women were asked at the pre-redundancy interview what they anticipated doing with their time if they did not find another job. Before the redundancy the women did not generally anticipate extending their existing domestic activities (only 15 per cent mentioned housework and none mentioned gardening), but rather initiating a new non-domestic occupation: voluntary work, or extending a creative occupation: knitting, sewing, and other craft work. Self-employment and vocational education were also listed more frequently in anticipation than in realisation. Table 5.3.1 shows how, before the redundancy, the unemployed women had anticipated spending their time if and when they became unemployed.

Table 5.3.1
Anticipated activities of unemployed following the redundancy

	Company					Total
	A (%)	B (%)	C (%)	D (%)	E (%)	(%)
Knitting/sewing/crafts	29	34	28	33	23	30
Voluntary work	12	8	38	14	18	20
Housework	12	24	14	10	9	15
Not know/dreading	21	21	12	5	5	14
Visiting family/friends	12	13	2	10	9	8
Home decorating	3	5	8	5	14	7
Assistance to parents/ relatives	6	11	4	14	–	7
Self-employed	3	3	12	–	–	5
Looking after relatives' children	3	11	2	–	–	4
Vocational education	–	3	4	5	9	4
Other	–	–	8	23	29	9
N	34	38	50	21	21	164

N = no. of women with experience of unemployment.
Percentage is that of women mentioning given activity.

The most frequently mentioned activity was thus knitting/sewing or other craft activity, mentioned by 30 per cent of women, followed by voluntary work, mentioned by 20 per cent. The infrequent mention of housework may have been because it was taken for granted by many women, but in the event the default activity was more important than anticipated.

As many as 20 per cent (thirty-three) of women mentioned before the redundancies that they planned to take up voluntary work; however, only 6 per cent (ten) did so, most of whom had been involved in voluntary work before becoming redundant. This was possibly because charity work is to some extent organized as a social occupation and normally requires the formation of appropriate networks before active involvement becomes a real possibility. The intention to become involved in voluntary work may be realized in due course, when such networks are established. At the present time, only three of the ten women involved had taken up voluntary work as a new activity; for the remainder it involved greater participation in organizations to which they already belonged. Eight women anticipated self-employment, but only one had fulfilled this ambition by the time of the second interview, and again the first steps had been taken before the redundancy. Only one woman out of the six who planned to return to vocational education had done so by the time of the second interview. In general, therefore, the expectations of taking up an activity other than housework and recreation were not fulfilled, except that additional time was spent on knitting/sewing and craft work.

The majority of women interviewed were housekeepers as well as employees. Although few women had young children to care for, only twenty-seven out of the 196 respondents to the second questionnaire had neither husband nor children living at home, and only eleven out of the ninety-one who were still looking for work.

Table 5.3.2
Employment status and household circumstances

Employment status	Husband/children living at home (%)	No husband/children living at home (%)	N
Looking for work	88	12	91
Permanently retired	92	8	14
Temporarily retired	88	12	34
Working full time	70	30	33
Working part time	100	0	23
Own business	0	100	1

Nearly all the women therefore had housekeeping duties to perform. It is therefore not surprising that the activity most often mentioned as replacing paid employment during the daytime was housework, mentioned by 68 per cent of women. In addition, the five activities most commonly mentioned, after housework, were those associated with traditional female domestic activities, with the possible exception of visiting and entertaining. (And even visiting and entertaining was often associated with fulfilling family responsibilities rather than recreation.) Table 5.3.3 summarizes the activities which replaced going out to work for unemployed women. The five most often mentioned activities were also those on which most time was likely to be spent. In short, more women spent more time doing housework than doing any other single activity.

Table 5.3.3
Activities replacing work for unemployed women (by company)

	Company					Total
	A (%)	B (%)	C (%)	D (%)	E (%)	(%)
Housework	77	47	68	81	77	68
Visiting/entertaining/going out with friends/relations	56	60	34	57	9	44
Gardening	50	32	28	33	32	35
Knitting/sewing/crafts	50	32	28	33	32	35
Home decorating	9	29	42	24	27	28
Shopping	6	26	16	19	9	16
Reading	9	18	16	10	23	15
Walking/walking dog	24	21	8	10	9	15
Sport/gym	6	16	14	10	5	11
Baking/jam making/freezing	6	21	4	5	18	10
Assisting relatives	6	8	4	5	9	6
Looking after relatives' children	6	10	6	5	9	6
Voluntary work	6	5	6	5	9	6
Hobbies n.e.c.	6	8	6	–	–	5
Looking after own children	3	5	4	–	9	5
Looking for work	6	5	4	9	–	5
Other	23	8	8	19	19	13
Average no. of activities mentioned	3.3	3.6	3.1	3.3	2.8	3.1
N	34	38	50	21	21	164

N = no. of women with experience of unemployment.
Percentage is that of women mentioning each activity. The women were permitted to mention up to six activities, the average number mentioned being 3.1.

The focus upon domestic tasks was characteristic of the most frequently mentioned activities in all case studies and, less predictably, was independent of marital status. Single, or married women without children, were no less likely than married women with children to mention housework as the activity which replaced paid employment. As they were mostly young women living with their mothers, their friends were usually at work during the day, and often their parents also: they assumed more responsibility for running the house than they had done previously. No fewer than 79 per cent of single and childless women mentioned housework as one of the major activities that replaced going out to work: 58 per cent mentioned knitting and sewing; 47 per cent mentioned gardening; 42 per cent mentioned visiting, entertaining, and going out; and 32 per cent mentioned home decorating.

Social activities as a pastime varied greatly between firms, possibly reflecting local cultural patterns, the women from the two northern towns mentioning visiting, entertaining, and going out with friends or relatives significantly more often than the women from the two Midlands towns. Variations in patterns of social contact are of some significance in assessing the impact of unemployment among women, as those women whose domestic lives are highly privatized are likely to be dependent upon going out to work for social contact. This aspect of unemployment is discussed in section 5.5. Knitting and sewing were mentioned most often by the garment workers from A, many of whom used their work skills in making garments for friends and relations and occasionally for private sale. Home decorating, an activity made possible by the availability of redundancy money, was much less likely to be mentioned by women from A than from the other four companies, redundancy payments in A having been small. It was most likely to be mentioned by women from company C, the firm with the largest redundancy payments.

Two of the most commonly mentioned activities, home decorating and gardening, mentioned by 28 and 35 per cent of unemployed women respectively, did not provide a regular occupation. Home decorating was initiated as a practical use for redundancy money, mostly involving repainting and re-wallpapering, often after tradesmen had completed building repairs or renovations. Once completed it would not need to be done again for some time. Gardening, one of the more popular activities, is to some extent seasonal, especially popular in summer time: a number of women mentioned in passing that, although unemployment might be bearable in the summer, they were dreading the winter when their activities would be further restricted.

Far fewer women mentioned activities undertaken solely for recreation: reading and visiting the library (15 per cent); walking and taking the dog for a walk (15 per cent); sport and gymnastics (11 per cent); baking, jam- and wine-making, and freezing (10 per cent). In addition, 16 per cent mentioned shopping, which may combine recreation and utility.

A final group of activities were again task-oriented: helping or looking after sick or elderly relatives was mentioned by 8 per cent, whilst looking after nieces, nephews, grandchildren, looking for work, charity work, and hobbies were each mentioned by 5 or 6 per cent of women. Only 4 per cent mentioned looking after their own baby or young children as a major activity, a reflection of the small number of women with young children. The remaining thirteen activities, mostly recreational, were each mentioned by only one or two women.

To a large extent the unemployed women simply spent more time when unemployed doing the things they had previously done during their non-work hours. However, we also asked the women which of their present activities they had started since becoming unemployed. A minority, 35 per cent, had started no new activities, although 29 per cent had initiated more than one and 7 per cent more than two. The activities most commonly mentioned as being new were: social (16 per cent); home decorating (13 per cent); gardening (9 per cent); knitting and sewing (9 per cent); walking/walking the dog (8 per cent); and reading (7 per cent). Amongst the two most commonly mentioned were the short-term activity, home decorating, and the seasonal activity, gardening. There were few indications of new activities replacing paid employment as a permanent means of spending time, much less of establishing a new identity.

The number of new activities did not increase with the time out of work; on the contrary, there was an inverse relationship, the average length of time out of work being longer for women who reported having no, or only one, new activity than for women who reported two or more. The availability of redundancy money may have heightened people's opportunities for a short period after the redundancy; home decorating, gardening, and knitting and sewing are all activities requiring at least a small outlay of money.

As well as documenting how the women spent the time they had available during unemployment, we were also interested to find out how they rated their activities subjectively: to discover whether they found their domestic activities as satisfying a way of spending time as they had their paid employment, or whether they missed the activities involved in paid employment. The particular value of being able to interview women immediately after the redundancy was that they were able to make a direct and immediate comparison between their domestic activities and those of their previous paid employment. The time available during the interview did not permit a detailed analysis of the rewards of the various specific activities with which the women filled the day: they were simply asked to rank each of the three activities on which they spent the most time according to whether they found the activity more or less interesting, or about the same, as the paid work they had been doing. Obviously, because of the multi-dimensional nature of the rewards of activities, not all ways of spending time are directly comparable: household activities involve autonomy and a degree of freedom in time and space, in addition to the intrinsic interest (or otherwise) of the tasks themselves; market employment provides opportunities for companionship, especially in the jobs in which the women were engaged. Moreover, different values were attributed to the activities: in domestic life, the knowledge that the activity is performed for the benefit of family, and in market employment the feeling of performing a socially and economically useful and recognized service, possibly make domestic and paid occupations difficult to compare. However, the feelings of subjective satisfaction gained from different activities, no matter how unlike, were in many instances comparable. The majority of women were able to make a comparison, although this varied according to which activity was being compared with market work, the routine task activity of housework being the most easily comparable, recreational activities the least.

Housework was the activity on which women spent the most time. It was also likely to be considered less interesting than their previous paid employment: as Table 5.3.4 shows, 52 per cent of women who included housework as one of their three major activities said that it was less interesting than their previous paid work, 18 per cent that it was about the same, and 10 per cent that it was more interesting. One women summed up her post-redundancy activities as 'just basic housework you know. Just completely bored. Nothing else. I'm not clever at anything else.' On the other hand, knitting and sewing, productive activities which produced articles for gifts or even for sale, were more likely

Table 5.3.4
Rating of most time-consuming activities

Activity	More interesting than paid work (%)	Less interesting than paid work (%)	About the same (%)	Not comparable (%)	Missing (%)	N
Housework	10	52	18	18	1	109
Social	30	28	15	26		53
Gardening	24	24	24	27		45
Knitting and sewing	30	12.5	27.5	30		40
Home decorating	24	36	12	27		33
Other	29	23	16	33		146

N = no. of respondents mentioning each activity as one of the three on which they spent the most time.

to be ranked the same as, or more interesting than, paid employment (the high proportion in the 'not comparable' category being due to the high proportion for whom knitting was a subsidiary activity, done while visiting, watching television, or resting). Social activities were regarded as only slightly more interesting than paid employment; some 'social' activities were considered as duty rather than recreation. Gardening ranked about equal with paid employment, and home decorating slightly below, the high rate of non-comparability in the latter case being due to the temporary and non-routine nature of home decorating as a task. 'Other' activities were mostly recreational and were likely, but only by a small margin, to be more interesting than the job, with a large proportion not comparable.

When comparing the satisfactions afforded by domestic activities with those afforded by paid activities, preference depends not only upon the intrinsic qualities of the activities, but also upon the environment within which they are carried out. However, differences in environment made little difference to the comparisons, if the women's occupational status and husband's income can be used as proxies for environmental differences. Preference for home activities was not linked to occupational status or husband's income. High status and high household income are likely to be associated with good conditions at work and at home: the privileged were comparing two privileged environments, the deprived two deprived environments.

Unemployment meant that women had time to fill which had previously been filled by going out to work. But the loss of a job also meant the loss of an income, which might have implied a curtailment of, rather than an increase in, recreational activities. However, in practice few women (25 per cent) had had to give up any activities, since most women had sufficient redundancy money to maintain their normal standard of living up to the time of the second interview. Before the redundancies the women's lives had centred upon work and domestic activities and they had probably spent little time or money on recreation. Moreover, having become accustomed to a work-oriented way of life, only 33 per cent of the women could think of activities which they would have liked to do on leaving employment, but could not because of lack of money.

The list of activities that the women had had to give up altogether was not large; eight women had given up going out for meals in a pub or restaurant, seven had given up going out for drives in the car, seven going out generally, five going out dancing, and four going out for a drink. Remaining activities given up were each mentioned by only one or two women. The major activity the women would have liked to take up, but felt unable to, was attendance at keep-fit classes or other ways of keeping fit, mentioned by nine women: four women were unable to afford sewing machines to do sewing at home. The remaining activities forgone were mentioned by only one or two women each.

Because of the small numbers involved, it was not possible to discern any pattern by age or occupational status among those women who felt constrained in their activities by lack of money. However, the evidence suggests that a significantly higher proportion of widowed, divorced, and separated women felt a financial constraint on their activities compared with married or single women.

Table 5.3.5

Women experiencing financial constraint on activities (by marital status)

Marital status	Percentage	N
Single	29	14
Widowed	43	7
Divorced/separated	70	13
Married	28	130
Total	33	164

More specific questions were asked on the extent to which the women had had to cut back their recreational activities, rather than cancel them altogether, and here change could be discerned: in general, activities involving significant expenditure were reduced, those involving little or no expenditure were increased. The women were given a list of seventeen activities and asked whether, after becoming unemployed, they undertook them more or less often or about the same, or had never done them at all. The first six activities listed were social: going out with friends to a pub or for a meal, visiting or entertaining relatives, having friends round for a drink or a meal. Taking the average of all answers on social activities 26 per cent gave answers signifying greater activity and only 12 per cent less, 42 per cent the same rate of activity, and 20 per cent the same absence of activity, as shown in Table 5.3.6. Social activities costing little or nothing became more common. Visiting and dropping in on friends and relatives informally was done more often, but having friends in for a meal or going with friends to a pub was likely to be done less, or had never been done.

Ten other recreational activities were also listed, which involved only the respondent or her immediate family. Of these, gardening, sewing and other personal hobbies, and reading were likely to be done more by a majority of women, watching television was likely to be done more by a large minority. Other recreations listed: sport, going to sports events, going to the theatre or to bingo were most likely not to have been done at all before or after the redundancy. There was no difference in regional patterns worth noting.

Table 5.3.6
Changes in social activities during unemployment

	More (%)	Less (%)	About same (%)	Never done (%)
Going with friends to pub	9	19	37	35
Going with friends for meal	6	30	31	34
Visiting relatives	51	4	41	3
Having relatives to visit	34	5	56	4
Friends dropping in	45	7	39	9
Having friends round for meal/drink	11	9	47	33

Table 5.3.7
Changes in other recreational activities: individual activities

	More (%)	Less (%)	About the same (%)	Never done (%)
Taking family on outing	18	9	43	30
Gardening, sewing, hobbies	67	2	25	6
Sports	18	4	22	56
Reading, bought	54	8	29	9
Reading, borrowed	41	2	21	35
Smoking	19	8	16	57
Watching television	37	9	51	3
Going to sports events	4	8	20	72
Going to cinema/theatre	4	12	23	61
Bingo	4	2.5	15	79
Having a bet	2	6	32	61

By transferring the household tasks previously done in the evenings and weekends to weekday hours, and extending them, and extending hours spent in visiting and entertaining friends and relations, the majority of women were able to find enough to do to fill in their time. However, a substantial minority, in all age groups and occupations, said that they found that they had time on their hands (30 per cent said that they had time on their hands nearly every day). Although most women found enough to do to fill in their time, they appeared to prefer the pattern of activities they had followed when going out to work: having more time available to do more housework was not generally considered an advantage. Nor was the opportunity to reorganize their time so that evenings and weekends were now free for recreation necessarily a sufficient advantage to compensate for the loss of their paid activity. The majority of women (70 per cent) agreed with the statement 'You get bored if you haven't a job, as Table 5.3.8 shows. There was no statistically significant difference in responses by age (0.679), marital status (0.835), or occupational status (0.761). As was suggested earlier, trade-offs between work and home activities tended to be similar for all ages and occupational statuses: those women who had the most interesting home activities tending also to have the most interesting jobs and vice versa.

Table 5.3.8
Responses to *You get bored if you haven't got a job*

	Company					Total
	A (%)	B (%)	C (%)	D (%)	E (%)	(%)
Agree	71	60	82	57	68	70
Disagree	26	35	18	34	32	27
No opinion	3	5	0	9	0	3
N	33	38	50	21	21	163

Table 5.3.9
Advantages of unemployment

Advantages	Percentage
Not being tied to a time, no pressure, no deadlines	54
Able to do things I want to do, weekends free	34
Nothing	28
More time to spend with family	8
Able to perform family duties more efficiently	3
Not having to get up early	5
Being my own boss/no harrassment	3
Other	10
N	163

Percentage is that of women giving each response.

The women saw some advantages in the change in their weekly routine, as Table 5.3.9 shows. They were asked whether, all round, considering the work they used to do and what they did now, there was anything they liked about their current way of life. Seventy-two per cent of women mentioned at least one advantage. Concepts of a slower pace and of autonomy, the freedom to allocate time according to preference and to perform activities without pressure, and the freedom to choose activities dominated the women's responses. One woman described the slower pace of her life: 'I like reading — my life. You are nice and relaxed. You can take life easier, you can go out and look at the shops when you want to, but the days do seem longer. I can have a lie in at home.' However, she added: 'I don't think I would like to do it much longer' (engineering assembly worker, Company C).

To summarize: the activities that most women reported as filling the time during which they had previously been employed were housekeeping, visiting friends and relations, gardening, knitting and sewing, and home decorating. The activities most often mentioned were domestic task activities, followed by social activities and some knitting and sewing done for private sale or exchange. Sixty-five per cent of women reported that they had begun at least one new activity, the most frequently mentioned as new being social activities (16 per cent), home decorating (13 per cent), gardening (9 per cent), knitting and sewing (9 per cent). Not all activities that replaced going out to work were comparable with paid activities. However, the most comparable activity was housework, which was generally regarded as less interesting than paid employment. There was little indication that loss of income had yet led to major changes in their activities for many women, only a small number of women saying that they had had to give up activities, or had not been able to begin activities, through lack of money. However, there were indications that the women were cutting down on activities that involved expenditure and increasing those that did not. In general, although most women found that they did not have time on their hands, the great majority of women associated unemployment with boredom.

5.4 The effects of unemployment on family life

In this section we discuss how the women's experience of unemployment affected their immediate families and relationships within the family. Since the research timetable did not allow time to interview husbands and children, we have had to rely on the women's own perceptions of their families' reactions to their change in status: there is no reason to presume that these perceptions were systematically distorted.

The section begins with an outline of changes in family size and in the employment status of family members. There was no evidence that the redundancies led the women to begin a family or to become pregnant. There were few changes in family circumstances between the first and the second interviews, and those changes that did occur were more likely to involve a contraction than an expansion in household size. There were both advantages and disadvantages for husbands and other family members in the women being unemployed; overall, 39 per cent of women believed that their husbands preferred them to be at home, and 62.5 per cent believed that their families appreciated their being at home more. These views contrasted with the women's own preference for going out to work, but the differences in view point did not appear to lead to conflict.

Women may use redundancy as an opportunity to make a not unwilling move from a work role to a family role, the only effect of redundancy being to move the date of the change forward. Pregnancies would therefore follow redundancy. However, for the women in our sample, redundancy came at a time in the life cycle when their households, and hence their family responsibilities, were shrinking rather than growing. Some women took the opportunity to retire permanently, but they were mainly older women, and none had retired permanently to start a family. Two women had given birth since the redundancy and two had become pregnant. However, for at least one woman the conjunction of the redundancy and pregnancy resulted in her being ineligible for either unemployment benefit or the maternity leave she had intended to take if the redundancy had not occurred – the conjunction was therefore unfortunate rather than otherwise.

Few households changed in size between the first and second interviews, only twenty. More households declined than increased. Hence twelve households declined in size, due either to children leaving (nine) or other relatives leaving (three). Eight households increased in size, either through children joining (three), other relatives joining (three) or births (two). In addition, two women had become pregnant. The number of women responsible for sick or elderly relatives had not changed: three women were no longer responsible and three had gained responsibilities. (In total twenty five women were responsible for sick or elderly relatives, a significant indication of major family responsibilities.)

Unemployment among husbands had not risen, but remained at 10 per cent of the total, the rate being the same for husbands of both unemployed and employed women. Unemployment had not become a family phenomenon: only 15 per cent of households had one or more other members unemployed. In general there had been no significant changes in family size nor in the employment status of other family members.

There was potentially both a negative and a positive side to families' attitudes regarding the wife working, making simple yes/no answers on the matter of preference inappropriate. It is most likely that families had mixed feelings about the benefits of the wife working, compared with the benefits of having her at home full time, and it is also likely that these feelings were not always accurately conveyed to the women. In order to get as accurate an impression as possible of the women's perceptions of both dimensions of their families' feelings an open-ended question was asked: 'What does your husband think about your current (unemployed) way of life?', followed later in the interview by the more precisely directed question: 'Do your family appreciate having you at home more?' Answers to the first question fell into four main categories: 'He is pleased that I am now home full-time'; 'He does not mind'; 'He is sorry about it for my sake or that of the family's economic interest'; 'He is sorry because I am hard to live with when unemployed.' Only 11 per cent gave comments outside this range. Forty-four per cent of husbands preferred their wives to work, 26.5 per cent for the positive reason of the benefit to herself and the family and 18 per cent because a non-working wife was hard to live with. Thirty-eight per cent of husbands preferred to have their wives at home and 6 per cent were either happy whatever their wives did or were indifferent as Table 5.4.1 shows. Although only 38.5 per cent of married women said that their husbands preferred to have them at home, a much larger proportion, 63 per cent, felt that their families appreciated having them at home more. Husbands' attitudes did not appear to be shaped by their wives' actual employment status; wives who had found work were as likely to think that their husbands preferred them at home as were unemployed or retired wives, although the numbers are too small to be anything but suggestive.

Table 5.4.1
Husband's attitude to wife's employment

	Percentage
Prefers wife to be at home	38.5
Prefers wife to work for benefit of herself/family	26.5
Prefers wife to work because otherwise she gets on his nerves	18
Doesn't mind/not bothered	6
Other comment	11
N	119

Most women thus felt that their families were pleased to have them at home full time. However, most women preferred to go out to work. How far the difference in attitude represented even a latent conflict of interest in some families is not clear. Thirty per cent of women who preferred to work said that their husbands preferred them to stay at home as Table 5.4.2 shows. However, only five women said that they felt under pressure from their husbands not to return to work, and only four from their children. Families' attitudes may have been largely shaped by a desire to make the best of a situation where a return to work was unlikely and to reassure the women that they still had a valued role. On the other hand, some women felt that their husbands did not understand how important their jobs had been to them. As one woman from the Midlands engineering factory said: 'He can't understand why I don't settle. He can't understand why I don't have a lie down. He can't understand why I miss the company at the factory. I was happy there, I'd go back tomorrow.

This was not the only direction in which a potential conflict of interest lay. Although they were only a small proportion of the total number of women interviewed, a substantial minority (40 per cent) of the women who preferred not to work felt that their husbands preferred them to work. Again, it did not seem that this difference was a serious source of conflict: only one woman said she had been under pressure from her husband to take a job she did not want. Put in more positive terms, the majority of married women appeared to have the support of their husbands and children in their return to full-time domesticity,

Table 5.4.2
Husbands' and wives' attitude to wife's unemployment

Husband's preference	Wife's preference			Total	N
	Prefer work (%)	Prefer home (%)	50/50 (%)	(%)	
Prefers wife to stay at home	30	44	73	38.5	44
Doesn't mind	8	3		26.5	31
Prefers wife to work for benefit of family/herself	28	28	9	18	21
Non-working wife gets on his nerves	22	12.5	9	6	7
Other comment	12	12.5	9	11	14
N	74	32	11	100	117

as did single women from their parents or other close relatives. There was no significant difference between married women with children living at home or with children under 15 and those with no children at home. The women who were most likely to feel that their family preferred them at work were those who had been divorced or separated from their husbands. Talking to the women involved it seemed that the stigma of unemployment as well as that of divorce or separation put a psychological strain on the women themselves, which in turn placed an emotional burden upon the remaining family, straining family relations. The need for work was not purely economic, because in many cases the money earned from going out to work was very little more than could be obtained from supplementary benefit. Paid work appeared to be particularly important for their self respect. The evidence is summarized in Table 5.4.3.

Other potential sources of tension within the family are the anxieties engendered by money problems with the loss of one income, and the wife's loss

Table 5.4.3
Responses to *Does your family appreciate having you at home more?*

	Marital status				Total	N
	Single (%)	Widowed (%)	Separated/ Divorced (%)	Married (%)	(%)	
Family appreciates	36	100	33	61.5	59	93
No, prefer not	18	–	42	8	11	17
No difference	36	–	16	15	17	27
Whatever makes me happy	–	–	–	11	9	14
Don't know	9	–	8	2	2.5	4
Husband no/Children yes	–	–	–	2	1	2
N	11	5	12	130		158

of financial independence, and the problems of sharing a house with another adult where an unemployed husband or parent had been used to having the house to themselves all day. However such problems occurred rarely. Only 17 per cent of the women said that their unemployment had caused tension within the family, 7 per cent saying that tension was due to loss of income and the remainder that it was due to the woman's own depression, the problems of sharing a house with other adults, or both. Although sharing a house with other adults was sometimes a cause of tension, having a non-working husband at home was not necessarily so: twenty-one of the women who experienced unemployment had non-working husbands, but only four mentioned tension in the family, caused by their being together too much.

In general, the women did not consider that their unemployment caused problems for their families, although financial problems had not yet had time to a rise. Only 24 per cent of the women could think of problems caused by their unemployment for family relations, and only three mentioned more than one. Eighty per cent of problems related to money: seven of the twenty-one who had non-working husbands mentioned money problems.

On the other hand the women mentioned a number of advantages their families derived from their being at home: 63 per cent of women mentioned at least one advantage, including 18 per cent who mentioned more than one, as shown in Table 5.4.4. With few exceptions, the advantages mentioned were instrumental and related to a higher standard of home comfort: tea could be on the table when the husband came in and husband and children did not have to help with housework. Since only a minority (30 per cent) of the women had children of school age or younger, for the majority of families the woman's presence in the home during the day only made a difference to family communal life to the extent that more chores could be done during week days, leaving evenings and weekends free for relaxation together. However this was mentioned specifically by only one woman. Four women also said that they could now visit housebound relatives, who were sick, elderly, or had young babies. Single women, most of whom lived with their parents, were as likely to mention advantages to their family in their being at home full time as were married women; however, separated and divorced women were less likely: only 36 per cent could think of any advantage compared to an overall 63 per cent. Numbers are too small to be significant, but are suggestive.

The benefits of having a woman at home full time were at least as important to the other adults in the house as to the children. Women who had no children under 15, and women who had no children at home were as likely to feel that their family appreciated having them at home as those who had children. A slightly higher proportion of those who had children at home felt that their families preferred to have them at work and a higher proportion of women who had no children at home felt that their families wanted them to do whatever the woman herself wanted. The presence of children at home or children under 15 made no difference in general to the women's perceptions of the advantages to their family of their being at home full time. For families with children under 15 the financial advantages of having the wife work would weigh more heavily than for families where children had grown up, cancelling out the extra need that a household with children might feel for a full-time housekeeper.

Table 5.4.4
Advantages to the family in being home full time (by marital status)

	Single (%)	Widowed (%)	Divorced/Separated (%)	Married (%)	Total
One or more	64	80	36	65	63
None	36	20	64	35	37
N	11	5	11	131	158

($p = 0.263$)
Missing = 6 (no family to be affected).

Although a majority of women believed that their family appreciated their being at home full time, this did not necessarily mean that the women themselves were more satisfied with their own performance in running, or helping to run, the household. Women who had had a period of unemployment before returning to work were particularly unlikely to think that their quality of housekeeping had improved in that interim period. Only the permanently retired were more satisfied with their housekeeping. Fewer women felt that their domestic performance had improved than felt that their family enjoyed advantages by their being at home. The difference, from general impressions, lay less in the women's modesty than in their feeling that their additional provision of home comforts when at home full time was unnecessary.

Table 5.4.5
Satisfaction with housekeeping standards during unemployment (by employment status)

	Employment status					Total	N
	Looking for work (%)	Permanently retired (%)	Temporarily retired (%)	Working full time (%)	Working part time (%)	(%)	
More satisfied	34	77	30	18	6	32.5	53
Less satisfied	4.5	–	6	–	18	5.5	9
No difference	55	23	54.5	82	76.5	57	92
No housekeeping	7	–	3	–	–	4	7
Other	–	–	6	–	–	2	2
N	89	13	34	11	17		164

($p = 0.025$)

To summarize: the second interview took place too soon after the redundancy to investigate fully the problems caused to the women's families by the loss of their income from work or major deterioration in family relations brought about by financial worries. A majority of women were unhappy about having to adapt to a new way of life, but only a few felt that their unhappiness had affected family relations; on the contrary, most women had been made to feel that their families appreciated having them at home full time. The obviously supportive attitude of most husbands to their wives' return to full-time domestic life was shared by the parents of single women, possibly because many single women took over domestic roles in the household on becoming unemployed. The only group containing a majority of women who did not feel that they had family support for their return to a full-time domestic life was that of separated and divorced women: unfortunately the number of women in this group, thirteen, was too small to allow detailed analysis of why this was so, or whether divorced and separated women in general feel less support for their domestic role than do widowed women, of whom there were only five in our sample. However, it is likely that their own feelings of the stigma of divorce compounded by the stigma of unemployment affected their relations with their families (as Goode (1956) suggested in his classic study of divorced women).[1]

A latent, but not obviously overt, source of tension lay in the difference between husbands' and wives' attitudes to the wives' employment. Thirty per cent of women who preferred to work felt that their husbands preferred to have them at home, including some women who had returned to work after the redundancy. However, only five women felt that they had been put under pressure by their husbands not to return to work, and none of the temporarily or permanently retired mentioned family pressure as a reason for retirement, although some mentioned family responsibilities. In positive terms, families' support for the women's domestic role (which included single women) meant that very few women felt stigmatized by unemployment, only 6 per cent (nine) of women saying that they were worried that their families might think less of them if they could not get work, and of these three were divorced and one widowed. None of the unemployed single women felt that their families would think less of them if they could not get work.

5.5 The effect of unemployment on social life and social contact

We now turn to describing the changes that occurred in the women's contact with society outside their own families; the relevance to the women of the social contact they had had at work, the changes brought about by unemployment, and the women's attitudes to those changes.

The time-consuming commitments of full-time employment and housekeeping responsibilities may have caused some women to lose touch with people in their neighbourhood. A majority of women said that they knew many people in their neighbourhood; however, a large minority (41 per cent) said that they did not. Knowing local people did not depend upon whether the women were born in the area or not. Only a minority of women saw more of their husbands, children, neighbours, or other friends after they were redundant, but a majority saw more of other family members such as parents and siblings. Work had been a significant source of social contact for the women. Nearly all women had made at least one friend at work, and 20 per cent said that most of their friends came from work. The likelihood that most of their friends were made at work increased the lower the occupational status. Most women kept in touch with their friends from work after becoming unemployed, and 48 per cent continued to see ex-work friends regularly. Although they kept in touch with their work friends, the women had less social contact on ceasing work. There appeared to be some regional variation in feelings of loneliness on stopping work, women from the Midlands and South Eastern factories being more likely to feel socially deprived by the loss of their jobs than women from the North Western factories. Feelings of loneliness were associated with suffering periods of depression following unemployment. However, the women did not feel that being unemployed lowered their status in the eyes of the community.

Most of the women in our sample lived in small households, and, although most of them were married, among the unemployed women only 30 per cent had children under 15 and only 52 per cent had children living at home. Since most of the husbands were working and most of the children were at school, in practice a large number of the unemployed women were at home alone during the day, and an even larger proportion at home alone during school hours. The change in the pattern of social contact following redundancy was therefore considerable. Moreover, some of the women commented that the pressure of work and domestic responsibilities had left them little time to form social networks outside work and family. Forty-one per cent said that they did not know many people in their own neighbourhood.

We had expected that the women would spend more time with their family and non-work friends on ceasing work and that this would to some extent replace the loss of social contact from work. The women were asked if they saw more of their neighbours, friends, husband, children, and other family on ceasing work. Only 12 per cent said that they did not see more of any of the groups mentioned. A minority of women (32 per cent) said that they saw more of neighbours and non-work friends after ceasing work, but most women maintained the same level of contact both with neighbours and with other friends, as Tables 5.5.1 and 5.5.2 show. A large proportion of the people whom the women knew locally were at work during the day. Moreover fortuitous contact between frields and acquaintances occurs rarely in metropolitan areas, and contact between friends often requires money for fares or the ownership of a car and money for petrol, expenditure which the women may have considered inessential and been unprepared to meet after losing their income.

Unemployment did not necessarily mean that all women saw more of their immediate families: only 40 per cent saw more of their husbands or boy-friends and 37 per cent more of their children, as Tables 5.5.3 and 5.5.4 show. The twenty-one women who had non-working husbands and the cleaners who had previously worked the 'unsocial' hours of evening or early morning when the family were at home saw more of their immediate family on becoming unemployed. But most husbands were at work during the day and children working

Women and Unemployment

Table 5.5.1
Contact with neighbours since leaving work

	A (%)	B1 (%)	B2 (%)	C1 (%)	C2 (%)	D (%)	E (%)	Total (%)
More	31	29	21	33	36	38	32	32
The same	69	62	79	67	64	62	64	66
Less		8					4	2
N	33	24	14	18	33	21	21	164

Table 5.5.2
Contact with other friends since leaving work

	A (%)	B1 (%)	B2 (%)	C1 (%)	C2 (%)	D (%)	E (%)	Total (%)
More	39	46	29	22	31	33	36	35
The same	42	50	71	67	56	67	59	57
Less	18	4	–	11	12.5	–	4.5	8.5
N	33	24	14	18	33	21	21	164

or at school. In this respect unemployed married women probably find their circumstances significantly different from those of unemployed married men, many of whom are likely to have their wives at home to provide company.

Since household chores could now be done during the day instead of when the family were at home, family contact may have improved in quality if not in quantity. However, patterns of family interaction are probably slow to change, and it is remarkable that few women mentioned increased family contact as one of the advantages of being out of work. Members of the immediate family were simply usually not present to provide an alternative to the social contact of the work-place during the day. As Tables 5.5.4 and 5.5.5 show, women were likely to see the same or more of husbands, boy-friends, and children following the redundancies, very few reporting less contact. However, only a minority actually reported increased contact, 40 per cent with husbands and 37 per cent with children.

Table 5.5.3
Contact with husband/boy-friend since leaving work

	A (%)	B1 (%)	B2 (%)	C1 (%)	B2 (%)	D (%)	E (%)	Total (%)
More	33	54	38.5	44	30	43	45.5	40
The same	36	42	61.5	28	42	29	45.5	40
Less	–	–	–	11	9	5	4.5	4
No husband/ boyfriend	30	4	–	17	18	24	4.5	16
N	33	24	14	18	33	21	21	164

Working Women in Recession

On the other hand, a majority of women (54 per cent) tended to see more of their wider family, as shown in Table 5.5.5. Although 16 per cent of women had no husband or boyfriend and 29 per cent had no children, only 7 per cent had no other family; neighbourhood networks may atrophy from neglect when women go to work, but family ties can provide a permanent — if sometimes only latent — link that can be strengthened when circumstances require. Many women had retired parents, or mothers, sisters, and other adult female relations who did not go out to work, either because they had young children at home or because they belonged to an older generation when women were likely to stay at home. These women were available to provide company during the day.

Table 5.5.4
Contact with children since leaving work

	A (%)	B1 (%)	B2 (%)	C1 (%)	C2 (%)	D (%)	E (%)	Total (%)
More	27	42	29	50	33	33	50	37
The same	33	54	57	17	15	29	14	30
Less	3	—	7	11	3	5	4.5	4
No children	36	4	7	22	48.5	33	32	29
N	33	24	14	18	33	21	21	164

Table 5.5.5
Contact with other family since leaving work

	A (%)	B1 (%)	B2 (%)	C1 (%)	C2 (%)	D (%)	E (%)	Total (%)
More	42	71	43	28	76	57	45.5	54
The same	40	21	50	61	24	33	50	38
Less	6							1
No other family	12	8	7	11	—	9	4.5	7
N	33	24	14	18	33	21	21	164

Only 20 per cent of women said that most of their personal friends came from work. However, the advantage of social contact in the work-place is that it is easily accessible, whilst a private friendship network is normally limited by constraints of time and distance and often unable to provide day to day company. Nearly all the women had found their work-groups congenial, 86 per cent of the unemployed women saying that the atmosphere in their work group was normally good or very good in the interview before the redundancies, and only three women referring to work-group relationships as poor. Nearly all of the women had some personal friends among their work-mates — 83 per cent had at least one and 74 per cent had more than one. Moreover, work provided social contact which, although not described as personal friendship, was nevertheless considered valuable in itself.

The likelihood that most friends came from work increased slightly the lower the occupational status, except for the relatively small group in occupational status 5, who were mostly part-time cleaners and had few work-mates, with whom they spent relatively little time: the data is summarized in Table 5.5.6. The inverse relationship between job status and work friendships may have reflected the varying opportunities within each status to cultivate friends: the higher the status the more likely that the woman worked for much of the time on her own in a competitive situation and under pressure, under conditions that did not encourage the cultivation of many personal friendships.

Table 5.5.6
Source of majority of respondents' friends (by occupational status)

	Occupational status					Total
	1 (%)	2 (%)	3 (%)	4 (%)	5 (%)	(%)
From work	7	14	21	32	27	20
From outside work	87	75	64	65	64	68
50/50	7	11	15	3	9	11
N	15	44	91	34	11	195

N = all women interviewed twice.

Although there were differences between occupational statuses in the extent to which women drew most of their friends from work, the differences were only slight and the only difference between occupational status groups in feelings of social deprivation on leaving work was that women in status 4, the caterers, hand-sewers, and storewomen, who were the most likely to make most of their friends at work (32 per cent), were more likely to feel isolated on leaving work (63 per cent) than other occupational statuses.

The proportion of women with personal friends at work was similar in six of the seven factories, as was the proportion of women who said most of their friends came from work: only in factory E did a large minority of women have no friends at work. In cross-tabulations by factory the small numbers in each group make minor variations insignificant: see Table 5.5.7.

To some extent the unemployed women were able to maintain the friendships they had made at work after the redundancies. Sometimes even the entire friendship network from work groups continued to meet, although it cannot be estimated how long work contacts would be maintained once the common interests arising from work had begun to fade. Some of the women from Company A, which was located in a market town with only one large shopping centre, made a practice of having coffee together in their original work-groups on Fridays when they went in to do the weekend shopping and go to the Job

Centre. This meant that they could meet without having to spend extra money on fares. However, the chief common interest appeared to be swapping experiences in job-hunting, and this particular interest was unlikely to be maintained over a long period of time. On the other hand, if friends did not live within walking distance and meetings could not be fitted in with necessary journeys the cost of the transport required was likely to make the survival of such friendships difficult. As a result, fewer than half of the unemployed women still saw their friends from work regularly, although 68 per cent kept in some sort of touch, as shown in Table 5.5.8. There was substantial variation between factories in the proportions of women who kept in touch with their work-mates regularly after the redundancy, ranging from 66 per cent in C2 to 36 per cent in B2, but we do not know how far this was due to differences in ease of access, or a reflection of the value the women placed upon their work-based friendships.

Table 5.5.7
Friends from work (by factory)

Factory	Number of friends from work			N
	At least one (%)	More than one (%)	Most friends come from work (%)	
A	81	70	26	32
B1	92	87	21	24
B2	79	64	9	14
C1	94	88	28	18
C2	85	76	24	33
D	90	90	15	21
E	54	41	10	22
Total	83	74	20.5	164

N = unemployed women.

Table 5.5.8
Contact between unemployed women and former work-mates

Factory	Regularly (%)	Occasionally only (%)	Telephone only (%)	Any contact (%)	N
A	47	0	6	53	32
B1	54	8	8	70	24
B2	36	0	36	72	14
C1	39	5	11	55	18
C2	66	21	6	93	33
D	57	9	14	80	21
E	50	9	14	73	22
Total	48	8	12	68	164

Stage in the life cycle, and possibly also regional cultural patterns probably influenced the degree to which women relied upon the work-place for companionship, and therefore the effect of unemployment on social contact. Women are likely to have different patterns of social contact depending upon whether they are young and single or middle-aged and married: social life for the former often revolves around courting and going out with friends at night, for the latter the extent to which most non-work social contact revolves around family, meeting with other women during the day, or going out and visiting with husband and other couples during evenings and weekends probably varies considerably from one group to another.

Changes in the amount of social contact after the redundancy show variations by marital status and stage of life cycle. Single and younger women were thus likely to say that they had the same amount of social contact after the redundancy as they did before, although a substantial minority (43 per cent) had less, as indicated in Table 5.5.9. Some lived with retired parents or a non-working mother and therefore were not alone during the day, and for most the focus of their social life was going out with friends or boy-friend at night, activities which appeared to increase, not diminish, on redundancy. As mentioned before, married women were likely to be alone in the house during the day: the large majority of married women and women over 35 therefore said they had less social contact on becoming unemployed. Married women were also the most likely to say they felt more isolated: 55 per cent of married women said that they felt more isolated as compared with only 27 per cent of single women.

Table 5.5.9
Social contact on leaving work (by marital status)

Marital status	Social contact				N
	More (%)	Less (%)	The same (%)	Other comment (%)	
Single	29	43	29	0	14
Widowed/Separated/ Divorced	20	40	40	0	20
Married	24	63	11.5	1.5	130
Total	24	58.5	16.5	1	164

($p = 0.046$)

Differences in age were slightly more significant statistically than differences in marital status, few women under 25 saying they had less social contact on leaving work, as shown in Table 5.5.10.

The women were invited to comment generally on the changes they perceived in their social life and contacts since ceasing work: 34 per cent could not think of any major changes, 13 per cent mentioned more than one. A minority of comments, 19 per cent, centred on the enrichment of general social life, and a

Table 5.5.10
Social contact on leaving work (by age)

Age	Social contact				N
	More (%)	Less (%)	The same (%)	Other comment (%)	
18–24	40	20	20	20	5
25–34	17	55	28		29
35–44	20	61	17	2	59
45–54	29	59	12		51
55–59	25	65	10		20
Total	24	58.5	16.5	1	164

($p = 0.031$)

further 9 per cent on the enrichment of family life: among this group the main points commented upon were that it was possible to see more of friends in the daytime, to stay out late at night without having to get up early, to get out and about in general, and to meet local people in the streets and shops.

You are just freer, you have more freedom. You have no social life when you are working – it's limited, so you are freer to choose when you're not working. It could be a dinner dance during the week you can go to now because you don't have to worry about being tired the next day. (Valve assembler from B1)

Being at home and around the shops you bump into local people much more and see more of different members of the family – you can be more useful to your relatives at home. (Engineering assembler from C2)

I'm closer to my family but I spend more time on my own during the day than I've ever done. That's a mixed blessing, sometimes I'm glad of it, sometimes not. (Machinist from A)

A further 10 per cent of comments related to a change in social life without any implication of impoverishment or deterioration: mixing with a different group of people, spending more time with elderly neighbours, mixing less with men, no longer going to the pub with workmates.

The majority of comments (61 per cent) related to a deterioration in social life, some demonstrating extreme loneliness and feelings of losing touch with society.

I feel as though I'm drifting – it's only when I'm working with people that I feel I have a purpose to life or a pattern to life. I can't come to terms with the life I lead, doing housework over and over, sometimes you think of things – you haven't got anyone to talk them over with. (Machinist from A)

You can become in a little world of your own, nobody to say hello to. You get very lonely. I've been out for a walk around just to see another person. (Engineering assembler from C1)

Others related to a deterioration in the quality of social life, or to a social world that had begun to shrink:

I see less of everyone except my husband. We've always got on well but since we are both not working I feel we *might* get on each other's nerves. (Machinist from A)

The home is always here – you know everything everyone is going to say. (Cleaner from E)

I think you get out of touch – like in the morning I used to sit with the men for my lunch and it's surprising the worldly conversation, and things you learn. You would hear other opinions when at home you have only yourself to think about and no one really to talk to all day. (Valve assembler from B1)

The common use of the word 'social' to mean contact with other people in a recreational context only rather than all contexts including work and family resulted in some ambiguity over questions which were designed to discover the extent and quality of changes in the women's contacts with other people in general. When asked directly about whether they felt from their own experience that unemployment led to loneliness and increased isolation, the majority of answers were affirmative: 67 per cent of women agreed that 'you often get lonely when you haven't a job', and 52 per cent said that they felt more isolated on leaving work. Fewer women felt that the quality of their social life had deteriorated: only 32 per cent said their social contact was less satisfactory, and 35 per cent that their circle of acquaintance was more restricted. That the social contact previously provided by their work environment was important to the women even if it was not a major source of personal friendships is apparent from the responses from factory E. Only 10 per cent of the women from that factory said that most of their friends came from work, and only 54 per cent said they had any personal friends at work, but 82 per cent agreed that 'you often get lonely if you haven't got a job.' Nearly all the women missed the company they had enjoyed at work: when asked what they missed most about their jobs 80 per cent of all the unemployed women mentioned missing the company of their work-mates.

There were differences between factories in the proportions of women who felt more socially isolated as a result of unemployment, suggesting a regional pattern. The women from the two West Midland towns and the South East were more likely to feel socially isolated than women from the three Northern towns. Table 5.5.11 shows the proportional variations from the average for each factory in answers to the questions on whether they had less social contact, whether it was more restricted and less satisfactory, and whether they in general felt more isolated on leaving work.

There were no significant differences in feelings of social isolation between different occupational statuses, although women from lower statuses had been more likely to draw most of their friends from work; women from statuses 1 and 2 were just as likely to say that unemployment led to loneliness, that their social life and contacts were less satisfactory and they felt more isolated. The numbers are too small to be significant, but the twelve unemployed women from status 1 were more likely than average to say that they felt more isolated (75 per cent), that their social life and contacts were less satisfactory (50 per cent) and that their circle of acquaintance more restricted (42 per cent). This suggests that the value of association with others in the work environment is independent of the number of personal friendships made.

Married women were significantly more likely to say they had less social contact on leaving work than single women. It is therefore not surprising that they were more likely to feel that unemployment led to loneliness. Sixty-nine per cent of married women agreed that unemployment led to loneliness, compared with 46 per cent of single women, as shown in Table 5.5.12.

Table 5.5.11
Social deprivation on leaving work (by factory)

Factory	Less contact in general (%)	More restricted (%)	Less satisfactory (%)	Feel more isolated (%)	Total
C2	+ 3	+ 9.5	+ 19.5	+ 15	+ 47
C1	+ 14	+ 8	+ 1	+ 9	+ 32
A	+ 8	+ 11	+ 5.5	+ 1	+ 25.5
E	+ 1	− 4	− 5	− 2	− 10
D	− 10	+ 2	− 8	− 9	− 25
B2	− 1	− 15	− 25	− 2	− 43
B1	− 12	− 24	− 10	− 14.5	− 46
Base (%)	58.5	36	32	52	

Table 5.5.12
Responses to *Unemployment leads to loneliness (by marital status)*

	Marital status			Total
	Single (%)	Separated/Widowed/Divorced (%)	Married/Cohabiting (%)	(%)
Agree	46	65	69	67
Disagree	46	35	28	30
No opinion	8	–	2	2.5
N	13	20	130	163

($p = 0.038$)

There is a risk of injuring people's pride in asking questions about the extent to which they suffer any form of deprivation: people often blame themselves for their misfortunes. In asking the women about their subjective feelings of isolation as a result of unemployment we ran the risk not only of offending them but of their answers being biased by pride or a feeling that it showed weakness to complain. People are likely to be particularly sensitive about questions to do with their own success or failure in maintaining social contact. We tried to deal with this problem by asking the women to compare their post-redundancy with their pre-redundancy life where possible, rather than make any absolute assessment of their present life, and also asking some questions impersonally: whether they agreed or disagreed with statements that are 'sometimes said' about unemployed people in general rather than themselves personally. A higher proportion of women (67 per cent) said that they agreed with the statement that 'you often get lonely when you haven't a job' than said that they themselves were 'more isolated' (52 per cent) or 'had less social contact' (58.8 per cent). This leaves us with no way of knowing whether some women answered the impersonally phrased questions according to how they considered the majority would feel, whilst excepting themselves, or whether more women were likely to reveal their true feelings when questions were phrased obliquely rather than directly. We can say that a minimum of 52 per cent of women felt 'more isolated' and a smaller proportion, 32 per cent, felt that their social life and contacts were 'less satisfactory' since leaving work.

The answers to these questions do not reveal how serious a deprivation the women felt this to be. There is, however, a strong association between a decline in social contact and the incidence of self-reported periods of depression following the redundancy, and an even stronger association between depression and feeling that social life and contacts were less satisfactory; 72 per cent of depressed women said that they had less social contact compared with 48 per cent of women who were not depressed, as is shown in Table 5.5.13.[2] General health and state of mind of the unemployed women are discussed at greater length in section 5.6.

Table 5.5.13
Proportions of women who reported feeling depression and decline in social contact

Change in social contact on leaving work	Depressed (%)	Not depressed (%)	Total (%)
More	19	28	24
Less	72	48	58.5
The same	7	24	16.5
More with family, less other	3	–	1
N	70	93	163

($p = 0.023$)

Although most women clearly felt that being unemployed had reduced their contact with society, it is less clear how far the women felt that being unemployed had altered their status in the eyes of their family and acquaintances. Much has been written about the stigma of unemployment for men. However, it is not possible to make comparisons on a quantitative basis with our sample, comparability in such matters as the level of local unemployment and the precise nature of the questions being vital but unobtainable. Many married women doubted their right to work in a period when there were not enough jobs for the major breadwinner in each family. Only a minority of women felt that people in general respected them more if they went out to work: 29 per cent of the sample at the first interview. At the second interview, when asked of unemployed women only, this proportion was lower, 23 per cent of unemployed women feeling that men respected them more if they worked and 19.5 per cent that women respected them more. There were insignificant differences in responses by age or marital status — but numbers among young or single women were too small to provide any real guide. Such evidence suggests that unemployment was not felt as a social stigma by the women.

To summarize: work had been a source of friendship for most of the women; whether or not they made most of their friends from work was inversely correlated with occupational status. More importantly, work provided a means of social contact for all women, although the degree to which they were dependent upon work for social contact varied according to area and marital status. The women from the Midlands and the South East were more likely to feel socially isolated by unemployment than the women from the North West, and married or once married women were more likely to feel isolated and lonely than single women. Although lower-status women were more likely to say that most of their friends came from work, higher-status women were just as likely as lower-status women to think that unemployment caused loneliness, and women from status 1 were more likely than lower-status women to think that the quality of their social contacts had deteriorated on becoming unemployed. A majority of women said that they had less social contact on leaving work, women with reduced social contact also being the most likely to feel depressed by unemployment. Only a minority of women thought that people respected them less if they did not have a job.

5.6 The effects of unemployment upon health

In this section we are concerned with the effects of redundancy and unemployment upon physical and psychological health. The data are derived from the comments of the respondents themselves: obviously, we did not have access to the medical records of the women involved. In general, more women reported an improvement in their physical health than reported a deterioration: amongst women who had been out of work for three months or more, 29 per cent reported that their health had improved, and only 16 per cent reported that their health had deteriorated. The accuracy of self-reported mental illness is difficult to assess. Nevertheless, there was more extensive reporting of mental illness than of physical illness: 43 per cent of women reported feeling at least mildly depressed, and 34 per cent reported feeling under stress. There is thus some indication that unemployment leads to an improvement in the physical health of women, but a deterioration in mental health.

5.6.1 *The effect of unemployment on physical health*

More women reported an improvement than reported a deterioration in general health, the improvement being due usually to being less physically tired and no longer under the pressure of doing piece work and of having to complete household duties in non-work hours. In chapter 2 we reported that many women had agreed that 'looking after a family and doing paid work as well is too tiring' and more than half the unemployed women referred to having more time, fewer deadlines, and less pressure as major advantages of being unemployed. Company B, the valve-assembly plant, had the highest proportion of women reporting an improvement in physical health, and work in that company was sedentary, monotonous, and paced, and, while not unhealthy, probably not conducive to good health. Altogether, among those women who had been unemployed three months or longer (141), 29 per cent reported that their health had improved, 10 per cent significantly and 19 per cent slightly.

Table 5.6.1.1
Physical health since leaving work

	Company					Total
	A (%)	B (%)	C (%)	E (%)	E (%)	(%)
Deteriorated	21	–	22	15	21	16
The same	59	57	49	61.5	58	55
Improved	21	43	29	23	21	29
N	29	35	45	13	19	141

($p = 0.168$)
N = women unemployed for three months or more.

Changes in general health were not significantly related to age, but it is worth noting that those in the oldest age group were more likely than others to say their health had deteriorated on leaving work, and some of the older women commented that a decrease in physical activity had resulted in a worsening of minor rheumatic or arthritic disorders: five out of the eighteen women in the 55–9 age group reported a deterioration in general health. However, the same number reported an improvement. Other illnesses reported as being induced or exaggerated by unemployment were nervous illnesses and were attributed by the women to the strain of leaving their job. Thus, two women said that they suffered from depression serious enough for them to describe it as an illness, five from 'nerves', one from acute loss of appetite, one from acute weight gain, and one from temporary partial paralysis of the legs.

We were of course unable to obtain official diagnoses of the women's complaints – only that they were severe enough for the women to consider themselves ill. All of the women (196) interviewed a second time were asked if they had had specific 'serious or relatively serious' health problems since leaving work, and twenty-six mentioned an illness that they considered serious: all except three had been ill for over a month. It was not possible with the information available to estimate whether this was a greater number than average for women of a comparable age. However, in view of the current debate on the effects of unemployment on health, we considered it worth while to record the incidence and type of health problems reported among the women who had been unemployed for three months or longer and where health had deteriorated after becoming unemployed. This category does not include those women whose health had detiorated before the redundancy through the stress of anticipating unemployment.

Table 5.6.1.2
Illnesses reported by women after redundancy

Illness	N
Depression	2
'Nerves'	2
Bronchitis	1
Back disorder	2
Pagett's disease	1
Rheumatism in hands	1
Arthritis	1
Loss of appetite	1
Sudden weight gain	1
Phlebitis	1
Partial paralysis of legs	1
Total	15

5.6.2 The effect of unemployment on mental health

In considering mental health we focused on two conditions, stress and depression. We also considered the effect of unemployment on self-respect. We expected that the reorganization of an established pattern of life and the search for a new job could be stressful for at least some of the women and the loss of identity brought about by the loss of an occupational role could result in depression and low self-esteem.

The term 'stress' is generally used to describe a state of anxiety which produces uncomfortable symptoms, caused through endocrine induced arousal. Lazarus and Averill[3] offers a definition of stress as being 'an emotion based on the appraisal of threat' and 'an anticipatory reaction to a future possibility'. Stress therefore can be considered a symptom that occurs while a person still has hopes and searches for a way out. Depression, on the other hand, is typically caused by the irretrievable loss of a major source of value or reward where no satisfactory alternative is perceived to exist (Beck).[4] Symptoms of depression described by Beck include feeling sad, loss of appetite, sleeplessness, and feelings of worthlessness which are generally ill founded and do not reflect the opinion that others have of the depressed person.[5]

Fewer women reported feeling under stress (34 per cent) than reported feeling depressed (43 per cent), reflecting, no doubt, an acceptance by most that there was little they could do about their position in the present state of the job market. As might be expected, the women from the two companies A and C, where most conflict was experienced over the closure, were those most likely to report feelings of stress.

Table 5.6.2.1
Proportion of women who reported feeling under stress after the closure (by company)

Company	Percentage	N
A	41	32
B	21	38
C	52	48
D	15	20
E	23	22
Total	34	160

($p = 0.031$)

Stress was also significantly related to employment status, with temporarily retired women and women who were working part time being the most likely to report feeling under stress (see Table 5.6.2.2). It is possible that these two groups of women were those among whom feelings of conflict about their role were the strongest: they were women who found it difficult to come to terms with conflicting pressures to stay at home or go out to work. Most women had recovered from their feelings of stress by the time of the second interview, only 11 per cent reporting still feeling under stress; the remainder had either 'come to terms' with the closure, or other activities, worries, or commitments had taken their minds off it.

A greater number of women reported suffering from periods of depression, and forty-two women, 26 per cent of those who had experienced unemployment, said they still suffered from depression at the time of the second interview. Nearly half of those still looking for work at the time of second interview said that they had been depressed. The women suffered varying degrees of depression, 12 per cent reporting feeling very depressed, and 6 per cent reporting feeling depressed every day. By the time of the second interview, 40 per cent of those who had experienced depression reported recovering, or beginning to recover, and 10 per cent reported that their depression had intensified over time.

We have already suggested that the majority of women preferred being employed to being at home full time, and that this preference was indepedent

Table 5.6.2.2
Proportion of women who reported feeling under stress (by employment status)

Employment status	Percentage	N
Looking for work	33	90
Permanently retired	21	14
Temporarily retired	41	32
Now working full time	18	11
Now working part time	47	17
Total	34	164

Table 5.6.2.3
Proportion of women who reported being depressed (by employment status)

Employment status	Percentage	N
Looking for work	49	90
Permanently retired	14	14
Temporarily retired	47	32
Now working full time	2	11
Now working part time	41	17
Total	43	164

($p = 0.262$)

Table 5.6.2.4
Degree and frequency of depression

	Percentage		Percentage
Very depressed	12	Every day	6
Depressed	13	Often	11
Mildly depressed	18	Occasionally	26
Total	43	Total	43
N	164	N	164

of occupational status, age, or marital status. It is therefore not surprising that depression as a result of unemployment was not associated with prior occupational status, age, or marital status. Nor was depression associated with financial circumstances: there was no relation with husband's income, and the highest incidence of depression was found among the women from Company C, whose redundancy payments had been the largest. Sixty-seven per cent of women from C1 reported feeling depressed, and 51 per cent from C2. Only 19 per cent of depressed women said that they found it difficult or impossible to manage financially.

As we have shown earlier, depression was strongly associated with reduced social contact, and it was even more strongly associated with feelings of increased isolation, less satisfactory social contact and loneliness. Depression was also strongly associated with boredom, 92 per cent of depressed women agreeing that 'you get bored without a job', compared to only 51 per cent of non-depressed women.[6]

We have shown that 43 per cent of women said that they had periods of depression as a result of being unemployed, the women themselves defining the condition of depression. We also gave the women who had been unemployed for three months or more a list of the various conditions associated with depression (Beck, 1967) and asked whether such feelings had started or increased since becoming unemployed. The most commonly noted changes were feeling less independent, feeling frustrated, insecure, worthless, isolated, and experiencing changing sleep patterns. Women who said that they were depressed were significantly more likely to report changes than those who were not depressed, in particular to report increased feelings of frustration. Seventy-three per cent of depressed women reported feeling frustrated compared to only 14 per cent of non-depressed women. Only one symptom, loss of independence, was also reported by a large proportion (46 per cent) of non-depressed women.

Table 5.6.2.5

Symptoms of depression among unemployed women, starting or increasing after they became unemployed

	Reported depression (%)	Not depressed (%)	All (%)
Lack of concentration	40	16	27
Changed sleep patterns	60	14	35
Feeling useless	54	11	31
Lethargic and listless	49	5	25
Losing confidence	48	8	26
Feeling isolated and alone with problems	57	9	31
Feeling less independent	78	46	61
Feeling frustrated	73	14	41
Feeling insecure	60	14	35
Thinking yourself worthless	36	1	29
N			140

N = women unemployed for three months or more.

The unemployed women were also asked indirect questions about self-esteem. We showed earlier that more women tended to give answers indicating loneliness when asked indirectly whether they thought unemployment led to loneliness than when asked questions directly related to their own condition. Similarly, although only 31 per cent of women said that they themselves felt useless, a larger number, 43.5 per cent, agreed with the statement: 'You feel useless if you haven't got a job.'

In contrast to the small proportion of women who considered that working raised their status in the eyes of the community, most women, 60 per cent, felt that paid employment was important for their self-respect. If the thirteen women who had retired permanently are excluded, 71 per cent of women who were still in the labour market, or had withdrawn only temporarily, felt that work was important for their self-respect. Among those women who had temporarily withdrawn from paid employment, 79 per cent said that work was important for their self-respect.

Table 5.6.2.6

Proportions of women who felt that going to work was important for their self-respect (by employment status)

	Employment status					Totals
	Looking for work (%)	Permanently retired (%)	Temporarily retired (%)	Now working full time (%)	Now working part time (%)	(%)
Yes	70	23	79	73	65	68
No	29	77	15	18	35	35
Don't know	1	–	6	9	–	2
N	90	14	32	11	17	164

($p = 0.004$)

It is puzzling why so many women felt that paid employment was important for their self-respect, since the women plainly did not feel any moral pressure from their families or from society to go to work – more commonly the contrary seems to have been the case. It does point to a possible conflict in the women's minds regarding what they felt from their own experience made them more useful citizens and how they felt society as a whole measured their contribution. Significantly, 79 per cent of women who had retired temporarily from work said that going out to work was important for maintaining self-respect, suggesting a conflict between roles which had been resolved in a less than fully satisfactory manner. Women who reported feeling depressed were particularly likely to say that work was important for their self-respect (80 per cent, $p = 0.029$).

A large minority, 46 per cent of the 104 women who had signed on at the Job Centre, agreed with the statement that 'you feel ashamed of having to sign on at the benefit office', and 19 per cent felt embarrassed telling people they were out of work.

To summarize: a minority of women (34 per cent) reported feeling under stress as a result of the closures, and only 11 per cent still felt under stress at the time of the second interview. A larger minority (43 per cent) reported having periods of depression, and 49 per cent of those who were looking for work reported periods of depression. The incidence of depression was not related to occupational status, age, marital status or financial circumstances. Most of the women who were depressed said that they felt unemployment caused boredom (92 per cent), loneliness (81 per cent), and 'made you feel useless' (69 per cent); they considered work to be important for their self-respect (80 per cent). This suggests that almost half the women looking for work found their work role necessary for the social contact and interesting activity it provided and also for their self-respect. The proportion may in fact be larger: there was an understandable tendency for women not to label themselves in terms that could be associated with failure — for example, to say that they felt socially isolated or useless — whilst agreeing to similar concepts couched in less direct terms — 67 per cent of all unemployed women agreed that 'you often feel lonely if you haven't got a job', 70 per cent that 'you get bored', and 68 per cent that going to work was important for their self-respect.

5.7 Women's general attitudes to unemployment

This section considers women's general attitudes to unemployment: whether they preferred going out to work to staying at home and the attributes that distinguish those who preferred working from those who did not. We also examine what women liked about not going to work and what they missed about their jobs. The majority (64 per cent) of women preferred working; a preference for going out to work was unrelated to age, marital status, occupational status, or husband's financial status. The majority of women who had retired temporarily preferred to work, but all except one of those who had retired permanently preferred to be at home. Seventy per cent of those looking for work said they preferred to work. Those who preferred to stay at home averaged a higher proportion of home activities that they preferred to work activities, and a higher proportion said that they had the same, or more, social contact on becoming unemployed than when they were at work. This suggests that a preference for staying at home is related to the existence of a satisfactory alternative domestic role in the form of a range of activities and a social network equally valued, or preferred to those provided by their employment.

The things the women liked about unemployment were not being tied to a strict time schedule (24 per cent), having more time to devote to their family (15 per cent) and their household duties (11 per cent), and having more time for themselves (15 per cent). However, 43 per cent of women said that there was nothing they liked about being unemployed. The things women mainly missed about their job were the company, interest, and activity that the work provided, and the money. Relative priorities for these cannot be given as responses varied according to the context in which they were asked, which suggests that all three are important.

In the first interview 87 per cent of the women who were to experience unemployment said that they were happier going to work than they would be staying at home, and 6 per cent said that they had no preference. We suggested that the overwhelming preference for going to work might be the result of a general tendency for people to rate their own activities favourably. This proved correct in part: when asked their preferences on becoming unemployed, a smaller proportion of women said that they preferred work, but the proportion was still a majority. Hence 64 per cent of the total number of respondents who had experienced unemployment or retirement said that all round they preferred going to work, 25 per cent said that they preferred staying at home (or would if they had sufficient money to manage), and 9 per cent said that they were happy to do either. If those who had permanently retired are eliminated the proportion who would prefer to stay at home falls to 18 per cent and those who are happy to do either to 8 per cent.

Table 5.7.1
Preference for staying at home (by employment status)

Employment status at 2nd interview	Preferred to work (%)	Preferred to stay home (%)	Happy either way (%)	Missing (%)	N
Looking for work	70	18	8	4	89
Permanently retired	7	79	14	0	14
Temporarily retired	59	35	6	0	34
Now working full time	64	9	27	0	11
Now working part time	87.5	6	6	0	16
Total	64	25	9	2	164

It might be argued that the continuing high proportion of women who preferred work was due to their not having yet accepted, or begun to identify fully with, their change in status; after a period of adjustment a preference for domestic life would develop. However, there was no indication of a reconciliation to unemployment amongst the longer-term unemployed. There was a slight, but not statistically significant, tendency for those unemployed for a longer period to be more likely to prefer work: 70 per cent of the twenty-seven women who had been unemployed for five to seven months and 67 per cent of the nine who had been unemployed for over seven months said that they preferred to work, compared with an overall percentage of 64 per cent.

As many as 59 per cent of women who had voluntarily dropped out of the labour market and considered themselves temporarily retired would have preferred to work. This represents twenty out of the thirty-four women who referred to themselves as temporarily retired. Only four of the twenty dropped out through discouragement alone, the remainder giving a variety of other main reasons, mostly related to family responsibilities. On the other hand, only one of the permanently retired women would have preferred to work, although eight of the fourteen permanently retired women interviewed were under 55 and therefore well below normal retiring age. The only permanently retired woman who would have preferred to work was over 55. It could be concluded then that most women who refer to themselves as permanently retired have

Table 5.7.2
Reasons for temporarily dropping out of the labour market

	Prefer to work (N)	Prefer to stay home (N)	Happy to do either (N)
To have a baby	7		1
Discouraged/no jobs around	4		1
Illness	3		1
Family responsibilities, undefined	2		
Needed a rest	2	7	
Husband's benefit affected	1		
Still getting pay in lieu		1	
Retraining	1	3	
Total N	20	11	3

dropped out of the labour market because of age or through free choice interpreted in the strictest possible sense.

Fourteen of the sixteen women who had found part-time jobs said that they preferred working to staying at home, indicating that going to work was an important part of their life for most of this group. The relatively high proportion of part-time women who said they preferred to work suggests that the motivation for part-time work could be as much a need for purposeful activity as for a supplement to the family income. Although the total number of women in this group is too small for the figures to be anything but suggestive, impressions gathered during interviews with part-time women throughout the total project lend support to this view.

An explanation for the reasons governing the minority's preference for staying at home is elusive, as it was not associated with any significant pattern of age, occupational status, age of children, length of time out of work, or husband's income. However, numbers in the lower age brackets and in the highest and lowest occupational-status categories were too small for figures to be illuminating. A preference for work was unrelated to whether the husband was working or not — fourteen women who had unemployed, retired, or invalided husbands preferred to be at work, six preferred to be at home, and one was happy either way — proportions similar to those for women whose husbands were employed.

From personal impressions based on over 200 interviews, a preference for domestic life rather than paid employment seemed to depend upon a combination of factors resulting in some individuals finding, almost fortuitously, a social network and set of unpaid activities that suited them: these were not associated with any particular age, income, or social status. Women who preferred to stay at home listed, on average, a higher proportion of home activities which they preferred to their paid employment, naming an average of 1.2 activities preferred, compared with only .48 for those who preferred work, the overall average being .7. Women who preferred home life were also much more likely than those who preferred work to say that the social contact they had on becoming unemployed was as much as, or more than, they had when employed. Sixty-three per cent of those who preferred home life said that they had as much, or more, social contact when unemployed as when working, whereas only 29 per cent of those who preferred work said that they had as much, or more, social contact when unemployed ($p = 0.001$). Of course, it is impossible to say whether the prior existence of the activities preferred led to a preference for staying at home, or whether a preference for staying at home led to the activities – or indeed, whether both were caused by a third factor.

The women were asked about the general advantages of being unemployed. The answers were very similar to those given to questions on the advantages of the activities undertaken when unemployed (see above, pp. 238–9). As Table 5.7.3 shows, the largest single group, 43 per cent, saw no advantages; 24 per cent of women mentioned being freed from pressure, 15 per cent mentioned more time to devote to their family, and the same number more time to devote to themselves.

Table 5.7.3
Advantages of not going to work

	Percentage
Not being tied to timetable/no pressure	24
More time for family	15
More time for self	15
Better housekeeper	11
Better health, more relaxed	7
Can see non-work friends more	2
No advantages	43
N	164

Percentage of women mentioning each advantage.

The advantages of not going out to work thus fell into two main categories: not having to do things under pressure, and having the time for activities forgone, or carried out less effectively, when they went out to work. However, the major conclusion is that, for the women themselves, the advantages of unemployment were limited: 43 per cent saw no advantages and only twenty-eight women, 17 per cent, mentioned more than one advantage.

The women were also asked, in the context of questions on activities, what they missed about their former work. Later in the interview they were asked what they missed about their former jobs in general. The range of responses given to both questions was the same, and covered a liking for the work itself, the money, and the company. However, the proportion of women giving each response differed on the two occasions, depending upon the context in which the question was asked. When the women were asked 'Considering the work you used to do and what you do now, what don't you like about your current way of life?' in the context of questions on activities, the highest proportion of women referred to the boredom, a smaller proportion of women to the lack of company, and a slightly smaller proportion to the lack of money (see Table 5.7.4). When the women were asked later in the interview, following questions on social contact and health, what they missed most about their jobs, the overwhelming majority said the company, a much smaller proportion the money, and the work itself was the third most frequently mentioned.

Table 5.7.4
Responses to *What don't you like about being out of work?*

	Percentage
Boredom, lack a purpose in life, not achieving anything	45
Lack of company, not a part of society, miss work-mates	35
Miss the money	30
Miss independence, security	4
Other	6
Like being out of work	9
N	164

Percentage is that of women giving each response.

Table 5.7.5
Responses to *What do you miss most about your job?*

	Percentage
Company	80
Money	47
Work itself, interest	29
Independence	5
Identity, a sense of belonging	5
Responsibility	2
Nothing	3
N	164

Percentage is that of women giving each response.

The financial disadvantages of unemployment will probably be given greater importance when redundancy and other special moneys have run out. But the different priorities given to company and the work itself, depending upon the precise context, may demonstrate that both are of equal importance: the priority given to each of the advantages of paid employment — money, company, and purposeful activity — will depend upon the immediate need uppermost in the person's mind, but we have no firm evidence on which to allocate absolute priorities. Most of the women missed going to work, even though for the time being they had enough money to maintain their normal standard of living.

5.8 Attitudes towards Government

Experience of redundancy and unemployment might be expected to influence both the degree of interest in politics, and the content of political beliefs. The experience might be expected to produce either increased apathy, or increased interest. On the one hand, redundancy and unemployment might be expected to lead to demoralization and cynicism about government, resulting in political apathy and cynicism towards politicians. On the other hand, direct experience of the way in which broad economic and political trends influence individual experience (of how, in Wright-Mills's words, public issues become private problems) might be expected to increase interest in politics.

Since the focus of the study was upon specific changes in women's attitudes towards employment and unemployment, and in general the women interviewed were suspicious of political questions which seemed marginal to the study's major concerns, we could undertake only limited investigation into the effects of redundancy upon political attitudes. We asked whether the experience of the redundancy had changed their views on politics and whether, since the redundancy, they had taken more interest in politics than before. The responses showed that the redundancies had led to a 'radicalization' and to an increased interest in politics among only a small minority of the women: only 10 per cent had changed their views (all described their change in terms of a shift to the left) and 16 per cent had begun to take more interest. On the other hand, the redundancy had not produced a significant change in the direction of increased apathy: only 4 per cent of the women said that since the redundancy their interest in politics had decreased.

Table 5.8.1

Responses to *Has your experience of redundancy changed your views on politics?*

	Company					Total	N
	A (%)	B (%)	C (%)	D (%)	E (%)	(%)	
Changed	17	10	11	–	7	10	19
No change	57	66	66	71	62	64	126
Not interested in politics	26	24	23	29	31	26	51
N	42	41	53	31	29		196

($p = 0.562$)

Table 5.8.2

Responses to *Since the redundancy, have you taken more interest in politics than you used to?*

	Company					Total	N
	A (%)	B (%)	C (%)	D (%)	E (%)	(%)	
Yes	33	12	13	6.5	10	16	31
No change	43	66	58.5	64.5	62	58	114
Never interested	19	22	24.5	19	28	22	44
Less interested	5	–	4	10	–	4	7
N	42	41	53	31	29		196

($p = 0.067$)

As the tables show, a major change occurred amongst the clothing workers, whose experience of redundancy had involved the sharpest conflict with previous experience, with the breakdown of a pattern of traditional, paternalist attitudes leading to disillusion both with management and with trade unionism. As one clothing worker commented, '[redundancy] tends to make you more aware. You go along in your own little world and think everything is alright. It's only when it affects you that you think.'

The detailed explanations for changes in political interests varied widely and, since there were so few changes, are not worth analysing statistically. However, the women who had changed had changed in the direction of becoming more left wing, with either previously Conservative supporters becoming disillusioned and unwilling to continue helping the party, or with previously 'middle-of-the-road' women becoming critical of the government for seeming to encourage redundancies. Only a small minority of women had changed their political views: but that minority had uniformly become more hostile to the Conservative Party.

Although the experience of redundancy had led to a minority of women becoming more left wing, the majority of women did not believe that the government was responsible for their losing their jobs, or for failing to find alternative employment. As was shown in Chapter 3, it was recognized that redundancies were caused by a combination of factors, including changes in product markets and in technology, as well as management and government action (or inaction). As Table 5.8.3 shows, the women did not blame any particular institution or group for their difficulties in finding work. The most frequent specific reference was to no one. Although the government received the next most frequent mention, it was mentioned by only 22 per cent; 14 per cent blamed the recession, and 11 per cent blamed themselves.

Although the majority of women did not blame the government for their failure to find work, the majority did believe that the government should introduce a deliberate policy to provide work for all who wanted it: 80 per cent. This is hardly surprising: the women were asked about the policy in isolation,

Table 5.8.3
Responses to *Do you blame anyone for your failure to find another job?*

	Company					Total	N
	A (%)	B (%)	C (%)	D (%)	E (%)	(%)	
No one	33	56	36	67	35	43	57
Government	12.5	14	33	17	29	22	29
Respondent herself	12.5	8	9	8	11	11	14
Recession	16	11	14	8	18	14	18
Foreign Imports	4	8	–	–	–	3	4
Other	12.5*	3	–	–	–	4	4
Don't know	8	–	7	–	–	4	5
	24	36	42	12	17		131

*Previous firm.

rather than in the context of specific alternative policies, each of which might have undesirable as well as desirable consequences – the political equivalent of asking for a vote in favour of virtue. However, not all women believed that the government should act: only 67 per cent of women aged under 35 thought that the government should follow policies designed to maximize employment. There was also a slight difference between occupational-status groups, women in the slightly and unskilled-manual groups being more inclined to believe that the government should maximize employment. The women did not distinguish between the right to work of women and men: only 3 per cent said that government policy should provide for men only, 77 per cent saying that the government should follow policies designed to provide employment for both women and men.

From the interviews it is difficult to gauge the extent to which the women blamed their experiences upon government policy. There was considerable personal anxiety caused by redundancy and unemployment, and an awareness that unemployment caused serious difficulties for society in general. Unemployment was blamed for a range of social ills, including vandalism. Although there were few young women in the group, there was special anxiety about youth unemployment, which was already or in the immediate future likely to involve their own children. As one women electronics worker put it, 'Being out of work is so degrading; that's the cause of the trouble with the youngsters – nothing to interest themselves with.' Unemployment was seen as likely to undermine the desire for work. As one Midlands engineering worker said, 'I think if they worked it would give people more of an incentive to. They get used to it; on the dole you get used to that and you don't want to work. It's especially bad for the young ones who've never done a whole 7–5 day.' The solutions most frequently mentioned were earlier retirement and reduced hours of work, either through a shorter day or through a shorter working week. Despite the depth of feeling about the ill effects of unemployment, shown in the explanations given for their opinions on the extent to which the government should pursue policies to maximize employment, there was no great optimism that the government would act.

There was also considerable uncertainty about the extent to which the unemployed should act together to draw attention to this situation. Forty-five per cent thought that the unemployed should act together, but only 21 per cent of respondents had specific ideas on how the unemployed should draw attention to their situation, for example by getting together and petitioning MPs, and only 5 per cent counselled rallies and protest marches. Five per cent of women felt that communal action would be useless and 28 per cent that it would be undesirable, 21 per cent having no opinion. However, although the overall picture is unclear, there was a clear contrast between the views of non-manual and manual workers: non-manual workers were much more likely than manual workers to believe that the unemployed should not act together. Hence 53 per cent of professional, administrative, and supervisory women did not believe that the unemployed should act together, and 32 per cent of clerical workers; comparable figures for manual workers were 29 per cent of semi-skilled women, 15 per cent of slightly skilled workers, and 9 per cent of unskilled workers. The contrast between occupational groups was more striking than the contrast between firms. However, more support for combined action by the unemployed was shown by women in case study A, who had been partially 'radicalized' by their experience of redundancy, and in case study E, where the women were more inclined to relatively 'radical' views before the redundancy.

The second interviews were held, at the latest, seven months after the redundancy. There was thus insufficient time for fundamental changes in attitudes towards broad political and employment issues to have occurred. Moreover, attitudes will be heavily influenced by subsequent employment experience. The experience of redundancy and unemployment had led to a change in political views, involving an increase in interest in politics, for only a minority of women. This minority was heavily concentrated in the South East clothing-industry study, where there was considerable disillusion with both management and unions. For this group redundancy and unemployment had led to an increased interest in politics, and a slight 'radicalization'.

5.9 Conclusion

The women defined as unemployed comprised 83 per cent of those interviewed twice, and 59 per cent of the original sample — 164 women. The length of time out of work ranged from one to thirty-three weeks, the majority (87 per cent) of women being out of work for three months or more: the average time unemployed was twenty weeks.

Although this period was sufficiently long for the women to feel the effects of loss of the activities involved in market employment, and of the companionship of their work-mates, it was not long enough for them to feel the full effects of a drop in income. The loss of a regular income was cushioned by redundancy and related payments. Redundancy pay averaged £847 in Company A, £3124 in Company B, £3535 in Company D, £3545 in E, and £4019 in C. Only 16 per cent of women received under £1000 and 70 per cent received £2000 or more. In addition, 54 per cent of unemployed women received unemployment benefit.

Only a small proportion of women, 5 per cent, used their redundancy payment solely as a substitute for wages; 29 per cent put all redundancy payments into savings accounts, 17 per cent spent all redundancy payments on specific items or outstanding debts, the remaining 48 per cent using their money in various combinations of saving, current expenditure, and purchase of nonroutine items. Items of specific expenditure most frequently mentioned as a use for redundancy money were home improvements (25 per cent); home furnishings or consumer durables (21 per cent); holiday (17 per cent); and outstanding bills (14 per cent).

Through the receipt of redundancy payments, together with tax rebates, payment in lieu of notice and unemployment benefit most women had sufficient money to maintain their normal standard of living for several months after becoming redundant: 34.5 per cent of women unemployed for three months or more said that they were able to manage financially without difficulty, and 49 per cent that they could manage, but without much money to spare, only 16 per cent reporting serious financial difficulties. As prospects for re-employment were bleak the women were reluctant to use up their capital. Forty-six per cent of women had begun to make economies, for example in clothes, entertainment, and food.

The redundancies led to an unanticipated disruption of the women's established pattern of activities: 65 per cent of women had worked for their pre-redundancy employers for ten years or more, and 70 per cent had intended to continue to work without a break until retirement. Few women had planned a range of new activities to replace market employment, the most frequently anticipated new activity being voluntary work, mentioned by 33 per cent of the women who were to become unemployed. In the event only ten unemployed women were doing voluntary work at the time of the second interviews. In general, the women filled the time previously occupied in market work by extending their existing domestic and social activities — housework, social visiting, or entertaining, gardening, knitting, sewing or craft work. Domestic activities were mentioned as frequently by single as by married women. The activities most commonly mentioned as being new were also domestic and social activities: social visiting and entertaining (16 per cent), home decorating (13 per cent), gardening (9 per cent), knitting and sewing (9 per cent). The activity on which most time was spent, housework, was regarded by the majority of women as less interesting than market work.

Only 25 per cent of women said they had had to give up recreational activities because of reduced income. Activities forgone were mostly social activities involving expenditure – having meals out or going to the pub or dances. Social activities not involving expenditure – dropping in on friends or relatives or having friends of relatives in for a chat – had increased.

Most of the women found enough to do to fill in the time, only 39 per cent saying that they had time on their hands. However, whether because their domestic activities were intrinsically less interesting or because many of them were carried out in isolation, 70 per cent of women associated unemployment with boredom. On the other hand the majority of women (72 per cent) were able to find some advantages in their new pattern of activities, the most frequently mentioned advantages relating to a more relaxed schedule and freedom from pressure.

Unemployment had not led to increased tensions in family life: only 17 per cent of women said that unemployment had caused tension in their families. The majority of women (59 per cent) felt that their families appreciated having them at home more, and only 11 per cent that their families did not do so. There was little difference between the responses of married and single women, although separated and divorced women were significantly more likely to feel that their families did not appreciate having them at home more. Sixty-three per cent of women mentioned advantages to their family in their being at home, the advantages mentioned being primarily enhanced comfort; 38.5 per cent of married women felt that their husbands preferred them to be at home rather than going out to work. On the other hand, the women themselves were not especially likely to feel that unemployment led them to improve their standards of housekeeping, only 32.5 per cent saying that they were more satisfied with the way they ran their households.

The women tended to associate unemployment with loneliness, 67 per cent of women agreeing with the statement 'You often get lonely if you haven't got a job.' Eighty per cent of unemployed women mentioned missing their work-mates as one of the things they most missed about their jobs. Married women were more likely to feel socially isolated than were single women, older women than younger, and women in the Midlands and South East than women in the North West. A minority of women saw more of their husbands, children, neighbours, and non-work friends on ceasing work, but a majority had increased contact with parents, sisters and other relatives; some women pointed out that they were now able to devote more time to the needs of their elderly or housebound relations. Most of the women had made friends at work but only 48 per cent were able to keep in touch with them regularly after ceasing work.

Unemployment was more likely to produce an improvement than a deterioration in physical health, a finding that is not surprising in view of the report by 44 per cent of the women that combining household duties with market employment was 'too tiring'. The large number of women who mentioned release from pressure and from the tyranny of deadlines as one of the advantages of unemployment lends support to the view that many women had found their daily schedule during employment physically taxing, especially women engaged in piece work. (However, it cannot be concluded that their schedule was more exhausting than that of men in similar occupations.)

A substantial minority of women reported a decline in mental health: 34 per cent reported feeling under stress as a result of becoming redundant, and 43 per cent reported periods of depression. Stress tended to be short-lived: only 11 per cent were still feeling under stress at the time of the second interview, compared with 26 per cent still feeling depressed. Reported depression was associated with feelings of boredom, loneliness, frustration, changed sleep patterns, loss of independence, insecurity, and loss of self-respect. Although few women felt that going to work enhanced their status in the eyes of their family and acquaintances, a large majority of women (68 per cent) felt that going to work was important for their own self-respect.

The majority of women preferred market employment to full-time domestic life in general. The women missed the work itself, the company, and the money earned. The most frequently mentioned advantage in not going out to work was the lack of pressure.

The redundancies led to a small, but perceptible, change in women's interest in, and views on, politics, especially in Company A: the women became slightly more interested in politics and slightly more radical in their views. No widespread blame was attached to the government for the redundancies, or for their failure to find alternative employment. On the other hand, a substantial majority believed that the government should introduce policies designed to provide work for all who wanted it — men as well as women.

Notes

1. W. J. Goode, *Women in Divorce* (New York: The Free Press, 1956).
2. There was no relationship between self-reported feelings of stress and decline in social contact ($p = 0.402$), which is as would be expected, stress being a reaction to the imminence of a testing situation, while depression is most generally associated with irretrievable loss. This suggests that answers were given thoughtfully and were not simply the outcome of a tendency by those women who did not like being unemployed to give indiscriminate answers which might indicate a general decline in the quality of life.
3. R. S. Lazarus and J. R. Averill, 'Emotion and Cognition with special reference to Anxiety', in Charles Spielberger (ed.) *Anxiety, Current Trends in Theory and Research* Vol. 11 (Academic Press, 1972).
4. A. T. Beck, *Cognitive Theory, the Emotional Disorders* (New York: International Universities Press, 1976), p. 129.
5. A. T. Beck, *Depression, Clinical Experimental and Theoretical Aspects*, (Harper & Row, 1967), pp. 14–32.
6. Feelings of depression were, of course, self-reported. However these findings have some support from medical research. According to Brown and Harris (1979), psychiatric disorder is 'common' among working-class women in London and is predominantly depressive. From a study in Camberwell he estimated that 15 per cent of women were suffering from a definite affective disorder and a further 18 per cent were borderline cases. He also found that women who were employed were less likely to suffer from depression than those who were not employed. This implies that depression may be related to not having a job as well as to losing a job. As most of the women in our study were from urban areas, similar findings could be expected. (G. W. Brown and T. Harris, *Social Origins of Depression*, Tavistock, 1978.) We are grateful for the assistance of Mr Michael White, of the Policy Studies Institute, in this area.

6

CONCLUSION: WORKING WOMEN IN RECESSION

Research into women and work has traditionally focused on the relation between work and family roles, and the possible tensions produced by attempting to reconcile the demands of each. According to this view, women's experience of, and attitudes towards, work are seen as conditioned by their position in the household. For women, going out to work is an ancillary activity, desirable as a means of earning extra income, primarily to embellish the home, or as a source of social satisfaction, but not a basis of social identity, or even a means of enhancing social status.[1] Moreover, the kinds of jobs undertaken by women are conditioned by traditional female roles, involving the sale in the labour market of the caring and 'expressive' (in the Parsonian sense) qualities fostered within the family — hence the predominance of women in the caring professions, in primary education, in service industry, and in service occupations in manufacturing industry.[2] Going out to work has modified women's adult lives, but has not fundamentally altered them.

More recently, feminist writers, especially Marxist feminists, have examined women's position in employment in terms of patriarchy both in the household and in the labour market.[3] In this same tradition Veronica Beechey has argued that female employment experience is ultimately determined by the same factors as determine male employment experience, notably the labour requirements of advanced capitalism, although the means by which women are led to satisfy capital's needs are different from those that affect men.[4] Although we have not adopted Beechey's Marxist analysis, we have operated from similar assumptions, namely that the starting-point for the examination of women's employment experience should *not* be women's position in the household: there should be no presumption that gender is the primary determinant of employment experience. Instead, women workers should be treated as workers as well as women. This does not necessarily involve disregarding gender as an influence upon employment experience and attitudes, since there are many differences between female and male employment; it does necessarily involve adopting the terms used in analysing male employment in analysing female employment. The effects of gender cannot be analysed without comparison, and comparison is impossible without a common language. Gender interacts with other attributes in determining employment experience and attitudes. We anticipated — and found — differences in employment experience and attitudes amongst women associated with differences in occupational status and region, as well as marital status and position in the life cycle. Similar findings are reported from research into male employment, different groups of male workers having different orientations to work — as Goldthorpe and his colleagues showed in their widely quoted *Affluent Worker* studies.[5] Since domestic and labour market situations differ between different groups of women, and between women and men, employment experiences and attitudes are likely to differ, some groups of women having similar experiences and attitudes to those of some groups of men, others having significantly different ones.

Following this logic, in this concluding chapter we summarize our findings on employment, redundancy, and unemployment in turn, drawing comparisons with other research, including relevent research on men, where possible.

The majority of women interviewed were marginal members of the primary labour market, sharing a similar labour-market position to the broad mass of semi- and unskilled male manual workers and routine non-manual workers in large-scale manufacturing industry.[6] The majority of women were employed in 'permanent' jobs in large-scale manufacturing industry, and as such enjoyed the benefits of working in large organizations — trade-union membership, paid holidays, subsidized welfare facilities, and in some cases contributory pension schemes. They also, of course, experienced the disadvantages of working in large organizations — bureaucratization and routinization. (Employees in the clothing factory were in a different position, since they were employed in a relatively small, previously independent factory which had been taken over by a larger organization: many of the employment practices of small organizations were continued.[7]) The extent to which the women participated in promotion hierarchies differed: women in status group 1 recognizably belonged to promotion hierarchies, whilst some clerical workers and semi-skilled manual workers were able to move from less to more desirable jobs of a broadly similar type. Finally, the women had acquired limited property rights in their jobs through long service. However, membership of the primary labour market conferred fewer benefits than writers in the early 1970s assumed. As the redundancies studied showed, 'permanent' jobs were not permanent: even major national and multinational corporations were unable to cushion themselves against the effects of recession. Moreover, job segregation confined the women to a limited range of occupations in four of the five companies, whilst in the fifth women, for historical reasons, were not distributed randomly amongst jobs, despite a genuine policy of integration. The skills and experience the women acquired were thus limited and, amongst manual workers especially, largely firm specific (except for sewing-machinists). The women had thus built up 'human capital' in skills and experience, but that capital was largely 'sunk' in their pre-redundancy employment: its value was severely reduced by the redundancies.

The women's attitudes to work were in some ways similar to, and in other ways different from, those of male workers. Like the affluent male manual workers studied by Goldthorpe et al., the women went out to work for instrumental reasons. Hence 89 per cent of women asked mentioned money as one of the three major reasons for going out to work. Although the financial circumstances of the women differed widely, for domestic as well as employment reasons, there were no differences between different groups of women in the likelihood of mentioning financial reasons for going out to work. This is hardly surprising: at the most general level, going out to work for financial reasons is so pervasive as to represent a cultural norm. Money was important as a means of raising the household's material standard of living and as a source of financial independence for the women concerned, 79 per cent of women agreeing that women needed to go out to work because having their own money provided financial independence. However, money was only one reason for going out to work – 69 per cent of women spontaneously gave additional reasons for going out to work. Hence 38 per cent of the women asked mentioned broadly 'intrinsic' reasons for going out to work – because of the interest of the job itself or, more negatively, to avoid boredom – and 27 per cent mentioned 'company'.

For women, as for men, the financial reasons for going out to work are so commonplace as to be taken for granted. But it is difficult to establish the intensity of the incentive. Financial pressures depend upon the availability of alternative sources of income, upon perceptions of financial commitments, and upon tastes. Evidence on alternative sources of income is notoriously difficult to acquire and to interpret, and financial commitments depend upon personal preferences – one woman's luxury is another woman's necessity. However, very few women, only 10 per cent, described themselves as earning 'extras' for their households, the majority of women, 55 per cent, classifying themselves as 'joint breadwinners'. Similarly, 55 per cent of women interviewed regarded a 'good rate of pay' as essential or very important in a job – the fourth most frequently mentioned attribute (compared with 72 per cent placing friendly people to work with, the most frequently mentioned item in the same category). In short, financial reasons were the major reason for going out to work in the first place, but a good rate of pay was not the most frequently sought attribute of a good job – working with friendly co-workers was more frequently sought. Like the women in the biscuit factory interviewed by Beynon and Blackburn, the women's 'reasons for working were typically a combination of economic and social considerations ... their economic interest was to some extent based on fundamental necessity but ... the actual level of income were [sic] less important for the women than for their husbands.'[8]

Women workers are thus very similar to male workers in their reasons for undertaking employment, although less economistic in the qualities sought for in particular jobs. For them, as for adult male workers, going out to work had become a routine: 89 per cent had been going out to work for ten years or more at the time of the interviews, and 65 per cent had been in their pre-redundancy jobs for ten years or more. But there were major differences between the work histories of the women and those of male manual workers. Most importantly, the majority of women had spent part of their adult lives out of the labour market: 69 per cent had had a break in their working lives, including 12 per cent who had had more than one break. The effect of interrupted employment was to inhibit movement up the promotional ladders associated with the primary labour market, although our evidence on occupational mobility is insufficiently extensive to demonstrate the effects of the disruption conclusively.[9] Overall, there was a slight drop in the average occupational status of the women interviewed between their initial entry into the labour force and the time of the interviews; there were fewer women in the central-status category, a slight increase in the higher-status category, and a larger increase in the lower-status categories. This would be consistent with the disruptive effects of broken employment, a suggestion made more plausible by the fewer breaks in employment recorded by non-manual than by manual women workers. The break in employment also meant that women, unlike men, had a way of adult life, full-time child-rearing and housekeeping, to compare with going out to work. The ability to make comparisons between full-time domestic life and going out to work may have influenced the relative importance attached to different job attributes, leading to increased emphasis upon company; unlike men, the women had a realistic appreciation of the potential isolation of domestic life, especially in the absence of young children.

A second difference between the women interviewed and male workers was that the majority of women had not intended to work throughout their adult lives when they had first gone out to work. Hence 13 per cent said that they had intended to work until retirement age, and 10 per cent until retirement with a break for bringing up children. The belief that going out to work was to be only an interlude was, of course, likely to inhibit the acquisition of skills and experience helpful to upward occupational mobility. In the event, going out to work filled more of the women's adult lives, and probably had acquired more importance, than they had expected when first going out to work. It is hardly surprising that the majority of women would thus have done something different at the age of 16 if they had the chance to begin their work-lives again.

There were thus similarities in, and differences between, the women interviewed and male workers in their attitudes towards employment in general, reflecting the influence of gender and gender-related characteristics on the women interviewed. On the other hand, we did not expect that gender, or gender-related characteristics, would influence attitudes towards specific jobs; we expected that attitudes towards specific jobs would be more profoundly influenced by the jobs themselves. This expectation was largely confirmed: differences in jobs, rather than differences in marital status, life-cycle position, or age, influenced attitudes towards specific jobs. Hence there were few differences between married, single, and divorced women in job satisfaction. There was some slight evidence that women who had children aged under 15 were less satisfied with their jobs than others, which may have been due to unfavourable comparison with the greater satisfaction they would have obtained from looking after their children at home, or may have been due to the practical difficulties involved in combining responsibilities for looking after dependent children with going out to work, and resulting tiredness. But far more substantial differences were associated with differences between women in different occupational statuses. The majority of women, 95 per cent, were at least reasonably satisfied with their jobs. However, non-manual workers, especially professional, administrative, and supervisory workers, were more positive about their jobs than manual workers; engineering assembly workers, and electronics assembly workers, were least satisfied with their jobs. Such findings parallel similar findings amongst men.[10] Moreover, women in different occupations stressed the importance of different job attributes: women were likely to regard as important those qualities likely to be provided by the jobs they were doing. Hence women in professional, administrative, and supervisory jobs were more likely to stress the importance of intrinsically interesting work than women in the other four groups (84 per cent regarding interesting work as essential or very important, compared with 50 per cent of women in occupational status group 5). Women in clerical jobs, and in semi-skilled and slightly skilled jobs were more likely to stress the importance of friendly people to work with, whilst women in unskilled jobs were more likely to stress pay and autonomy. Whether the stress upon certain values preceded or followed the experience of doing the jobs involved, it is, of course, impossible to say: the women's priorities were realistically congruent with the rewards afforded by the jobs they were doing. More specifically, an emphasis upon sociability and friendly work-groups, which some sociologists have seen as characteristic of women workers, did not receive the same priority from all women workers; women in high-status jobs were considerably less likely than other workers to stress the importance of 'friendly people to work with'.[11]

Although the five redundancies studied involved men as well as women, the research focused upon women's experiences and attitudes. In view of the absence of relevent evidence relating to women, and the practical trade-off which had to be made between obtaining extensive evidence on women and securing comparable evidence on men, this seemed a justifiable restriction. All five redundancies were total or, in the electronics case study unit, closures, involving declaring all (or nearly all) affected workers redundant; it was therefore impossible to obtain evidence as to the extent to which women were more likely to be declared redundant than men, if at all. Such evidence as we were able to obtain suggested that location in the division of labour was more important than gender in determining the chances of being declared redundant. In turning to the reactions to the redundancies, it has been suggested that women are more likely than men to accept redundancies as inevitable, partly because of fatalism and partly because of lower commitment to specific jobs — women are seen as being more optimistic than men about the prospects of obtaining comparable jobs elsewhere.[12] We found no evidence to support such views, and some evidence to counter them. The women interviewed were no more — and no less — acquiescent in the redundancies in their plants than men similarly employed. Where meetings were held and protests organized, women participated, and the majority of women said that they would have been willing to take part in strike action against the redundancies if they had been asked to do so by their unions. All workers, female and male, are placed on the defensive by redundancies, and find difficulty in exercising a significant influence upon events: the five redundancies studied were no exceptions. The weakness reflects general trade-union weakness, unrelated to gender.[13] Moreover, the majority of women believed (rightly) that they would have difficulty in finding jobs as good as the jobs held before the redundancies, and, where possible, took steps to secure such jobs as were available.

Very few women obtained jobs following the redundancies — only 29 per cent. Non-manual workers were more successful in obtaining work than manual workers: 31 per cent of professional, administrative, and supervisory women obtained jobs, 34 per cent of clerical workers, 27.5 per cent of semi-skilled, 26.5 per cent of slightly skilled, and 18 per cent of unskilled manual workers obtained jobs. Non-manual workers succeeded largely in obtaining jobs similar to the ones they had had before the redundancy (although often less conveniently located): manual workers were likely to obtain only part-time work, primarily in service occupations — the only group finding work in the manufacturing sector being the South East clothing workers. The limited success in obtaining jobs was not because of unrealistic aspirations — earnings aspirations were lower than the level of earnings the women had had before the redundancies: nor was it because of family restrictions — 85 per cent said that they had no family commitments which limited their job choice; nor was it because of lack of effort in looking for jobs — job search was both persistent and comprehensive. The reason for the lack of success was the absence of suitable jobs; even in the most favoured travel to work area, in the South East, there were 5.17 unemployed workers for every notified vacancy.

The redundancies transferred women from the primary labour market into the secondary labour market, into unemployment, or out of the labour market altogether. This transfer was the result of the large-scale contraction of manufacturing industry, especially the engineering industry, reinforced by technological obsolescence in one case. This change affected men as well as women. Re-employment was possible, in a limited number of cases, because the public-sector and service industries proved more resilient than manufacturing industry during the recession. Women's expulsion from the primary labour market occurred because of their position in the division of labour in the manufacturing sector: women manual workers were concentrated vertically and horizontally in the sectors most exposed to competitive pressures. Women non-manual workers were affected by the closure of the manufacturing firms in which they were employed. However, if job segregation resulted in the exposure of women to redundancy, it also helped their re-employment prospects: the majority of women did not feel that they were competing for jobs with men, since men and

Conclusion 285

women were employed in different types of jobs, and the women who secured re-employment did so in 'non-masculine' jobs. No engineering assembly worker obtained a similar job.

At the time of the second interview 84 per cent of redundant women had experienced some unemployment, and 71 per cent were not working when interviewed, including 7 per cent who had permanently retired and 17 per cent who had temporarily retired. The women were interviewed, on average, twenty weeks after leaving their pre-redundancy jobs, and the long-term effects of unemployment had not yet begun to show themselves. In view of the slow pace of obtaining jobs it was likely that the women would remain unemployed for several further months; we were therefore seeing the early stages of long-term unemployment. There was no evidence of declining commitment to employment: more women applied for jobs in the last month before the interviews than in any month except the first month following the redundancy. Similarly, women who were interviewed after seven or eight months of unemployment were no more likely to be reconciled to unemployment than those interviewed three or four months after leaving work.

The unemployed women were cushioned from the full financial impact of unemployment in the short term by the special payments they received on being declared redundant; the women previously employed in the electronics and engineering plants received payments averaging between £3000 and £4000. In addition, the majority of women qualified for unemployment benefit, although its value declined in 1982 with the ending of earnings-related benefit and the reduction in the time period during which unemployment benefit was payable. In the long term married women might be cushioned by their husbands' earnings, although the loss of earnings had a substantial impact on the financial resources of the majority of households. At the time of the second interviews only a small number of women reported severe financial pressures as a result of their unemployment, 13 per cent of women out of work for three months or more saying that they were finding it difficult or impossible to manage financially.

Unemployment reinforced traditional female domestic preoccupations. Housework filled the time previously spent in going out to work for the majority of women. They did not find their time unoccupied: 61 per cent said that they never had any time on their hands, although a substantial minority, 31 per cent, said that they had time on their hands everyday. However, the activities that filled their time were regarded as less rewarding; the majority of women regarded housework as less interesting than going out to work, and agreed that 'you get bored if you haven't got a job'; 45 per cent of women specifically mentioned boredom, lack of purpose, or lack of a sense of achievement as disadvantages associated with unemployment. The majority of women had enjoyed the social contact of the work-place, and mentioned reduced social contact as one of the disadvantages of unemployment; married women especially felt more isolated when unemployed than when going out to work. The intensity of the feelings of boredom and isolation of course varied between women, but 43 per cent said that they had felt depressed at some stage during their unemployment: the depressions were sufficiently severe as to lead to loss of sleep and other physical symptoms in some cases. Depressed women were especially likely to feel socially isolated. Privatization thus led to feelings of social isolation, and in some circumstances contributed to depression. More generally, it reduced the opportunities for finding out about job vacancies, especially part-time vacancies which employers would often not bother to advertise.

Unemployment was not a total loss for all the women concerned. Hence 25 per cent of women who experienced unemployment said that they preferred being at home to going out to work, and a further 9 per cent were content to do either. Moreover, 9 per cent said that there was nothing they disliked about no longer going out to work. For a small number of women for whom work was not financially necessary the redundancies provided an opportunity to discontinue a routine which had lost its attractions. The absence of pressure was the major advantage the women saw in unemployment, mentioned by 54 per cent. The attractions of unemployment were not especially great for women who had been disadvantaged at work — there was no evidence that unemployment offered compensations for a deprived work environment. Women with the most resources to undertake interesting activities when unemployed were also likely to have had the most interesting jobs when employed. There was thus no difference in the evaluations of employment and unemployment by women of different occupational statuses; the privileged were comparing two relatively privileged situations, the deprived two relatively deprived situations. Although the majority of women saw some advantages in unemployment, as many as 43 per cent said that they could see no advantages in unemployment. Moreover, it is of course impossible to say how far expressions of satisfaction with unemployment reflected reconciliation to the inevitable.

Although unemployment was experienced as a personal deprivation by the majority of women, few women (17 per cent) reported that it led to increased tension within the family. Unemployment might have been expected to lead to increased family tension because of financial pressures, getting on top of each other, an increased feeling of dependence, or anxiety about loss of status. However, because of payments associated with the redundancies and other benefits, financial pressures had not yet become a major source of family tension: only 7 per cent of women with experience of unemployment said that tension had increased in their families because of the loss of their income. A further 10 per cent of unemployed women mentioned family tension, due to increased proximity, but for most of the women unemployment did not mean increased proximity because husband and children were out of the house all day at work or school. A majority of women (61 per cent) reported feeling a loss of financial independence as a result of unemployment, but this was not associated with increased tension within the family. Finally, unemployment did not lead the women to feel that their role within the family had been undermined, rather the reverse; 63 per cent of women said that their families 'appreciated' having them at home, and 38 per cent that their husbands preferred them at home.

Comparison between female and male experience of unemployment suggests that women suffer more from some aspects of job loss than men, and less from others. Although both women and men are likely to experience increased social isolation, the degree of privatization is likely to be greater for women than for men. Bunker and Dewberry document the process of privatization experienced by men and women in their appositely entitled paper, 'Unemployment Behind Closed Doors: Staying in and Staying Invisible', although previous surveys had not stressed this aspect of unemployment (for example, Daniel's 1974 survey did not suggest that loneliness was one of the worst aspects of unemployment).[14] As many as 35 per cent of women who had experience of unemployment mentioned loneliness as one of the worst aspects of being out of work, and the activities that replaced going out to work were largely privatized. Women are less likely to have their spouses at home than men, and are less likely to have access to their own transport, even if they are able to drive. On the other hand, women are less likely than men to be stigmatized for being out of work; few women we interviewed felt that they lost status in the eyes of others by being unemployed, although research amongst men has indicated that this was a major negative aspect of male unemployment.

Employment opportunities in the late 1980s are likely to be limited, especially for new entrants to the labour force — whether adolescents or married women looking for work after child rearing. More particularly, technological change, especially in the office, is likely to reduce women's employment opportunities especially sharply: for example, according to one estimate approximately 17 per cent of all typing and secretarial jobs will have been lost by 1990 as a result of the expansion of word processing.[15] The level of unemployment can be reduced either by a reduction in the size of the labour force, or by an increase in the number of jobs available. If the former strategy is followed the reduction can be formal (by bureaucratic manipulation, ceasing to count as unemployed groups who fail to satisfy certain criteria) or real. One possible source of reduction in the size of the labour force is for married women to drop out of the labour market, either because they wish to, or because they feel that the financial or other needs of men or single women are greater than their own, or because employment and fiscal policies are designed to encourage them to do so. As our project indicated, there is little evidence that employed women wish to drop out of the labour market, although some evidence of a preference for part-time, rather than full-time, work among manual workers. However, many women were unassertive about female employment, reflecting the still current ambivalence about female employment during periods of high unemployment. But it is easy to exaggerate the importance of such ambivalence. Although the women recognized the complexities involved in determining relative priorities in jobs, they also believed that men and women were not competing for the same jobs, and the practical effects of any belief in employment priorities for other groups is limited.

The financial burdens of unemployed married women may be less than those of unemployed married men, although the long-term financial consequences for the women interviewed were grave. The psychological consequences are also likely to be less because of the ambiguities surrounding female employment: care of a household is a legitimate female role — even for women without children. However, the women interviewed preferred going out to work, finding work rewarding both financially and personally, while the alternative role available was seen as less satisfying. Women, like men, find work the conventional way of participating in a common endeavour and, in Durkheim's terms, participating in the 'conscience collectif' on a day-to-day basis. Moreover, it is misleading to talk of a 'return' to a domestic role, since for the majority of women going out to work was the normal pattern of their adult lives, not a deviant one. Stopping going out to work was not a return to a 'natural' way of life, but a change to a new, more restricted, and less rewarding way of life. Even if it were possible to return to the pattern of female employment characteristic of the early 1950s, changes in attitudes and values since 1950 make it likely that reactions would differ. Employment policy should therefore be based on current values and attitudes, not on those of a largely illusory past.

Notes

1. e.g. Beynon and Blackburn comment: 'The demands made upon women by marriage and childbirth in our society have meant that women in general have tended to develop a much lower commitment to work than men. This tendency for women to centre their lives around their position in the home has been reinforced by severe discrimination against them in the labour market . . . it is not surprising that many women regard being a housewife and bringing up a family as more important and rewarding than the meaningless, alienating jobs that are available to them' (Beynon and Blackburn, op. cit., pp. 146–7).
2. For a convenient summary of the distribution of women in employment see Delamont, op. cit., p. 109; for one view of the mechanisms involved see T. S. Chivers, 'Gender Reproduction and the Labour Market', Paper presented to British Sociological Association Annual Conference, University of Manchester, April 1982, pp. 12–19.
3. S. Walby comments: '. . . we should look at patriarchal relations in order to explain these limits on women's paid employment . . . . There is a need to analyse patriarchal relations both within the labour market and within the household' (Sylvia Walby, *Women and Unemployment*, Lancaster Regionalism Group, Working Paper no. 5, 1981), p. 15. Walby draws attention to the need to take account of 'both patriarchal and capitalist relations in both the family and in the labour market' (p. 30).
4. V. Beechey, 'Women and Production: a critical analysis of some sociological theories of women's work', in (ed.) A. Kuhn and A. M. Wolpe, *Feminism and Materialism: Women and Modes of Production* (Routledge & Kegan Paul, 1978).
5. J. H. Goldthorpe, D. Lockwood, F. Bechhofer and J. Platt, *The Affluent Worker: Industrial Attitudes and Behaviour* (Cambridge University Press, 1968).
6. For a succinct summary of dual-labour-market theory see Barron and Norris, op. cit.
7. G. K. Ingham, *Size of Industrial Organization and Worker Behaviour* (Cambridge University Press, 1970).
8. Beynon and Blackburn, op. cit., p. 147.

9. For more extensive evidence on women's occupational careers see Martin and Roberts, op. cit., Ch. 10.
10. Cf. R. Blauner's famous study, *Alienation and Freedom* (Chicago University Press, 1964), based on different groups of manual workers.
11. S. Hill, *Competition and Control at Work* (Heinemann, 1981), p. 120: 'Not a lot is known about the orientations of women workers as distinct from men, because only a few industrial sociologists have distinguished between the genders. What is known is that women share much the same concerns as men, but that companionship may feature more prominently as a source of compensation for unsatisfying work. This is particularly so with women workers whose incomes are not essential for the support of themselves or their families, as is sometimes the case with married women working part-time.' Our findings are broadly consistent with this view.
12. Wood and Dey, op. cit., pp. 33–4.
13. Martin, *Employment Gazette,* 1984, forthcoming.
14. N. Bunker and C. Dewberry, 'Unemployment Behind Closed Doors: Staying In and Staying Invisible', *Journal of Community Education*, 1984.
15. Communications Studies and Planning Ltd., *Information Technology in the Office: the Impact on Women's Jobs* (Equal Opportunities Commission, 1980), p. 40.

APPENDIX

The major sources of data for the study were two interviews with women workers, which took place in 1981 and 1982. The case studies were carried out in the order indicated in the text. The first interviews in case study A were carried out in September and October 1981, in case study B in October and November 1981, in case study C in December 1981 and January 1982, in case study D in March–April 1982, and in case study E in April–May 1982. All initial interviews were carried out by the research team, Judith Wallace being primarily responsible for case studies A and D, and Jennie Dey case studies B, C, and E, although interviewing in all areas except D was shared between the researchers. The second interviews were carried out in 1982, case study A in April–May, B in June, C in September, D in August–September, and E in September–October. The second interviews in case studies A and D were carried out by Judith Wallace, and those in the remaining case studies by Public Attitude Surveys. The first interviews were carried out in the plants concerned, the second at home.

The data were analysed using P-Stat (S. Buhler et al., *P-Stat User's Manual*, P-Stat Inc., 1983) in the Oxford University Social Studies Faculty Computing and Research Support Unit. Judith Wallace was primarily responsible for data analysis, advised by Martin Range and Clive Payne.

The questionnaires used are not reproduced here because of their length and complexity. Interested scholars can obtain copies of the schedule from Professor R. Martin, Department of Social and Economic Studies, Imperial College of Science and Technology, 53 Prince's Gate, London SW7.

REFERENCES

Airey C. and A. Potts, 'Workplace Industrial Relations' (Unpublished report by Social and Community Planning Research for Department of Employment, 1981).
Allen S., *Women in Local Labour Markets* (SSRC Workshop on Research Initiatives on Local Labour Markets and the Informal Economy, SSRC, 1980).
Anthony P. D., *The Ideology of Work* (Tavistock, 1977).
Bakke E. W., *The Unemployed Man* (Nisbet and Co., 1933).
Barron R. and G. Norriss, 'Sexual Divisions and the Dual Labour Market', in ed. D. L. Barker and S. Allen, *Dependence and Exploitation in Work and Marriage* (Longman, 1976).
Baudoin T., M. Collin and D. Guillerm, 'Women and Immigrants: Marginal Workers?', in (eds) C. Crouch and A. Pizzorno, *The Resurgence of Class Conflict in Western Europe,* (Vol. 2) (Macmillan, 1978).
Beck A. T., *Depression: Clinical, Experimental and Theoretical Aspects* (New York: Harper and Row, 1967).
Beck A. T., *Cognitive Theory; the Emotional Disorders* (New York: International Universities Press, 1976).
Beechey V., 'Women and Production: a critical analysis of some sociological theories of women's work', in (ed.) A. Kuhn and A. M. Wolpe, *Feminism and Materialism: Women and Modes of Production* (Routledge and Kegan Paul, 1978).
Beechey V., 'Part-time Work and the Labour Process', (Mimeo) (University of Warwick, Department of Sociology, 1981).
Beechey V. and T. Perkins, 'Women's Part-time Employment in Coventry' (Unpublished, 1982).
Beynon H. and R. M. Blackburn, *Perceptions of Work: Variations within a Factory* (Cambridge University Press, 1972).
Blauner R., *Alienation and Freedom,* (University of Chicago Press, 1964).
Brayshaw P. and C. J. Laidlaw, *Women in Engineering* (Engineering Industry Training Board, 1979).
Breugel I., 'Women as a reserve army of labour: a note on recent British experience', *(Feminist Review,* 1979).
Brown G. W. and T. Harris, *Social Origins of Depression* (Tavistock, 1978).
Brown R. K., 'Women as Employees: some comments on research in industrial sociology', in (eds) D. L. Barker and S. Allen, *Dependence and Exploitation in Work and Marriage* (Longman, 1976).

Brown W. (ed.), *The Changing Contours of British Industrial Relations* (Basil Blackwell, 1981).
Buhler S. *et al.* P–Stat User's Manual (P–Stat Inc., 1983).
Bunker N. and C. Dewberry, 'Unemployment Behind Closed Doors: Staying In and Staying Invisible', *Journal of Community Education*, 1984.
Chivers T. S., 'Gender Reproduction and the Labour Market' (Unpublished paper presented to British Sociological Association Annual Conference, University of Manchester, 1982).
Communication Studies and Planning Ltd., *Information Technology in the Office: the Impact on Women's Jobs* (Equal Opportunities Commission, 1980).
Crosby F. J., *Relative Deprivation and Working Women* (Oxford University Press, 1982).
Daniel W. W., *Whatever Happened to the Workers in Woolwich? A Survey of Redundancy in South East London* (PEP, 1972).
Daniel W. W., *A National Survey of the Unemployed*, (PEP, 1974).
Delamont S., *The Sociology of Women* (George, Allen and Unwin, 1980).
Feldberg R. L. and E. N. Glen, 'Male and Female: Job Versus Gender Models in the Sociology of Work', in ed. R. Kahn-Hut, A. K. Daniels and R. Colvard, *Women and Work: Problems and Perspectives* (Oxford University Press, 1982).
Goldthorpe J. H., *Social Mobility and Class Structure in Modern Britain* (Clarendon Press, 1980).
Goldthorpe J. H., 'Women and Class Analysis: In Defence of the Conventional View', *Sociology*, 1983.
Goldthorpe J. H. and K. Hope, *The Social Grading of Occupations: a new approach and scale* (Clarendon Press, 1974).
Goldthorpe J. H., D. Lockwood, F. Bechhofer, and J. Platt, *The Affluent Worker: Industrial Attitudes and Behaviour*, (Cambridge University Press, 1968).
Goode W. J., *Women in Divorce* (New York: The Free Press, 1956).
Hakim C., *Occupational Segregation: a comparative study of the degree and pattern of the differentiation between men and women's work in Britain, the United States and other countries* (Department of Employment Research Paper no. 8, 1979).
Hayes J. and P. Nutman, *Understanding the Unemployed: the Psychological Effects of Unemployment* (Tavistock, 1981).
Heath A., *Social Mobility* (Fontana, 1981).
Hepple B. A. *et al.*, *Labour Relations: Statutes and Materials* (Sweet and Maxwell, 1979).
Herzberg F. *et al.*, *The Motivation to Work* (John Wiley, 1959).
Hill M. J., R. M. Harrison, A. V. Sargent, and V. Talbot, *Men Out of Work: A Study of Unemployment in Three English Towns* (Cambridge University Press, 1973).
Hill S., *Competition and Control at Work* (Heinemann, 1981).
Hurstfield J., *The Part-time Trap* (Low Pay Unit, 1978).
Institute of Manpower Studies, *Manpower Commentary No. 13: Redundancy Provisions Surveys* (2 volumes) (IMS, 1981?)
Ingham G. K., *Size of Industrial Organization and Worker Behaviour* (Cambridge University Press, 1970).
Jahoda M., *Employment and Unemployment: A Social Psychological Analysis* (Cambridge University Press, 1982).
Jahoda M., P. Lazarsfeld and H. Zeizel, *Marienthal: the Sociography of an*

Unemployed Community (Tavistock, 1972, first published 1933).
Jolly J., S. Creigh and A. Mingay, *Age as a Factor in Employment* (Department of Employment Research Paper, 1980).
Lazarus R. S. and J. R. Averill, 'Emotion and Cognition with special reference to Anxiety', in C. Spielberger (ed.), *Anxiety, Current Trends in Theory and Research,* Vol. 11 (Academic Press, 1972).
Loveridge R. and A. L. Mok, *Theories of Labour Market Segmentation* (University of Aston Management Centre Working Paper, December 1979).
Marsden D., *Workless* (Croom Helm, 1982).
Martin J. and C. Roberts, *Women and Employment: a Lifetime Perspective* (HMSO, 1984).
Massey D. and R. Meegan, *The Anatomy of Job Loss* (Methuen, 1982).
Miles I., *Adaptation to Unemployment?* (Science Policy Research Unit, University of Sussex, Occasional Paper no. 20, 1983).
Milkman R., 'Women's Work and the Economic Crisis: some lessons of the Great Depression' *Review of Radical Political Economy,* 1976.
National Economic Development Council, *Report of the Electronics Components Sector Working Party* (NEDC, 1981).
Pahl R., 'Family, Community and Unemployment', *New Society,* 1982.
Parker S. R., R. K. Brown and J. Child, *The Sociology of Industry* (George Allen and Unwin, 1967).
Pilgrim Trust, *Men Without Work* (Cambridge University Press, 1938).
Pollert A., *Girls, Wives, Factory Lives* (Macmillan, 1981).
Propper C., 'An Empirical Enquiry into the Nature of Clerical Work for Young Women' (Unpublished M.Phil thesis, University of Oxford, 1981).
Report of the Committee of Inquiry on Industrial Democracy (Bullock Committee), Cmnd. 6706 (HMSO, 1977).
Roberts K. *et al.,* 'Unregistered Youth Unemployment and Out-reach Careers Work', (Unpublished report, Department of Employment, 1981).
Sinfield A., *What Unemployment Means* (Martin Robertson, 1981).
Snell M., P. Glucklich and M. Povall, *Equal Pay and Opportunities: a study of the Equal Pay and Sex Discrimination Acts in 26 Organizations* (Department of Employment Research Paper no. 20, 1981).
Wadjman J., *Women in Control: Dilemmas of a Workers' Co-operative* (Open University Press, 1983).
Walby S., *Women and Unemployment* (Lancaster Regionalism Group, 1979).
West J. (ed.), *Work, Women and the Labour Market* (Routledge and Kegan Paul, 1982).
Wilkinson F. (ed.), *The Dynamics of Labour Market Segmentation,* (Academic Press, 1982).
Williams W. M., *Occupational Choice* (George Allen and Unwin, 1974).
Wood S., 'Redundancy and Female Employment', *Sociological Review,* 1982.
Wood S. and I. Dey, *Redundancy: Case Studies in Co-operation and Conflict* (Gower, 1983).

INDEX

Airey, C., 150
Allen, S., 49
Anthony, P. D., 10, 50
Averill, J. R., 278

Bakke, E. W., 50
Barker, D. L., 49
Barron, R., 49, 288
Baudouin, T., 49
Bechofer, F., 288
Beck, A. T., 278
Beechey, V., 49, 279, 288
Beynon, H., 49, 102, 281, 288
Blackburn, R. M., 49, 102, 281, 288
Blauner, R., 4, 49, 289
Brayshaw, P., 49
Breughel, I., 49
Brown, G. W., 278
Brown, R. K., 1, 49, 50
Brown, W., 150
Buhler, S., 290
Bullock Committee, 150
Bunker, N., 289

Child, J., 50
Chivers, T. S., 288
clothing, 103–4, 110, 117, 119
Collin, M., 49
Colvard, R., 102
Creigh, S., 51
Crosby, F. J., 5
Crouch, C., 49

Daniels, A. K., 102
Daniels, W. W., 5, 6, 7, 49, 50
Delamont, S., 49
Dewberry, C., 289
Dey, I., 49, 289

electronics, 104–7, 112–15, 117–18, 119
engineering, 107–9, 116, 118, 119
'entitlement' to work, 60–7

family circumstances and attitudes to work, 96–8

fatalism, 131, 143–5
Feldberg, R. L., 102

Glen, E. N., 102
Glucklich, P., 49
Goldthorpe, J. H., 24, 50, 51, 280, 281, 288
Goode, W. J., 278
Guillerm, D., 49

Hakim, C., 37, 49, 51
Harris, T., 278
Harrison, R. M., 50
Hayes, J., 6, 50
Heath, A. F., 24, 51
Hepple, B. A., 150
Herzberg, F., 102
Hill, M. J., 7, 50
Hill, S., 289
homeworking, 215–16
Hope–Goldthorpe Scale, 34–5
Hurstfield, J., 51

industrial conflict, 123–4
Ingham, G. K., 288

Jahoda, M., 8, 9, 50
job choice, 69–73
job search, 161–93
    application rates, 166–71
    female handicaps, 183–93
    methods used, 171–83
    timing, 162–8
job segregation, 36–9, 280, 284
jolly, J., 51

Kahn-Hut, R., 102
Kuhn, A., 288

labour markets, dual, 2, 280
    local, 218–22
    segmented, 2–4
Laidlaw, C. J., 49
Lazarsfeld, P., 8, 50
Lazarus, R. S., 278

length of service, 77
Lockwood, D., 288
Loveridge, R., 49

Marsden, D., 10, 50
Martin, J., 51, 289
Martin, R., 50, 289
Massey, D., 49, 150
Meegan, R., 49, 150
Miles, I., 8, 50
Milkman, R., 49
Mingay, A., 51
Mok, A. L., 49

Norris, G., 49, 288
Nutman, P., 6, 50

occupational careers, 73–7

Pahl, R., 11
Parker, S. R., 50
Perkins, T., 49
Pilgrim Trust, 6, 8, 50
Pizzorno, A., 49
Platt, J., 288
Pollert, A., 49
post-redundancy employment, 152–61, 193–213, 284
Potts, A., 150
Povall, M., 49
Propper, C., 102

Q Search, 49

redundancy, 5–6, 12–13, 117–49
  agreements, 127–31
  industrial relations, 124–7
  management decision-making, 117–18
  payments, 146–9
  women's reactions, 131–46
research strategy, 12–18, 103–50
reserve army of labour, 3
retail distribution, 50

retraining, 213–15
Roberts, C., 51, 289
Roberts, K., 102

sample characteristics, 19–46
  age, 19–21
  economic situation, 39–46
  education, 26–31
  family circumstances, 21–4
  length of working life, 31–4
  occupation, 34–7
  occupational status, 24–6
  social background, 24–6

Talbot, V., 50
trade unions, 118–21

Unemployment, 6–12, 155–61, 223–78, 285–8
  and activities, 233–43
  attitudes towards, 267–72
  and attitudes towards government, 272–5
  economic impact, 225–33
  and family life, 9–10, 243–9
  and health, 260–7
  and social contact, 249–60

voluntary work, 59

Wadjman, J., 6, 49
Walby, S., 49, 288
West, J., 49
White, M., 278
Williams, W. M., 102
Wilkinson, F., 49
Wolpe, A. M., 288
women and employment, 44–6, 77
Wood, S., 5, 49, 289
work attitudes, 81–96

Zeisel, H., 50